Advanced Paediatric Life Support

SIXTH EDITION

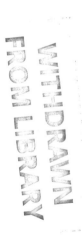

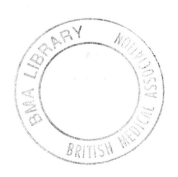

This new edition is also available as an e-book.
For more details, please see
www.wiley.com/buy/9781118947647
or scan this QR code:

Advanced Paediatric Life Support

A Practical Approach to Emergencies

SIXTH EDITION

Advanced Life Support Group

EDITED BY

Martin Samuels
Sue Wieteska

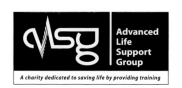

BMJ|Books

WILEY Blackwell

Contents

Clinical conditions list

Working group

Associate editors

A. Argent Paediatric Intensive Care, *Cape Town*

P. Arrowsmith Paediatric Resuscitation, *Liverpool*

A. Charters Paediatric Emergency Care, *Portsmouth*

E. Duval Paediatric Intensive Care, *Maastricht*

M. Hegardt-Janson Paediatric Surgery, *Lund*

S. Lewena Paediatric Emergency Medicine, *Melbourne*

T. Rajka Paediatric Intensive Care, *Oslo*

M. Samuels Paediatrics, *Stoke-on-Trent and London*

S. Smith Emergency Paediatrics, *Nottingham*

Working group

A. Argent Paediatric Intensive Care, *Cape Town*

P. Arrowsmith Paediatric Resuscitation, *Liverpool*

J. Brown Paediatrics, *Wellington*

A. Charters Paediatric Emergency Care, *Portsmouth*

E. Duval Paediatric Intensive Care, *Maastricht*

C. Ewing Paediatrics, *Manchester*

A. Hafeez Paediatrics, *Islamabad*

M. Hegardt-Janson Paediatric Surgery, *Lund*

A. Hutchison Paediatric Emergency Nursing, *Melbourne*

B. Kalkan Paediatrics, *Sarajevo*

S. Lewena Paediatric Emergency Medicine, *Melbourne*

K. Mackway-Jones Emergency Medicine, *Manchester*

J. Mestrovic Paediatric Intensive Care, *Split*

E. Molyneux Paediatric Emergency Medicine, Blantyre, *Malawi*

P. Oakley Anaesthesia/Trauma, *Stoke-on-Trent*

J. Paul Paediatric Emergency Medicine, *Trinidad*

B. Phillips Paediatric Emergency Medicine, *Liverpool*

P. H. Phuc Paediatric Critical Care, *Hanoi*

T. Rajka Paediatric Intensive Care, *Oslo*

M. Samuels Paediatrics, *Stoke-on-Trent and London*

J. Sandell Paediatric Emergency Medicine, *Poole*

S. Smith Emergency Paediatrics, *Nottingham*

G. Spyridis Paediatric Surgery, *Athens*

N. Turner Paediatric Anaesthesia and Intensive Care, *Utrecht*

C. Vallis Paediatric Anaesthesia, *Newcastle*

I. Vidmar Paediatrics, *Ljubljana*

S. Wieteska ALSG CEO, *Manchester*

S. Wood Paediatric Surgery, *Liverpool*

Contributors

Contributors to the sixth edition

S. Ainsworth Paediatrics and Neonatology, *Kirkcaldy*

R. Appleton Paediatric Neurology, *Liverpool*

A. Argent Paediatric Intensive Care, *Cape Town*

J. Armstrong Paediatric Anaesthesia, *Nottingham*

P. Arrowsmith Paediatric Resuscitation, *Liverpool*

A. Baldock Paediatric Anaesthesia, *Southampton*

K. Berry Paediatric Emergency Medicine, *Birmingham*

V. Bhole Paediatric Cardiology, *Birmingham*

D. Bramley Emergency Medicine, *Sunderland*

A. Burgess Paediatric ENT Surgery, *Southampton*

S. Bush Urgent Care, *Leeds*

A. Charters Paediatric Emergency Care, *Portsmouth*

R. Cheung General Paediatrics, *London*

F. Davies Emergency Medicine, *Leicester*

J. Davison Paediatric Metabolic Medicine, *London*

J. Doherty Paediatrics, *Dorchester*

I. Doull Paediatric Respiratory Medicine, *Cardiff*

E. Duval Paediatric Intensive Care, *Maastricht*

R. Fisher Paediatric Surgery, *Sheffield*

C. Fitzsimmons Paediatric Emergency Medicine, *Sheffield*

P-M. Fortune Paediatric Intensive Care, *Manchester*

J. Foster Paediatric Radiology, *Plymouth*

A. Gandhi Paediatric Cardiology, *Birmingham*

J. Grice Paediatric Emergency Medicine, *Liverpool*

G. Haythornthwaite Paediatric Emergency Medicine, *Bristol*

M. Hegardt-Janson Paediatric Surgery, *Lund*

M. Hellaby North West Simulation Education Network, *Manchester*

S. Hewitt Emergency Medicine, *Derby*

L. Hudson Paediatrics, *London*

P. Hyde Paediatric Intensive Care, *Southampton*

H. Ismail-Koch Paediatric ENT Surgery, *Southampton*

B. Ko Community Paediatrics, *London*

A. Lee Paediatric Trauma and Orthopaedics, *Reading*

S. Lewena Paediatric Emergency Medicine, *Melbourne*

C. Loew Anaesthesia, *Poole*

M. Lyttle Paediatric Emergency Medicine, *Bristol*

L. Mackintosh Community Paediatrics, *Bristol*

K. Mackway-Jones Emergency Medicine, *Manchester*

N. Makwana Paediatrics, *Birmingham*

W. Marriage Paediatrics, *Bristol*

P. McMaster Paediatric Infectious Diseases, *Manchester*

P. McQuillan Paediatric Intensive Care, *Portsmouth*

B. Mehta Paediatric Emergency Medicine, *Liverpool*

P. Oakley Anaesthesia, *Stoke on Trent*

B. Okoye Paediatric Surgery, *London*

F. O'Leary Paediatric Emergency Medicine, *Sydney*

L. Prentice Paediatric Anaesthetist, *Melbourne*

T. Rajka Paediatric Intensive Care, *Oslo*

T. Ralph Paediatric Resuscitation Training, *Sheffield*

G. Roberts Paediatric Allergy and Respiratory Medicine, *Southampton*

S. Roberts Paramedic; Pre hospital Trauma and Paediatric Care, *West Midlands*

M. Samuels Paediatrics, *Stoke-on-Trent and London*

D. Schenk General Paediatrics, *Newcastle*

N. Sen Emergency Medicine, *Manchester*

A. Simpson Emergency Medicine, *Stockton-on-Tees*

H. Smith Paediatrics, *Southampton*

S. Smith Emergency Paediatrics, *Nottingham*

E. Snelson Paediatric Emergency Medicine, *Sheffield*

K. Soanes Emergency Medicine, *Birmingham*

K. Thies Anaesthetics, *Birmingham*

R. Tinnion Neonatology, *Middlesborough*

Y. Tse Paediatric Nephrology, *Newcastle*

C. Vallis Paediatric Anaesthesia, *Newcastle*

A. Walker Paediatric Anaesthesia, *Glasgow*

L. Walton Paediatric Emergency Medicine, *Nottingham*

J. White Toxinologist, *Adelaide*

S. Wieteska ALSG CEO, *Manchester*

S. Wood Paediatric Surgery, *Liverpool*

J. Wyllie Neonatology, *Middlesbrough*

A. Young Paediatric Anaesthesia, *Bristol*

Contributors to previous editions

S. Agrawal Paediatric Intensive Care, *London*

R. Appleton Paediatric Neurology, *Liverpool*

A. Argent Paediatric Intensive Care, *Cape Town*

C. Baillie Paediatric Surgery, *Liverpool*

P. Baines Paediatric Intensive Care, *Liverpool*

I. Barker Paediatric Anaesthesia, *Sheffield*

D. Bickerstaff Paediatric Orthopaedics, *Sheffield*

R. Bingham Paediatric Anaesthesia, *London*

P. Brennan Paediatric Emergency Medicine, *Sheffield*

J. Britto Paediatric Intensive Care, *London*

G. Browne Paediatric Emergency Medicine, *Sydney*

C. Cahill Emergency Medicine, *Portsmouth*

H. Carty Paediatric Radiology, *Liverpool*

A. Charters Emergency Nursing, *Portsmouth*

M. Clarke Paediatric Neurology, *Manchester*

J. Couriel Paediatric Respiratory Medicine, *Liverpool*

P. Driscoll Emergency Medicine, *Manchester*

P-M. Fortune Paediatric Intensive Care, *Manchester*

J. Fothergill Emergency Medicine, *London*

P. Habibi Paediatric Intensive Care, *London*

D. Heaf Paediatric Respiratory Medicine, *Liverpool*

J. K. Heltne Anaesthesia, *Haukeland*

F. Jewkes Pre-Hospital Paediatrics, *Wiltshire*

E. Ladusans Paediatric Cardiology, *Manchester*

J. Leggatte Paediatric Neurosurgery, *Manchester*

J. Leigh Anaesthesia, *Bristol*

S. Levene Child Accident Prevention Trust, *London*

M. Lewis Paediatric Nephrology, *Manchester*

K. Mackway-Jones Emergency Medicine, *Manchester*

I. Maconochie Emergency Paediatrics, *London*

J. Madar Neonatology, *Plymouth*

T. Martland Paediatric Neurologist, *Manchester*

D. McKimm Paediatric Intensive Care Nursing, *Belfast*

E. Molyneux Paediatric Emergency Medicine, *Malawi*

S. Nadel Paediatric Intensive Care, *London*

D. Nicholson Radiology, *Manchester*

A. Nunn Pharmacy, *Liverpool*

E. Oakley Paediatrics, *Victoria*

P. Oakley Anaesthesia, *Stoke on Trent*

R. Perkins Paediatric Anaesthesia, *Manchester*

B. Phillips Paediatric Emergency Medicine, *Liverpool*

T. Rajka Paediatrics, *Oslo*

J. Robson Paediatric Emergency Medicine, *Liverpool*

I. Sammy Paediatric Emergency Medicine, *Trinidad*

M. Samuels Paediatric Intensive Care, *Stoke on Trent*

D. Sims Neonatology, *Manchester*

A. Sprigg Paediatric Radiology, *Sheffield*

B. Stewart Paediatric Emergency Medicine, *Liverpool*

J. Stuart Emergency Medicine, *Manchester*

L. Teebay Child Protection and Paediatric Emergency Medicine, *Liverpool*

J. Tibballs Paediatric Intensive Care, *Melbourne*

N. Turner Paediatric Anaesthesia and Intensive Care, *Utrecht*

J. Walker Paediatric Surgery, *Sheffield*

W. Whitehouse Paediatric Neurologist, *Nottingham*

S. Wieteska ALSG Group Manager, *Manchester*

M. Williams Emergency Medicine, *York*

B. Wilson Paediatric Radiology, *Manchester*

J. Wyllie Neonatology, *Middlesbrough*

S. Young Paediatric Emergency Medicine, *Melbourne*

D. Zideman Anaesthesia, *London*

Preface to the first edition

Advanced Paediatric Life Support: The Practical Approach was written to improve the emergency care of children, and has been developed by a number of paediatricians, paediatric surgeons, emergency physicians and anaesthetists from several UK centres. It is the core text for the APLS (UK) course, and will also be of value to medical and allied personnel unable to attend the course. It is designed to include all the common emergencies, and also covers a number of less common diagnoses that are amenable to good initial treatment. The remit is the first hour of care, because it is during this time that the subsequent course of the child is set.

The book is divided into six parts. Part I introduces the subject by discussing the causes of childhood emergencies, the reasons why children need to be treated differently and the ways in which a seriously ill child can be recognised quickly. Part II deals with the techniques of life support. Both basic and advanced techniques are covered, and there is a separate section on resuscitation of the newborn. Part III deals with children who present with serious illness. Shock is dealt with in detail, because recognition and treatment can be particularly difficult. Cardiac and respiratory emergencies, and coma and convulsions, are also discussed. Part IV concentrates on the child who has been seriously injured. Injury is the most common cause of death in the 1–14-year age group and the importance of this topic cannot be overemphasised. Part V gives practical guidance on performing the procedures mentioned elsewhere in the text. Finally, Part VI (the appendices) deals with other areas of importance.

Emergencies in children generate a great deal of anxiety – in the child, the parents and in the medical and nursing staff who deal with them. We hope that this book will shed some light on the subject of paediatric emergency care, and that it will raise the standard of paediatric life support. An understanding of the contents will allow doctors, nurses and paramedics dealing with seriously ill and injured children to approach their care with confidence.

Kevin Mackway-Jones
Elizabeth Molyneux
Barbara Phillips
Susan Wieteska
Editorial Board
1993

Preface to the sixth edition

The *Advanced Paediatric Life Support* (APLS) concept and courses have aimed from inception 23 years ago to bring a structured approach and simple guidelines to the emergency management of seriously ill and injured children. The manual was and continues to be an important part of the course, but it has also come to be used as a handbook in clinical practice. This has been a real tribute to the contributors of this text, both current and past editions.

The course has changed since the last edition to reflect the changes in health service provision, as well as the increasing evidence base of medical knowledge. Clinical practice has become more sophisticated and sub-specialised, and increasingly children with complex multisystem disorders are surviving. This has been accompanied by the need to develop increasingly expert teams to provide health care. As a result, providers of emergency care are no longer expected to possess the wide-ranging skills that were needed to treat children and young people 10–20 years ago. Trauma care has undergone the greatest revision and the importance of team working, utilising the skills of many different disciplines and knowing when and how to seek additional help are hopefully clearly reflected within the provider course.

The sixth edition of the manual reflects the pace of change of medical science and practice, the international nature of APLS and the increasing recognition of the importance of human factors in providing the best emergency care. This edition benefits from the latest guidelines for resuscitation from cardiac arrest by the International Liaison Committee on Resuscitation (ILCOR), published in October 2015.

Whilst the sixth edition is current, we hope that APLS providers will see the introduction of an app, paperless courses and an enhanced electronic learning resource with chronic and specialist conditions. Contributions and ideas are always welcome.

APLS is established in the United Kingdom, Australasia, the Caribbean, mainland Europe, the Middle and Far East, Scandinavia and South Africa. In addition, the Advanced Life Support Group (ALSG) has collaborated with many other agencies so that the course is now available in a number of resource-poor countries, either in its original form or modified for local use. To ensure this, ALSG has had to be responsive to the different styles, languages, cultures and clinical facilities found in many different countries. It is with the help of so many enthusiastic and dedicated local health professionals that APLS has flourished.

We hope that new as well as current providers of emergency paediatric practice appreciate the changes.

The material found in these sources, as well as in this manual, is all brought together by the increasing numbers of experts that have contributed to this update. We thank them and all our instructors, who have provided helpful feedback. We ask that this process does not stop, so that we can begin the process that will support the development of the next edition.

Martin Samuels
Sue Wieteska
Manchester 2016

Acknowledgements

A great many people have put a lot of hard work into the production of this book, and the accompanying advanced life support course. The editors would like to thank all the contributors for their efforts and all the APLS instructors who took the time to send us their comments on the earlier editions.

We are greatly indebted to Helen Carruthers, MMAA, Mary Harrison, MMAA and Kate Wieteska for producing the excellent line drawings that illustrate the text. The information in Table 6.1 is taken from *Lessons from Research for Doctors in Training* produced by the Meningitis Research Foundation. We would also like to thank Mark Hellaby, NW Simulation Education Network Manager for his input into the Human factors chapter.

ALSG gratefully acknowledge the support of the Royal College of Paediatrics and Child Health (UK). The Specialist Groups of the RCPCH agreed to advise on the clinical content of chapters relevant to their specialism. ALSG wish to thank the following:

Association of Paediatric Anaesthetists Dr A. Walker, Paediatric Anaesthesia, *Glasgow*
Association of Paediatric Emergency Medicine Dr K. Berry, Paediatric Emergency Medicine, *Birmingham*; Dr N. Sargant, Paediatric Emergency Medicine, *Bristol*
British Association for Paediatric Nephrology Dr Y. Tse, Paediatric Nephrology, *Newcastle*
British Association of Community Child Health Dr B. Ko, Community Paediatrics, *London*
British Association of Paediatric Surgeons – trauma committee Mr B. Okoye, Paediatric Surgery, *London*
British Inherited Metabolic Disease Group Dr J. Davison, Paediatric Metabolic Medicine, *London*
British Paediatric Allergy, Immunology and Infection Group Dr G. Roberts, Paediatric Allergy and Respiratory Medicine, *Southampton*; Dr P. McMaster, Paediatric Infectious Diseases, *Manchester* and Dr N. Makwana, Paediatrics, *Birmingham*
British Paediatric Neurology Association Dr R. Appleton, Paediatric Neurology, *Liverpool*
British Paediatric Respiratory Society Dr I. Doull, Paediatric Respiratory Medicine, *Cardiff*
British Society of Paediatric Radiology Dr J. Foster, Paediatric Radiology, *Plymouth*
Child Protection Special Interest Group Dr L. Mackintosh, Community Paediatrics, *Bristol*; Dr J. Doherty, Paediatrics, *Dorchester*; Dr H. Smith, Paediatrics, *Southampton*
Paediatric Intensive Care Society Dr P-M. Fortune, Paediatric Intensive Care, *Manchester*
Paediatricians with Expertise in Cardiology Special Interest Group Dr A. Gandhi, Paediatric Cardiology, *Birmingham*

We are also grateful to the following groups who have advised on the clinical content of chapters relevant to their specialism:

European Resuscitation Council: European Trauma Course Mr K. Thies, Anaesthetics, *Birmingham*
MARSIPAN group Dr L. Hudson, Paediatrics, *London*
Royal College of Surgeons: Advanced Trauma Life Support Dr H. Walmsley, Anaesthetics, *Eastbourne*; Dr A. Duby, Military Emergency Medicine, *Birmingham*; Mr S. Bush, Emergency Medicine, *Leeds*; Mr M. Bagnall, General Surgery, *Redhill*; Mr J. Hambidge, Trauma and Orthopaedics, *Romford*; Dr R. O'Donnell, Paediatric Emergency Medicine, *Cambridge*; Dr L. Zibners, Paediatric Emergency Medicine, *London*

Finally, we would like to thank, in advance, those of you who will attend the Advanced Paediatric Life Support course and other courses using this text; no doubt, you will have much constructive criticism to offer.

Contact details and further information

ALSG: www.alsg.org
BestBETS: www.bestbets.org

For details on ALSG courses visit the website or contact:
Advanced Life Support Group
ALSG Centre for Training and Development
29–31 Ellesmere Street
Swinton, Manchester
M27 0LA
Tel: +44 (0)161 794 1999
Fax: +44 (0)161 794 9111
Email: enquiries@alsg.org

Clinicians practising in tropical and under-resourced health care systems are advised to read *International Maternal and Child Health Care – A Practical Manual for Hospitals Worldwide* (www.mcai.org.uk) which gives details of additional relevant illnesses not included in this text.

Updates

The material contained within this book is updated on a 5-yearly cycle. However, practice may change in the interim period. We will post any changes on the ALSG website, so we advise that you visit the website regularly to check for updates (www.alsg.org/uk/apls). The website will provide you with a new page to download.

References

All references are available on the ALSG website www.alsg.org/uk/apls

On-line feedback

It is important to ALSG that the contact with our providers continues after a course is completed. We now contact everyone 6 months after their course has taken place asking for on-line feedback on the course. This information is then used whenever the course is updated to ensure that the course provides optimum training to its participants.

How to use your textbook

The anytime, anywhere textbook

Wiley E-Text

For the first time, your textbook comes with free access to a **Wiley E-Text: Powered by VitalSource** version – a digital, interactive version of this textbook which you own as soon as you download it.

Your **Wiley E-Text** allows you to:

Search: Save time by finding terms and topics instantly in your book, your notes, even your whole library (once you've downloaded more textbooks)
Note and highlight: Colour code, highlight and make digital notes right in the text so you can find them quickly and easily
Organize: Keep books, notes and class materials organized in folders inside the application
Share: Exchange notes and highlights with others
Upgrade: Your textbook can be transferred when you need to change or upgrade computers

The **Wiley E-Text** version will also allow you to copy and paste any photograph or illustration into assignments, presentations and your own notes.

To access your Wiley E-Text:

- Find the redemption code on the inside front cover of this book and carefully scratch away the top coating of the label. Visit **www.vitalsource.com/software/bookshelf/downloads** to download the Bookshelf application to your computer, laptop, tablet or mobile device.
- If you have purchased this title as an e-book, access to your **Wiley E-Text** is available with proof of purchase within 90 days. Visit **http://support.wiley.com** to request a redemption code via the 'Live Chat' or 'Ask A Question' tabs.
- Open the Bookshelf application on your computer and register for an account.
- Follow the registration process and enter your redemption code to download your digital book.

The VitalSource Bookshelf can now be used to view your Wiley E-Text on iOS, Android and Kindle Fire!

- **For iOS:** Visit the app store to download the VitalSource Bookshelf: **http://bit.ly/17ib3XS**
- **For Android and Kindle Fire:** Visit the Google Play Market to download the VitalSource Bookshelf: **http://bit.ly/BSAAGP**

You can now sign in with the email address and password you used when you created your VitalSource Bookshelf Account

Full E-Text support for mobile devices is available at: **http://support.vitalsource.com**

PART 1
Introduction

CHAPTER 1
Introduction

Learning outcomes

After reading this chapter, you will be able to:
- Describe the focus of the APLS course
- Identify the important differences in children and their impact on the management of emergencies

1.1 Introduction

Over the last two decades there has been a substantial reduction in childhood mortality across the world. This has been related to improvements in many areas such as maternal education, access to clean water, access to food, immunisation against an increasing number of infectious conditions, and improved access to healthcare services. Even conditions such as human immunodeficiency virus infections have potentially come under control with the development of highly effective antiretroviral therapeutic regimes. However, children across the world continue to suffer potentially life-threatening acute illness (sometimes on a background of chronic illness) and injury. The Advanced Paediatric Life Support (APLS) course is directed at training healthcare workers to recognise life-threatening illness or injury in children; provide effective emergency intervention; and ensure that children receive the appropriate definitive management of the condition as soon as possible. This approach is potentially applicable in many different settings across the world.

1.2 Principles

There are a number of principles that underpin this approach.

Physiological differences

Most clinical medicine is taught with the underlying assumption that adults best exemplify 'normal' in health. This is perhaps justified by the reality that in most parts of the world the majority of the population is made up of adults, but in poorer countries up to 40% of the population may be made up of children (depending on how children are defined). Thus it is important to highlight where children are different to adults in terms of physiology, pathophysiology and responses to various interventions (see Section 1.3). Among the most important differences are the substantially lower physiological reserves in children, particularly young children. A consequence of this is that in the face of injury or severe illness their condition may deteriorate more rapidly than would be expected for adult patients. Thus particular attention has to be paid to timeliness and effective support of the respiratory and cardiovascular systems.

Children come in a range of sizes, and a consequence of this is the constant requirement to adjust all therapy, interventions and selection of equipment or consumable to the size of the particular patient (see Table 1.1 in Section 1.3).

Advanced Paediatric Life Support: A Practical Approach to Emergencies, Sixth Edition. Edited by Martin Samuels and Sue Wieteska.
© 2016 John Wiley & Sons, Ltd. Published 2016 by John Wiley & Sons, Ltd.

Relationship between disease progression and outcomes

The further a disease process is allowed to progress, the worse the outcome is likely to be. The outcomes for children who have a cardiac arrest out of hospital are generally poor (this may be related to the fact that in children cardiac arrest is rarely related to cardiac arrhythmia, but more commonly is a sequel of hypoxaemia and/or shock with associated organ damage and dysfunction). By the time that cardiac arrest occurs, there has already been substantial damage to various organs. This is in contrast to situations (more common in adults) where the cardiac arrest was the consequence of cardiac arrhythmia – with preceding normal perfusion and oxygenation. Thus the focus of the course is on early recognition and effective management of potentially life-threatening problems before there is progression to respiratory and/or cardiac arrest (Figure 1.1).

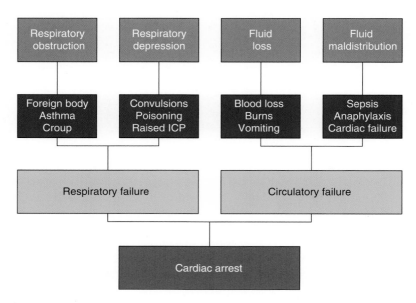

Figure 1.1 Pathways leading to cardiac arrest in childhood (with examples of underlying causes). [ICP, intracranial pressure]

Standardised structure for assessment and stabilisation

The use of a standardised structure for resuscitation provides benefits in many areas. Firstly it provides a structured approach to a critically ill child who may have multiple problems. The standardised approach enables the provision of a standard working environment, ensuring that all the necessary equipment is available as required. By focusing attention on life-threatening issues and dealing with those in a logical sequence it is possible to stabilise the child's condition as quickly as possible. The use of the standardised structure enables the entire team to know what is likely to be expected of them and in what sequence.

There may well be discussion around the optimum sequence of resuscitation, but in this course a particular approach has been accepted as being reasonable, and most in keeping with the available research information. It is likely that aspects of this approach will change over time, and in fact it may be appropriate to modify the approach in particular working environments and contexts.

Once basic stabilisation has been achieved, it is then appropriate to investigate the underlying diagnoses and proceed to definitive therapy. Occasionally, definitive therapy (such as surgical intervention) may be a component of the resuscitation.

Resource management

There is increasing realisation that provision of effective emergency treatment depends on the development of teams of healthcare providers who are able to work together in a coordinated and appropriately directed way (Figure 1.2). Thus part of training in paediatric life support must focus on understanding how the human resources available for a particular resuscitation episode can be utilised most effectively.

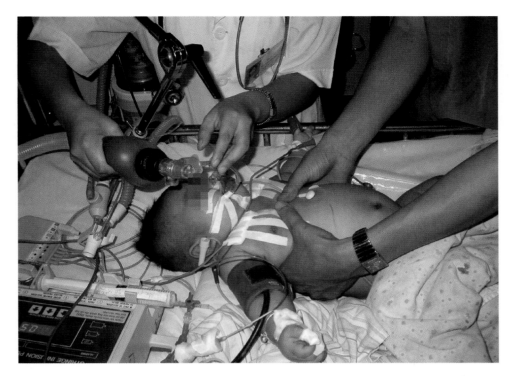

Figure 1.2 Advanced paediatric life support (APLS) in action

Early referral to appropriate teams for definitive management

It is clear that emergency areas are unlikely to be able to provide definitive management for all paediatric emergencies, and a component of stabilisation of critically ill or injured children is the capacity to call for help as soon as possible, and where necessary transfer the child to the appropriate site safely.

Ongoing care until admission to appropriate care

In most parts of the world it is impossible to transfer critically ill children into intensive care units or other specialised units within a short time of their arrival in the emergency area. Thus it is important to provide training in the ongoing therapy that is required for a range of relatively common conditions once initial stabilisation has been completed.

1.3 Important differences in children

Children are a diverse group, varying enormously in weight, size, shape, intellectual ability and emotional responses. At birth a child is, on average, a 3.5 kg, 50 cm long individual with small respiratory and cardiovascular reserves and an immature immune system. They are capable of limited movement, have immature emotional responses though still perceive pain and are dependent upon adults for all their needs. At the other end of childhood, the adolescent may be a 50 kg, 160 cm tall person who looks physically like an adult, often exhibiting a high degree of independent behaviour but who may still require support in ways that are different to adults.

Competent management of a seriously ill or injured child who may fall anywhere between these two extremes requires a knowledge of these anatomical, physiological and emotional differences and a strategy of how to deal with them.

Weight

The most rapid changes in weight occur during the first year of life. An average birth weight of 3.5 kg will have increased to 10 kg by the age of 1 year. After that time weight increases more slowly until the pubertal growth spurt. This is illustrated in the weight charts shown in Figure 1.3.

As most drugs and fluids are given as the dose per kilogram of body weight, it is important to determine a child's weight as soon as possible. Clearly the most accurate method for achieving this is to weigh the child on scales; however, in an emergency this may be impracticable. Very often, especially with infants, the child's parents or carer will be aware of a recent weight. If this is not possible, various formulae or measuring tapes are available. The Broselow or Sandell tapes use the height (or length) of the child to estimate weight. The tape is laid alongside the child and the estimated weight read from the calibrations on the tape. This is a quick, easy and relatively accurate method. Various formulae may also be used although they should be validated to the population in which they are being used.

(a)

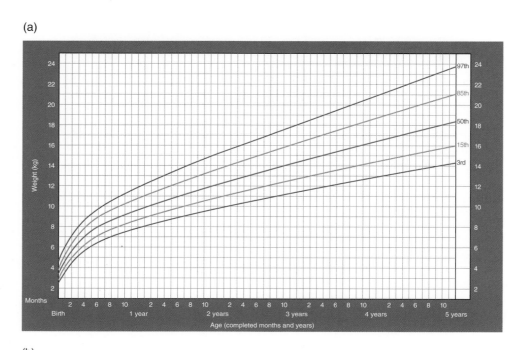

(b)

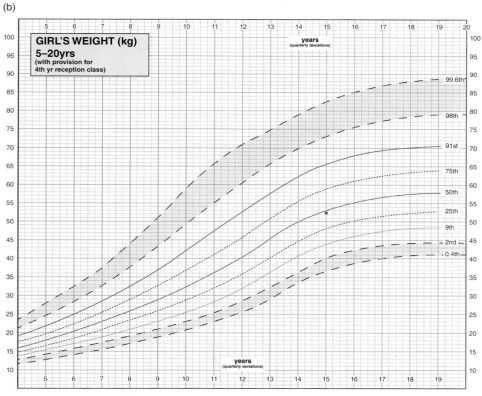

Figure 1.3 Centile chart for weight in (a) boys (0–5 years) and (b) girls (5–20 years)

If a child's age is known, the normal ranges table will provide you with an approximate weight (Table 1.1). This will allow you to then prepare the appropriate equipment and drugs for the child's arrival in hospital. Whatever the method, it is essential that the carer is sufficiently familiar with it to be able to use it quickly and accurately under pressure. When the child arrives, you should quickly review their size to check if it is much larger or smaller than predicted. If you have a child that looks particularly large or small for their age, you can go up or down one age group.

Table 1.1 Normal ranges: respiratory rate (RR), heart rate (HR) and blood pressure (BP)

Age	Guide weight (kg) Boys	Guide weight (kg) Girls	RR At rest Breaths per minute 5th–95th centile	HR Beats per minute 5th–95th centile	BP Systolic 5th centile	BP Systolic 50th centile	BP Systolic 95th centile
Birth	3.5	3.5	25–50	120–170	65–75	80–90	105
1 month	4.5	4.5					
3 months	6.5	6	25–45	115–160			
6 months	8	7	20–40	110–160			
12 months	9.5	9			70–75	85–95	
18 months	11	10	20–35	100–155			
2 years	12	12	20–30	100–150	70–80	85–100	110
3 years	14	14		90–140			
4 years	16	16		80–135			
5 years	18	18			80–90	90–110	111–120
6 years	21	20		80–130			
7 years	23	22					
8 years	25	25	15–25	70–120			
9 years	28	28					
10 years	31	32					
11 years	35	35					
12 years	43	43	12–24	65–115	90–105	100–120	125–140
14 years	50	50		60–110			
Adult	70	70					

Anatomical

As the child's weight increases with age the size, shape and proportions of various organs also change. Particular anatomical changes are relevant to emergency care.

Airway

The airway is influenced by anatomical changes in the tissues of the mouth and neck. In a young child the occiput is relatively large and the neck short, potentially resulting in neck flexion and airway narrowing when the child is laid flat in the supine position. The face and mandible are small, and teeth or orthodontic appliances may be loose. The tongue is relatively large and not only tends to obstruct the airway in an unconscious child, but may also impede the view at laryngoscopy. Finally, the floor of the mouth is easily compressible, requiring care in the positioning of fingers when holding the jaw for airway positioning. These features are summarised in Figure 1.4.

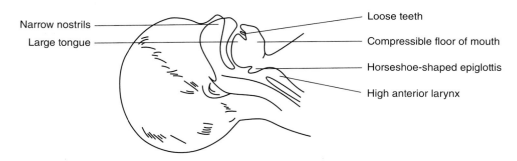

Narrow nostrils

Large tongue

Loose teeth

Compressible floor of mouth

Horseshoe-shaped epiglottis

High anterior larynx

Figure 1.4 Summary of significant upper airway anatomy

The anatomy of the airway itself changes with age, and consequently different problems affect different age groups. Infants less than 6 months old are primarily nasal breathers. As the narrow nasal passages are easily obstructed by mucous secretions, and as upper respiratory tract infections are common in this age group, these children are at particular risk of airway compromise. Adenotonsillar hypertrophy may be a problem at all ages, but is more usually found between 3 and 8 years. This not only tends to cause obstruction, but also may cause difficulty when the nasal route is used to pass pharyngeal, gastric or tracheal tubes.

In all young children the epiglottis is horseshoe-shaped, and projects posteriorly at 45°, making tracheal intubation more difficult. This, together with the fact that the larynx is high and anterior (at the level of the second and third cervical vertebrae in the infant, compared with the fifth and sixth vertebrae in the adult), means that it is often easier to intubate an infant using a straight-blade laryngoscope. The cricoid ring is oval in shape, and thus passage of a round endotracheal tube will almost always result in a leak around the tube. In fact, if there is not a leak at pressures of approximately 20 cmH$_2$O, it is likely that that tube is too large. Although uncuffed endotracheal tubes have been used preferentially in children, there is increasing evidence that cuffed endotracheal tubes may be advantageous in many settings. However, the use of a cuffed tube requires meticulous attention to size, to cuff pressure and to exact placement of the endotracheal tube in the correct position.

The trachea is short and soft. Overextension of the neck as well as flexion may therefore cause tracheal compression. The short trachea and the symmetry of the carinal angles mean that not only is tube displacement more likely, but a tube or a foreign body is also just as likely to be displaced into the left as the right main-stem bronchus.

Breathing

The lungs are relatively immature at birth. The air–tissue interface has a relatively small total surface area in the infant (less than 3 m²). In addition, there is a 10-fold increase in the number of small airways from birth to adulthood. Both the upper and lower airways are relatively small, and are consequently more easily obstructed. As resistance to flow is inversely proportional to the fourth power of the airway radius (halving the radius increases the resistance 16-fold), seemingly small obstructions can have significant effects on air entry in children. This may partially explain why so much respiratory disease in children is characterised by airway obstruction.

Infants rely mainly on diaphragmatic breathing. Their muscles are more likely to fatigue as they have fewer type I (slow-twitch, highly oxidative, fatigue-resistant) fibres compared with adults. Pre-term infants' muscles have even less type I fibres. These children are consequently more prone to respiratory failure.

The ribs lie more horizontally in infants, and therefore contribute less to chest expansion. In the injured child, the compliant chest wall may allow serious parenchymal injuries to occur without necessarily incurring rib fractures. For multiple rib fractures to occur the force must be very large; the parenchymal injury that results is consequently very severe and flail chest is tolerated badly.

Circulation

At birth the two cardiac ventricles are of similar weight; by 2 months of age the RV : LV weight ratio is 0.5. These changes are reflected in the infant's electrocardiogram (ECG). During the first months of life the right ventricle (RV) dominance is apparent, but by 4–6 months of age the left ventricle (LV) is dominant. As the heart develops during childhood, the sizes of the P wave and QRS complex increase, and the P-R interval and QRS duration become longer.

The child's circulating blood volume per kilogram of body weight (70–80 ml/kg) is higher than that of an adult, but the actual volume is small. This means that in infants and small children, relatively small absolute amounts of blood loss can be critically important.

Body surface area

The body surface area (BSA) to weight ratio decreases with increasing age (Figure 1.5). Small children, with a high ratio, lose heat more rapidly and consequently are relatively more prone to hypothermia. At birth the head accounts for 19% of BSA; this falls to 9% by the age of 15 years.

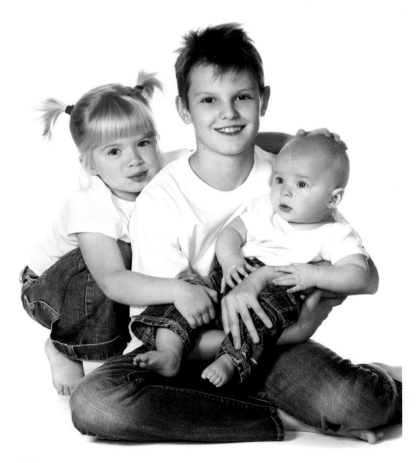

Figure 1.5 Differences in children

Physiological

Respiratory

The infant has a relatively greater metabolic rate and oxygen consumption. This is one reason for an increased respiratory rate. However, the tidal volume remains relatively constant in relation to body weight (5–7 ml/kg) through to adulthood. The work of breathing is also relatively unchanged at about 1% of the metabolic rate, although it is increased in the pre-term infant.

In the adult, the lung and chest wall contribute equally to the total compliance. In the newborn, most of the impedance to expansion is due to the lung, and is critically dependent on the presence of surfactant. The lung compliance increases over the first week of life as fluid is removed from the lung. The infant's compliant chest wall leads to prominent sternal recession when the airways are obstructed or lung compliance decreases. It also allows the intrathoracic pressure to be less 'negative'. This reduces small-airway patency. As a result, the lung volume at the end of expiration is similar to the closing volume (the volume at which small-airway closure starts to take place).

The combination of high metabolic rate and oxygen consumption with low lung volumes and limited respiratory reserve means that infants in particular will desaturate much more rapidly than adults. This is an important consideration during procedures such as endotracheal intubation.

At birth, the oxygen dissociation curve is shifted to the left and P_{50} (PO_2 at 50% oxygen saturation) is greatly reduced. This is due to the fact that 70% of the haemoglobin (Hb) is in the form of HbF; this gradually declines to negligible amounts by the age of 6 months.

The immature infant lung is also more vulnerable to insult. Following prolonged respiratory support of a pre-term infant, chronic lung disease of the newborn may cause prolonged oxygen dependence. Many infants who have suffered from bronchiolitis remain 'chesty' for a year or more.

Table 1.1 shows respiratory rate by age at rest.

Cardiovascular

The infant has a relatively small stroke volume (1.5 ml/kg at birth) but has the highest cardiac index seen at any stage of life (300 ml/min/kg). Cardiac index decreases with age and is 100 ml/min/kg in adolescence and 70–80 ml/min/kg in the adult. At the same time the stroke volume increases, as the heart gets bigger and muscle mass relative to connective tissue increases. As cardiac output is the product of stroke volume and heart rate, these changes underlie the heart rate changes seen during childhood (see Table 1.1). In addition, the average infant is only able to increase heart rate by approximately 30% vs the adult who may be able to increase heart rate under stress by up to 300%.

Normal systolic pressures are shown in Table 1.1.

As the stroke volume is small and relatively fixed in infants, cardiac output is principally related to heart rate. The practical importance of this is that the response to volume therapy is blunted when normovolaemic because stroke volume cannot increase greatly to improve cardiac output. By the age of 2 years, myocardial function and response to fluid are similar to those of an adult.

Systemic vascular resistance rises after birth and continues to do so until adulthood is reached. This is reflected in the changes seen in blood pressure (see Table 1.1).

Immune function

At birth the immune system is immature and, consequently, babies are more susceptible than older children to many infections such as bronchiolitis, septicaemia, meningitis and urinary tract infections. Maternal antibodies acquired across the placenta provide some early protection but these progressively decline during the first 6 months. These are replaced slowly by the infant's antibodies as he or she grows older. Infants may be particularly susceptible to infectious diseases in the period between waning of maternal antibodies and development of their own antibodies (sometimes in response to immunisation). Breastfeeding provides increased protection against respiratory and gastrointestinal infections.

Psychological

Children vary enormously in their intellectual ability and their emotional response. A knowledge of child development assists in understanding a child's behaviour and formulating an appropriate management strategy. Particular challenges exist in communicating with children and as far as possible easing their fear of the circumstances they find themselves in.

Communication

Infants and young children either have no language ability or are still developing their speech. This causes difficulty when symptoms such as pain need to be described. Even children who are usually fluent may remain silent. Information has to be gleaned from the limited verbal communication and from the many non-verbal cues (such as facial expression and posture) that are available. Older children are more likely to understand aspects of their illness and treatment and so be reassured by adequate age-appropriate communication.

Fear

Many emergency situations, and many other situations that adults would not classify as emergencies, engender fear in children. This causes additional distress to the child and adds to parental anxiety. Physiological parameters, such as pulse rate and respiratory rate, are often raised because of it, and this in turn makes clinical assessment of pathological processes such as shock more difficult.

Fear is a particular problem in the pre-school child who often has a 'magical' concept of illness and injury. This means that the child may think that the problem has been caused by some bad wish or thought that he or she has had. School-age children and adolescents may have fearsome concepts of what might happen to them in hospital because of ideas they have picked up from adult conversation, films and television.

Knowledge allays fear and it is therefore important to explain things as clearly as possible to the child. Explanations must be phrased in a way that the child can understand. Play can be used to do this (e.g. applying a bandage to a teddy first), and also helps to maintain some semblance of normality in a strange and stressful situation. Finally, parents must be allowed to stay with the child at all times (including during resuscitation if at all possible); their absence from the child's bedside will only add further fears, both to the child and to the parents themselves. But importantly, parents too must be supported and fully informed at all times.

1.4 Summary

The Advanced Paediatric Life Support course is focused on providing training for healthcare professionals in the recognition and management of life-threatening illness in children (in a way that is focused on the needs of the children); in recognition and initial management of important underlying conditions; and appropriate referral to teams that are able to provide definitive intervention. In this process it is also essential to remember the needs of the child's family and to support the clinical team.

You should also be aware that there are some important differences in children:

- Absolute size and relative body proportions change with age
- Observations on children must be related to their age
- Therapy in children must be related to their age and weight
- The special psychological needs of children must be considered

CHAPTER 2
Structured approach to paediatric emergencies

Learning outcomes

After reading this chapter, you will be able to:
- Describe the structured approach to paediatric emergencies
- Identify the approach to triage of a child
- Implement an approach to pain management in children

2.1 Introduction

The reception of a child with a life-threatening condition into the emergency department or the collapse of a child on the ward or in a GP clinic presents a major challenge to staff. The infrequent and, the often unforeseen, nature of the events adds to the anxiety for all. The structured approach will enable a clinician to manage emergencies in a logical and effective fashion and assist in ensuring that vital steps are not forgotten.

The structured approach focuses initially on identifying and treating any immediate threats to life: that is a closed or obstructed airway, absent or ineffective breathing, or pulselessness or shock. Clinical interventions to reverse these immediate threats comprise resuscitation. After resuscitation is commenced the next step is to identify the key features that in any serious illness or injury give the clinician a signpost to the likeliest working diagnosis. From this, the best emergency treatment can be initiated.

The final phase of the structured approach is to stabilise the child, focusing on achieving homeostasis and system control and leading on to transfer to a definitive care environment, which will often be the paediatric intensive care unit. Figure 2.1 shows the structured approach in diagrammatic form. Throughout this book the same structure will be used so that the clinician will become familiar with the approach and be able to apply it to any clinical emergency situation.

2.2 Preparation

If warning has been received of the child's arrival then preparations can be made:

- Ensure that appropriate help is available: critical illness and injury need a team approach
- Work out the likely drug, fluid and equipment needs

For unexpected emergencies, ensure that all areas where children may be treated are stocked with the drugs, fluid and equipment needed for any childhood emergencies.

Advanced Paediatric Life Support: A Practical Approach to Emergencies, Sixth Edition. Edited by Martin Samuels and Sue Wieteska.
© 2016 John Wiley & Sons, Ltd. Published 2016 by John Wiley & Sons, Ltd.

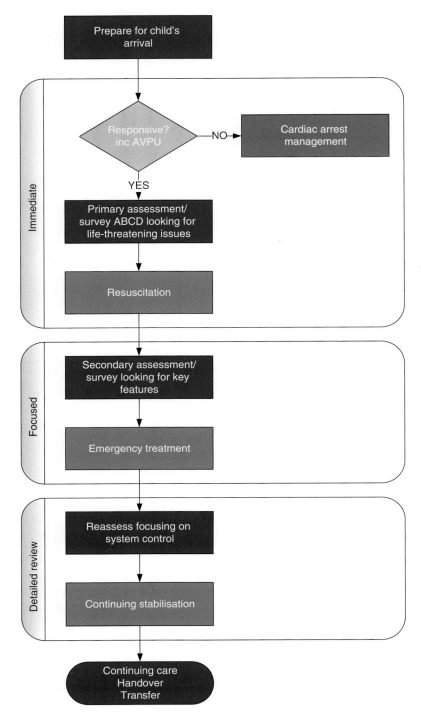

Figure 2.1 Structured approach to paediatric emergencies

2.3 Teamwork

Nowhere is a well-functioning team more vital than in the emergency situation. Success depends on each team member carrying out his or her own tasks and being aware of the tasks and the skills of other team members. The whole team must be under the direction of a team leader. Scenario practice by teams who work together is an excellent way to keep up skills, knowledge and team coordination in preparation for the 'real thing'.

2.4 Communication

In the previous chapter, issues about communication with the ill or injured child and their family were highlighted. Communication is no less important with clinical colleagues. When things have gone wrong, a fault in communication has often been involved. Structured communication tools may be useful in ensuring that all relevant information is conveyed to all the teams involved in the child's care. Contemporaneous recording of clinical findings, of the child's history and of test results and management plans seems obvious but in the emergency situation may be overlooked. A template for note keeping can be found in Chapter 11.

2.5 Triage

Introduction

Triage is the process whereby each child presenting with potentially serious illness or injury is assigned a clinical priority. It is an essential clinical risk management step, and also a tool for optimisation of resource allocation in any emergency.

In the United Kingdom, Canada and Australia, five-part national triage scales have been agreed. A scale is shown in Table 2.1. While the names of the triage categories and the target times assigned to each name vary from country to country, the underlying concept does not.

Table 2.1 Triage scale

Number	Colour	Name	Maximum time to clinician
1	Red	Immediate	0
2	Orange	Very urgent	10 min
3	Yellow	Urgent	60 min
4	Green	Standard	240 min
5	Blue	Non-urgent	N/A

We use triage to identify children who require urgent intervention. The priorities of triage may alter (for instance in an epidemic it may be as important to get potentially uninfected children away from possible infection as soon as possible). Never forget the need for repeated triage/reassessment – children may move from one category to another quite quickly and if there is no reassessment process, this may be missed.

Remember also that being triaged green does not mean that a child does not have a serious problem that requires specialist attention. It simply means that it can wait a little while.

It is important to make sure that the family understand the nature of the triage process (and why they are apparently being ignored while another child receives treatment).

Triage decision making

There are many models of decision making, each requiring three basic steps. These are: identification of a problem, determination of the alternatives and selection of the most appropriate alternative. The commonest triage method in the UK is that developed by the Manchester Triage Group. This method uses the following five steps:

1. *Identify the problem*
   This is done by taking a brief and focused history from the child, his or her parents and/or any pre-hospital care personnel. This phase is always necessary whatever the method used.

2. *Gather and analyse information related to the solution*

Once the presentation has been identified, discriminators can be sought at each level. Discriminators, as their name implies, are factors that discriminate between patients such that they allow them to be allocated to one of the five clinical priorities. They can be general or specific. The former apply to all patients irrespective of their presentation, whilst the latter tend to relate to key features of particular conditions. Thus severe pain is a general discriminator, but cardiac pain and pleuritic pain are specific discriminators. General discriminators would include life threat, pain, haemorrhage, conscious level and temperature.

- *Life threat*
  To an advanced paediatric life support (APLS) provider life threat is perhaps the most obvious general discriminator of all. Any cessation or threat to the vital (ABC) functions means that the patient is in the immediate group. Thus the presence of an insecure airway, inspiratory or expiratory stridor, absent or inadequate breathing, or shock are all significant.

- *Pain*
  From the child's and parents' perspectives pain is a major factor in determining priority. Pain assessment and management is dealt with later in this chapter. Children with severe pain should be allocated to the very urgent category, while those with moderate pain should be allocated to the urgent category. Any child with any lesser degree of pain should be allocated to the standard category.

- *Haemorrhage*
  Haemorrhage is a feature of many presentations, particularly those following trauma. If haemorrhage is catastrophic, death will ensue rapidly unless bleeding is stopped. These children must be treated immediately. A haemorrhage that is not rapidly controlled by the application of sustained direct pressure, and that continues to bleed heavily or soak through large dressings quickly, should be treated very urgently.

- *Conscious level*
  All unresponsive children must be an immediate priority, and those who respond to voice or pain only are categorised as very urgent. Children with a history of unconsciousness should be allocated to the urgent category.

- *Temperature*
  Temperature is used as a general discriminator. It may be difficult to obtain an accurate measurement during the triage process; however modern rapid-reading tympanic membrane thermometers should make this aim attainable. A hot child (over 38.5°C) is always seen urgently; children who are cold (less than 32°C) are seen very urgently, as are hot infants.

3. *Evaluate all alternatives and select one for implementation*

Clinicians collect a huge amount of information about the children they deal with. The data are compared to internal frameworks that act as guides for assessment. The presentational flow diagrams developed by the Manchester Triage Group provide the organisational framework to order the thought process during triage.

4. *Implement the selected alternative*

As previously noted there are only five possible triage categories to select from and these have specific names and definitions (see Table 2.1). The urgency of the patient's condition determines their clinical priority. Once the priority is allocated, the appropriate pathway of care begins.

5. *Monitor the implementation and evaluate outcomes*

Triage categories may change as the child deteriorates or gets better. It is important, therefore, that the process of triage (clinical prioritisation) is dynamic rather than static. To achieve this end all clinicians involved in the pathway of care should rapidly assess priority whenever they encounter the child. Furthermore, any changes in priority must be noted and the appropriate actions taken.

Secondary triage

It may not be possible to carry out all the assessments necessary at the initial triage encounter – this is particularly so if the workload of the department is high. In such circumstances the necessary assessments should still be carried out, but as secondary procedures by a receiving nurse. The actual initial clinical priority cannot be set until the process is finished. More time-consuming assessments (such as blood glucose estimation and peak flow measurement) are often left to the secondary stage.

2.6 Managing pain

Introduction

The adequate management of pain is integral to all emergency care and is therefore covered in an early section of the manual so it is considered in the reading of all subsequent sections. Attention to control of pain is not only more humane but it enhances care, as inadequate analgesia can be detrimental to the critically ill child. Bronchoconstriction and increases in pulmonary vascular resistance caused by pain can lead to hypoxia, whereas good pain control facilitates the assessment of the severity of illness.

Recognition and assessment of pain

There are three main ways in which we recognise that a child is in pain:

1. Firstly, listening to the child for statements that they are in pain.
2. Secondly, observing the child's behaviour and physiology for things such as crying, guarding of the injured part, facial grimacing, pallor, tachycardia and tachypnoea.
3. Thirdly, anticipating pain because of the event the child has experienced, such as fracture, burn or other significant trauma.

The purpose of pain assessment is to establish, as far as possible, the degree of pain experienced by the child so as to select the right level of pain relief. Additionally, reassessment using the same pain tool will indicate whether the pain management has been successful or whether further analgesia is required – the assess, treat and reassess cycle. The use of pain tools and protocols in the emergency setting has been shown to shorten the time to delivery of analgesia.

Pain assessment at triage in the emergency situation is unique and therefore a pain assessment tool, specifically designed for this situation, is desirable. The anxiety associated with a sudden and unexpected presentation in pain confounds the ability of an individual, especially a child, to make a satisfactory self-assessment of pain that can be used to guide analgesic requirements. Therefore, an observational pain scale appears to be more appropriate in this setting. The Alder Hey Triage Pain Score is one such tool that has been developed specifically for this situation and is shown to have some validity as well as good levels of inter-rater reliability (Table 2.2). It is an observation-based pain score, which is quick and easy to use.

Other commonly used pain scales are self-assessment tools, for example a faces scale or pain ladder (Figure 2.2). Self-assessment tools, however, were primarily developed for use with children where there was the opportunity for explanation of the scale prior to the painful event (e.g. before surgery). This is clearly not the case in the emergency department.

Table 2.2 The Alder Hey Triage Pain Score: reference scoring chart

Response	Score 0	Score 1	Score 2
Cry/voice	No complaint/cry	Consolable	Inconsolable
	Normal conversation	Not talking negative	Complaining of pain
Facial expression	Normal	Short grimace <50% time	Long grimace >50% time
Posture	Normal	Touching/rubbing/sparing	Defensive/tense
Movement	Normal	Reduced or restless	Immobile or thrashing
Colour	Normal	Pale	Very pale/'green'

Guidance notes for the use of the score can be found at the end of this chapter.

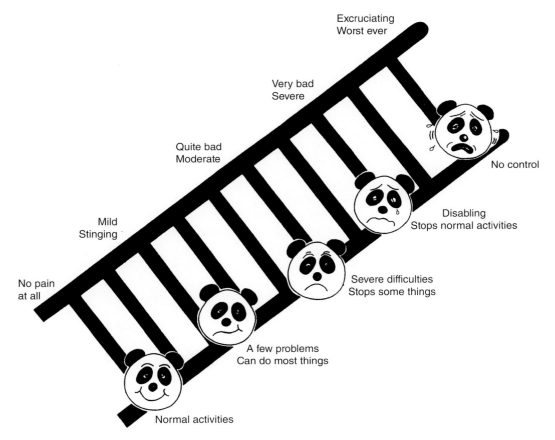

Figure 2.2 Faces scale and pain ladder

All or any of these tools can be used to assess the pain experienced by the child and help, in the setting of the specific clinical situation, to guide the need for the level and route of analgesia. The tools can then be used again to assess the efficacy of the intervention and to guide further analgesia.

Pain management

Environment

The emergency department and the treatment room of the paediatric ward can be frightening places for children. Negative aspects of the environment should be removed or minimised. This includes an overly 'clinical' appearance and evidence of invasive instruments. An attractive, decorated environment with toys, mobiles and pictures should be substituted.

Preparation

Except in a life-threatening emergency or when dealing with an unconscious child, an explanation of the procedure to be undertaken and the pain relief planned should be given to the child and the parents. If time permits, they should contribute to the pain management plan by relating previous pain experiences and successful relief measures. If a play therapist is available they may be able to assist with the preparation and the procedure.

Physical treatments: supportive and distractive techniques

The presence of parents during an invasive procedure on their child is important. In one study almost all children between the ages of 9 and 12 years reported that 'the thing that helped most' was to have a parent present during a painful procedure. Parents need some guidance on how to help their child during the procedure beyond just being present. Studies suggest that talking to and touching the child during the procedure is both soothing and anxiety relieving. Other distractive strategies include:

- Looking at pop-up books or interactive toys
- Listening through headphones to stories or music

- Blowing bubbles
- Video or interactive computer games
- Moving images projected onto a nearby wall, e.g. fish swimming or birds flying
- The presence of transitional objects (comforters), e.g. favourite blanket or soft toy

Pharmacological treatment

Local anaesthetics: topical on intact skin

Ametop gel   This contains tetracaine (amethocaine) base 4%.

- It is used under an occlusive dressing
- Analgesia is achieved after 30–45 minutes
- Anaesthesia remains for 4–6 hours after removal of the gel
- Slight erythema, itching and oedema may occur at the site
- Not to be applied on broken skin, mucous membranes, eyes or ears
- Can cause sensitisation on repeated exposure
- Not recommended for a patient under 1 month of age

EMLA   A mixture of lidocaine 2.5% and prilocaine 2.5% can be used in a similar fashion where sensitivity to Ametop occurs. EMLA, however, takes around 60 minutes to work effectively and tends to cause vasoconstriction rather than vasodilatation.

Ethyl chloride spray   This works immediately.

Local anaesthetics: infiltrated

Lidocaine (lignocaine)   1% lidocaine is used for rapid and intense sensory nerve block.

- The onset of action is significant within 2 minutes and is effective for up to 2 hours.
- It is often used with adrenaline to prolong the duration of sensory blockade and to limit toxicity by reducing absorption (adrenaline concentration 5 micrograms/ml). Adrenaline-containing local anaesthetic should not be used in areas served by an end artery, such as a digit.
- The maximum body dose is 3 mg/kg for plain solutions and 7 mg/kg for solutions that contain adrenaline.

Bupivacaine   This local anaesthetic is used – at a concentration of 0.25% or 0.5% – when longer lasting local anaesthesia is required, such as in femoral nerve blocks. L-Bupivacaine used in the same dose is associated with less toxicity.

- The onset of anaesthesia is for up to 15 minutes but its effects last up to 8 hours.
- Maximum body dosage is 2 mg/kg.

Local anaesthetics are manufactured to a pH of 5 (to improve shelf-life) and are painful for this reason. A buffered solution and the use of smaller needles will lessen the pain associated with infiltration, but local adrenaline cannot then be used because the bicarbonate buffer inactivates it.

Overdose or inadvertent injection of local anaesthetics into an artery or vein may result in cardiac arrhythmias and convulsions. Resuscitative facilities and skills must therefore be available wherever and whenever these drugs are injected.

Non-opioid analgesics

These drugs exhibit varying degrees of analgesic, antipyretic and anti-inflammatory activity.

Paracetamol   Paracetamol is probably the most widely used analgesic in paediatric practice. It may be administered by the oral, rectal and intravenous routes. It is thought to work through inhibiting cyclo-oxygenase in the central nervous system but not in other tissues, so that it produces analgesia without any anti-inflammatory effect. It does not cause respiratory depression. It is very safe when administered at the recommended dose although overdosage in a large single dose or too frequent smaller doses may cause hepatotoxicity. Higher loading doses have been shown to improve pain control (see Appendix G).

Non-steroidal anti-inflammatory drugs (NSAIDs)   These are anti-inflammatory and antipyretic drugs with moderate analgesic properties. They are less well tolerated than paracetamol, causing gastric irritation, platelet disorders, bronchospasm and renal impairment. They should therefore be avoided in children with a history of gastric ulceration, platelet abnormalities and dehydration or renal problems. Their advantage is that they are especially useful for post-traumatic pain because of the additional anti-inflammatory effect. Ibuprofen is given by mouth, and if rectal administration is necessary then diclofenac can be used.

Opiate analgesics

Morphine   Administered intravenously, morphine produces a rapid onset of excellent analgesia and remains the treatment of choice in many situations. It may be titrated to effect and reversed if necessary. Side effects include respiratory depression, nausea and vomiting. Cardiovascular effects include peripheral vasodilatation and venous pooling, but in single doses it has minimal haemodynamic effect in a supine patient with normal circulating volume. In hypovolaemic patients it will contribute to hypotension but this is not a contraindication to its use and merely an indication for cardiovascular monitoring and action as appropriate. Opioids produce a dose-dependent depression of ventilation primarily by reducing the sensitivity of brain-stem respiratory centres to hypercarbia and hypoxia. This means that a patient who has received a dose of an opioid requires observation and/or monitoring and should not be discharged home until it is clear that the effects of the opiate are significantly reduced. The nausea and vomiting produced in adults by morphine seems to be less common in children.

The intranasal route for the administration of opiates such as diamorphine and fentanyl has been shown to be a safe and effective route and is becoming increasingly popular for children. It also has the advantage of being quick and easy, avoiding the trauma of an intravenous cannula.

Opiate antagonists

Naloxone   Naloxone is a potent opioid antagonist. It antagonises the sedative, respiratory-depressive and analgesic effects of opioids. It is rapidly metabolised and is given parenterally because of its rapid first-pass extraction through the liver following oral administration. Following intravenous administration, naloxone reverses the effects of opiates virtually immediately. Its duration of action, however, is much shorter than the opiate agonist. Therefore, repeated doses or an infusion may be required if continued opiate antagonism is wanted.

Inhalational analgesia

Entonox   Nitrous oxide is a colourless, odourless gas that provides analgesia in subanaesthetic concentrations. It is supplied in premixed cylinders at a 50% concentration with oxygen or at a concentration of up to 70% with oxygen via a blender. Delivery devices either act on a demand principle, i.e. the gas is only delivered when the patient inhales and applies a negative pressure, or via a free-flowing circuit. The latter delivery system requires a scavenger circuit. Generally during nitrous oxide therapy, the patient has to be awake and cooperative to be able to inhale the gas; this is an obvious safeguard with the technique.

- Because nitrous oxide is inhaled and has a low solubility in blood, its onset of effect is very rapid. It takes 2–3 minutes to achieve its peak effect. For the same reason, the drug wears off over several minutes, enabling patients to recover considerably quicker than if they received narcotics or sedatives. Laryngeal protective reflexes do not always remain intact.
- Nitrous oxide is therefore most suitable for procedures where short-lived intense analgesia is required, e.g. dressing changes, suturing, needle procedures such as venous cannulation, lumbar punctures and for pain relief during splinting or transport. It is also of benefit for immediate pain relief on presentation until definitive analgesia is effective.
- Using a free flow circuit, nitrous oxide can be used by children as young as 2 years of age, although children will need to be 4 or 5 years of age before they can trigger the demand valve of a premixed cylinder.
- Nitrous oxide may cause nausea, vomiting, euphoria and disinhibition. Prolonged exposure to high concentrations can cause bone marrow depression and neuronal degeneration.
- Nitrous oxide is contraindicated in children with possible intracranial or intrathoracic air because gas diffusion into the confined space may increase pressure.

Sedative drugs

In addition to analgesics, psychotropic drugs may also be useful when undertaking lengthy or repeated procedures. Sedatives relieve anxiety but not pain and may reduce the child's ability to communicate discomfort and therefore should not be given in isolation. The problems associated with the use of sedatives are those of side effects (usually hyperexcitability) and the time required for the child to be awake enough to be allowed home if admission is not necessary.

Midazolam   This is an amnesic and sedative drug. It can be given intravenously, intramuscularly, orally or intranasally (although this is unpleasant). It has an onset time of action of 15 minutes after an oral administration and recovery occurs after about an hour. It may cause respiratory depression, necessitating monitoring of respiratory function and pulse oximetry. A few children become hyperexcitable with this drug. Whilst its action can be reversed by flumazenil, intravenously this is rarely necessary and can precipitate seizures.

Ketamine   Ketamine is a potent anaesthetic agent that has an established place in paediatric procedural pain relief in many emergency settings. It causes a dissociative anaesthesia, which is amnesic and analgesic, but has little effect on breathing and maintaining protective airway reflexes. Side effects include hypersalivation, tachycardia and hypertension, but previous concerns with regard to increasing intracranial pressure are no longer valid. Laryngospasm is a rare complication that may be precipitated by instrumentation of the upper airway.

Ketamine should be considered as an anaesthetic agent and used with all the precautions generally associated with anaesthesia. Emergence phenomenon can be treated with midazolam if necessary but are much less common in paediatric than in adult practice.

Specific clinical situations

Severe pain

Children in severe pain (e.g. major trauma, femoral fracture, significant burns, displaced or comminuted fractures, etc.) should receive IV morphine at an initial dose of 0.1–0.2 mg/kg infused over 2–3 minutes (see Appendix G). A further dose can be given after 5–10 minutes if sufficient analgesia is not achieved. The patient should be monitored using pulse oximetry and electrocardiography.

Head injuries

There is often concern about giving morphine to a patient who has had a head injury and who could therefore potentially lose consciousness secondary to the head injury. If the patient is conscious and in pain, then the presence of a potential deteriorating head injury is not a contraindication to giving morphine. First, an analgesic dose is not necessarily a significant sedative; second, if the child's conscious level does deteriorate, then the clinician's first action should be to assess airway, breathing and circulation, intervening where appropriate. If these are stable, then a dose of naloxone will quickly ascertain whether the diminished conscious level is secondary to morphine or (as is much more likely) represents increasing intracranial pressure. There are significant benefits for the head-injured patient in receiving adequate pain relief as the physiological response to pain may increase intracranial pressure.

In the common situation of the patient who has an isolated femoral shaft fracture and a possible head injury, a femoral nerve block may be an effective alternative (see Chapter 23).

Emergency venepuncture and venous cannulation

At present the management of this problem is difficult as topical anaesthetics take up to an hour to be effective. Inhaled nitrous oxide given by one of the methods described earlier gives excellent results. Alternatives in an emergency include ethyl chloride spray, an ice cube inside the finger of a plastic glove placed over the vein to be cannulated or local anaesthetic infiltration (1% buffered lidocaine) using a very fine gauge (e.g. 29 gauge) needle.

2.7 Summary

You should now be able to:

- Describe the structured approach to paediatric emergencies
- Identify the approach to triage of a child
- Implement an approach to pain management in children

Explanatory notes of the Alder Hey Triage Pain Score

Cry/voice

Score 0   Child is not crying and, although may be quiet, is vocalising appropriately with carer or taking notice of surroundings

Score 1   Child is crying but consolable/distractible or is excessively quiet and responding negatively to carer. On direct questioning says it is painful

Score 2   Child is inconsolable, crying and/or persistently complaining about pain

Facial expression

Score 0   Normal expression and affect

Score 1   Some transient expressions that suggest pain/distress are witnessed but less than 50% of time

Score 2   Persistent facial expressions suggesting pain/distress more than 50% of time

Grimace: open mouth, lips pulled back at corners, furrowed forehead and/or between eyebrows, eyes closed, wrinkled at corners.

Posture

This relates to the child's behaviour to the affected body area.

Score 0   Normal

Score 1   Exhibiting increased awareness of affected area, e.g. by touching, rubbing, pointing, sparing or limping

Score 2   Affected area is held tense and defended so that touching it is deterred; non-weight-bearing

Movement

This relates to how the child moves the whole body.

Score 0   Normal

Score 1   Movement is reduced or child is noted to be restless/uncomfortable

Score 2   Movement is abnormal, either very still/rigid or writhing in agony/shaking

Colour

Score 0   Normal

Score 1   Pale

Score 2   Very pale 'green', the colour that can sometimes be seen with nausea or fainting – extreme pallor

CHAPTER 3
Human factors

Learning outcomes

After reading this chapter, you will be able to:
• Describe how human factors affect the performance of individuals and teams in the healthcare environment

---

3.1 Introduction

The emphasis on the management of paediatric emergency care has traditionally concentrated on knowledge of the treatment process, for example when to give a specific intervention, drug or aliquot of fluid. An often over-looked element is how in these high pressure situations individuals from a variety of different professional and specialty backgrounds come together to form an effective team that minimises errors and works actively to prevent adverse events.

This chapter provides a brief introduction to some of the human factors that can affect the performance of individuals and teams in the healthcare environment. Human factors, also referred to as ergonomics, is an established scientific discipline and clinical human factors has been described as:

> *Enhancing clinical performance through an understanding of the effects of teamwork, tasks, equipment, workspace, culture and organisation on human behaviour and abilities and application of that knowledge in clinical settings.* (Catchpole, 2010)

3.2 Extent of healthcare error

In 2000 an influential report entitled *To Err is Human: Building a Safer Health System* (Catchpole, 2010) suggested that across the USA somewhere between 44 000 and 98 000 deaths each year could be attributed to medical error. A pilot study in the UK demonstrated that approximately one in 10 patients admitted to healthcare experienced an adverse event.

Healthcare has been able to learn from a number of other high-risk industries including the nuclear, petrochemical, space exploration, military and aviation industries about how team issues have been managed. These lessons have been slowly adopted and translated to healthcare.

Specialist working groups and national bodies have been instrumental in promoting awareness of the importance of human factors in healthcare. They aim to raise awareness and promote the principles and practices of human factors, identify current human factor activity, capability and barriers, and create conditions to support human factors being embedded at a local level. One such example of this in the UK is the Human Factors Clinical Working Group and the National Quality Board's concordat statement on human factors.

Advanced Paediatric Life Support: A Practical Approach to Emergencies, Sixth Edition. Edited by Martin Samuels and Sue Wieteska.
© 2016 John Wiley & Sons, Ltd. Published 2016 by John Wiley & Sons, Ltd.

3.3 Causes of healthcare error

Consider this example of an adverse event:

A child needs to receive an infusion of a particular drug. An error occurs and the child receives an incorrect drug. What are the potential causes of this situation?

Potential causes of our example drug error	
Prescription error	Wrong drug prescribed
Preparation error	Correct drug prescribed but misread
Preparation error	Contents mislabelled during manufacture
Drawing up error	Incorrect drug selected
Administration error	Patient ID mix-up, drug given to wrong patient

Q. What one thing links all of these errors?
A. The humans involved – these are all examples of human errors.

Humans make mistakes. No amount of checks and procedures will mitigate this fact. In fact the only way to completely remove human error is to remove all the humans involved. It is vital therefore that we look to work in a way that, wherever possible, minimises the occurrence of mistakes and ensures that when they do occur the method minimises the chance of the error resulting in an adverse event.

3.4 Human error

It has been suggested that these human errors can be further categorised into: (i) those that occur at the sharp end of care by the treating team and individuals; and (ii) those that occur at the blunt or organisational level, typically through policies, procedures, staffing and culture. These errors can be further subdivided (Table 3.1).

Table 3.1 Types of errors

		Explanation	Example
Sharp errors that occur with the team/individuals treating the patient	Mistake	Lack or misapplication of knowledge	Not knowing the correct drug to prescribe
	Slip or lapse	Skills-based mistake	Knowing the correct drug but writing another one
	Violation	Deliberate action that may be routine or exceptional	Not attempting to get a drug second checked as there are no staff available
Blunt/organisational errors		Policies, procedures, infrastructure and building layout that has errors embedded	Different drugs used by different specialities and departments for same condition

It is typically found that the latent/organisational issues often coexist with the sharp errors; in fact it is rare for an isolated error to occur – often there is a chain of events that results in the adverse event. The 'Swiss cheese' model demonstrates how apparently random, unconnected events and organisational decisions can all make errors more likely (Figure 3.1). Conversely, a standardised system with good defences can capture these errors and prevent adverse events.

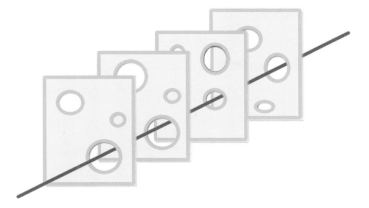

Figure 3.1 The 'Swiss cheese' model

Each of the slices of Swiss cheese represents barriers that, under ideal circumstances, would prevent or detect the error. The holes represent weaknesses in these barriers; if the holes align the error passes through undetected.

Reconsider the example of drug error using the Swiss cheese model. The first slice is the doctor writing the prescription, the second slice is the organisation's drug policy, the third is the nurse who draws up the drug and the fourth is the nurse who second checks the drug.

Now consider the following: What if the doctor is very junior and not familiar with that area or drugs used? – his slice of cheese has larger holes. What if the organisation has failed to develop a robust drug policy that is fit for purpose? – this second slice is considerably weakened or may even be removed completely. What if the nurse is a bank nurse who does not normally work on this ward and is not familiar with commonly used drugs? – her slice has also got larger holes. What if this area is always short of staff so other staff do not routinely attempt to get the drug second checked? – this slice is completely removed.

The end result is that multiple defences have been weakened or removed and error is more likely, and the error is more likely to cause harm. Also be aware of the different types of error with potential gaps in knowledge, a latent/organisational error (no effective policy and possibly an issue with nurse staffing) and a routine violation.

3.5 Learning from error

Historically, those making mistakes have been identified and singled out for punishment and/or retraining, in what is often referred to as a culture of blame. With our example drug error blame would most likely have fallen on the shoulders of the nurse administering and/or the doctor incorrectly prescribing. Does retraining these individuals make it safer for other or future patients? That clearly depends on the underlying reasons. If it was purely a knowledge gap, possibly, but does the same knowledge gap exist elsewhere? Potentially all the other issues remain unresolved. Moreover such punitive reactions make it less likely for individuals to admit mistakes and near misses in the future.

The focus is now on learning from error and, in shifting away from the individual, is much more focused on determining the system/organisational errors. Once robust systems, procedures and policies that work and are effective are in place, then errors can be captured. Of course issues will still need to be addressed where individuals have been reckless or lacked knowledge – but now reasons why the individuals felt the need to violate, or had not been given all the knowledge required, can be looked at.

For this to work health services need to learn from errors, adverse events and near misses. This requires engagement at both the individual level, by reporting errors, and the organisational level, investigating and feeding back the error using a systematic approach. It is also key that information is cascaded through the organisation and across the health service to raise awareness and prevent similar situations.

Violation may be indicative of the failure of systems, procedures or policies or other cultural issues. It is important that policies, procedures, roles and even our buildings and equipment are all designed pro-actively with human factors in mind so things do not have to be fixed retrospectively when adverse events occur. This means that all members of the organisation must be aware of human factors, not just the front-line clinical staff.

Improving team and individual performance

Having discussed the magnitude of the problem of healthcare error, the rest of this chapter will focus on how the performance of teams and individuals can be developed.

Raising awareness of the human factors and being able to practise these skills and behaviours within multi-professional teams allows the development of effective teams in all situations. Simulation activity allows a team to explore these new ideas, practise them and develop them. To do this we need feedback on our performance within a safe environment where no patient is at risk and egos and personal interests can be set aside. Consider how you developed a clinical skill. It was something that needed to be practised again and again until eventually it started to become automatic and routine. The same applies for our human factor behaviours. In addition, recognising our inherent human limitations and the situations when errors are more likely to occur, we can all be hyper-vigilant when required.

3.6 Communication

Poor communication is the leading cause of adverse events. This is not surprising; to have an effective team there needs to be good communication. The leader needs to communicate with the followers, and followers communicate with leaders and other followers. Communication is not just saying something – it is ensuring that information is accurately passed on and received. We all want to ensure effective communication at all times. Remember there are multiple components to effective communication (Table 3.2).

Table 3.2 Elements of communication				
Sender	**Sender**	**Transmitted**	**Receiver**	**Receiver**
Thinks of what to say	Says message	Through air, over phone, via email	Hears it	Thinks about it and acts

When communicating face-to-face a lot of the information is transmitted non-verbally, which can make telephone or email conversations more challenging. Communication can be more difficult when talking across professional, specialty or hierarchal barriers as we do not always talk the same technical language, have the same levels of understanding, or even have a full awareness of the other person's role.

There are a variety of similar tools to aid communication, like SBAR (Situation Background Assessment and Recommendation). Find out what your organisation uses and practise using it; look out for other staff using it too. SBAR is designed for acute clinical communications. It facilitates the sender to plan and organise the message, make it succinct and focused, and provide it in a logical and expected order. It is also an empowerment tool allowing the sender (who may be more junior) to request an action from a more senior individual. While these tools are useful, they tend to be reserved for certain situations, whereas we want to establish effective communication as the routine not the exception. One method to routinely improve communication is to incorporate a feedback loop.

Effective communication with a feedback loop

Errors can occur at any level or multiple levels. Consider a busy clinical situation and the team leader shouts '*We need an ECG connecting*' while looking at the blood pressure – what happens? The majority of times nothing – nobody goes to connect the ECG! So how can this be improved? Most obviously an individual can be identified to perform the task, by name: '*Michael can you please connect the ECG?*' If Michael says '*yes*' effective communication might be assumed; but not always. What has Michael heard and what will he do? At the moment we do not really know what message has been received. Michael might dash over with a cup of tea as this is what he thought he heard. This may seem a slightly strange thing to happen; but how often in a clinical emergency have you asked for something and been presented with something else? People are less likely to ask questions in emergencies as everyone is busy. This could be the catalyst for an error or precipitate a missed task. So how do we find out what message Michael received? The easiest way is to include a feedback loop.

> Now the conversation goes:
>
> Team leader: 'Michael, can you please connect the ECG?'
> Michael: 'Okay, just connecting the ECG'

We now know that the message has been transmitted and received correctly. For this process to work both parties (the sender and receiver) need to understand and expect it – again demonstrating the need for us to practise and train together.

3.7 Team working, leadership and followership

At a basic level a team is a group of individuals with a common cause. Historically we have tended to train individually or in professional silos; the risk here is that we are making a 'team of experts' rather than an 'expert team'. Often within healthcare our teams form at short notice and often arrive at different times. Much emphasis has previously been given to the role of the leader, but a leader cannot be a team on his or her own. As much emphasis should be given to developing the other team members, the active followers. A good leader will be able to swap from the role of leader to follower as more senior staff arrive and agree to take over.

The leader

The leader's role is multifaceted and includes directing the team, assigning tasks and assessing performance, motivating and encouraging the team to work together, and planning and organising. All leadership skills and behaviours need to be developed and practised. There are different leadership styles and the leader needs to choose an appropriate style for that situation. Effective communication is key and should be reviewed and reflected upon regularly. Constructive feedback should both be given and sought in order to facilitate continuously improving performance.

Who is the leader?

It is vitally important to have a clearly identified leader. There can be times when people come and go, or different specialties arrive, creating a situation where it may not be clear who the leader is. In some situations or institutions individuals will wear tabards or other forms of identification to mitigate against this uncertainty. If there is a scribe recording events they should record who is leading and any changes to the leader.

Physical position of the leader

As soon as the leader becomes hands on, and task focused, they are primarily concentrating on the task at hand. This becomes the focus of their thoughts and they lose situation awareness, their objective overview of the situation (see Section 3.8). The leader should be standing in an optimal position where they can gather all the information and ideally view the patient, the team members and the monitoring and diagnostic equipment. This enables them to recognise when a member is struggling with a task or procedure and support them appropriately.

Clear roles

Ideally the team should meet before the event and have the opportunity to introduce each other, and clarify roles and actions in emergencies. Sometimes this can be facilitated at the beginning of a shift but at other times it is impossible to predict or arrange. It is important, therefore, that individuals identify themselves to the leader as they arrive and roles are agreed, allocated and understood. A lot of the time their role may be determined purely in relation to the specific bleep the individual carries, but it is important that team members are flexible, for example if three airway providers are first on the scene we would expect other tasks to also be undertaken.

Followership

The followers have roles that are as mission critical as the leader. Followers are expected to work within their scope of practice and take the initiative. No one would expect to turn up at a ward emergency and have a neat row of staff against the wall waiting for instructions. It is important to think about the level of communication required between the leader and followers. If it is obvious we are doing a task, this does not need to be communicated. There is a risk that followers can overwhelm the leader with verbal communications where, in fact, the key is to communicate concerns or abnormal things. In the Formula

One pit lane during a tyre change, the crew communicate (visually) as tasks are completed; they also signal if they have a problem, they do not communicate every expected step.

Hierachy

Within the team there needs to be a hierachy. This is the power gradient; the leader is at the top of this as the person coordinating, directing and making the decisions. However, this should not be absolute. There is much discussion in the literature about the degree of the hierarchical gradient. If it is too steep the leader has a massive position of power, his or her decisions are unquestionable and the followers blindly follow the orders. This is not safe because leaders are humans too and also make errors – their team is their safety net. Safe practice is achieved where the followers feel they can raise concerns or question instructions. This must always be understood by the leaders as much as by the followers. One way to reduce the hierarchy is for the leader to invite the team's thoughts and concerns, particularly around patient safety issues. It is also important for the follower to learn how to raise concerns appropriately.

One method that is sometimes used to raise concerns appropriately is PACE (probing, alerting, challenging or declaring an emergency). The probing question allows diplomacy and maintenance of the hierarchy whilst raising a point.

Stage	Level of concern
P – Probe	*I think you need to know what is happening*
A – Alert	*I think something bad might happen*
C – Challenge	*I know something bad will happen*
E – Emergency	*I will not let it happen*

These stages are described with examples below:

- **Probe** – this is used where a person notices something they think might be a problem. They verbalise the issue, often as a question. 'Have you noticed that this child is cyanosed?'
- **Alert** – the observer strengthens and directs their statement and suggests a course of action. 'Dr Brown, I am concerned, the child is deeply cyanosed, should we start BVM ventilation?'
- **Challenge** – the situation requires urgent attention. One of the key protagonists needs to be directly engaged. If possible the speaker places him- or herself into the eye line of the person they wish to communicate with. 'Dr Brown, you must listen to me now, this patient needs help with his ventilation.'
- **Emergency** – this is used where all else has failed and/or the observer perceives a critical event is about to occur. Where possible a physical signal or physical barrier should be employed together with clear verbalisation. 'Dr Brown, you are overlooking this child's respiratory state, please move out of the way as I am going to ventilate him.'

The PACE structure can be commenced at any appropriate level and escalated until a satisfactory response is gained. If an adverse event is imminent then it may be relevant to start at the declaring 'emergency' stage, whereas a much lower level of concern may well start at a 'probing' question.

Some industries have also additionally adopted organisation-wide critical phrases that convey the importance of the situation, e.g. 'I am concerned', 'I am uncomfortable' or 'I am scared'.

3.8 Situation awareness

A key element of good team working and leadership is to be fully aware of what is happening; this is termed situation awareness. It not only involves seeing what is happening, but also captures how this is interpreted and understood, how decisions are made and ultimately to plan ahead.

Typically, three levels of situation awareness are described:

Level 1 – What is going on?
Level 2 – So what?
Level 3 – Now what?

Consider **Level 1** – the basic level – we are prone to errors even at this level. This is an active process, the risk seen is what is expected to be seen, rather than what is there. Figure 3.2 shows the similar package design of two different medications, making errors more likely. It is important to really concentrate on seeing what is actually there.

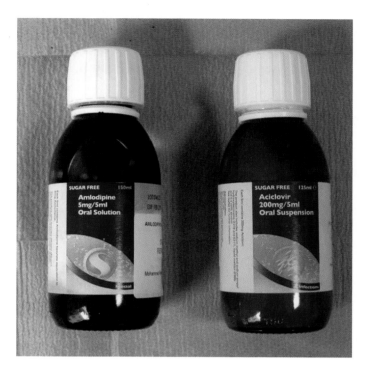

Figure 3.2 Similar package design of two different medications

Distraction

Within healthcare distractions become the norm to such an extent individuals are often not even aware of them. The risk is that mistakes are made and information is missed. It is important to try to challenge interruptions when doing critical tasks, and when they do occur restart the task from the beginning, rather than from where it is considered the interruption occurred. Some organisations are looking at specific quiet areas for critical tasks. Whatever the local set up, the key is to develop and maintain everyone's awareness of how distraction greatly increases the chance of error.

Level 2 captures how someone's understanding forms from what has been seen. To minimise level 2 errors consideration is needed as to how the human brain works, recognises things and makes decisions and choices. This level of detail is beyond the scope of this introductory chapter, and therefore this section will focus on a part of this – the decision making that leads into Level 3.

On the face of it the practice of decision making is familiar to everyone. However, to understand the factors that can compromise this process it is important to understand the factors that will influence the decision made. To make a good decision a person needs to assess all aspects of a problem, identify the possible responses to the problem, consider the consequences of each of those responses and then weigh up the advantages and disadvantages in order to draw a conclusion. Having completed this, they then need to communicate their decision to their team.

Good situation awareness is a basic prerequisite of this process. To achieve this, the decision maker must ensure they have all the key information. The whole team should be on the alert for ambiguities or conflicting information. Any inconsistent facts should be treated as a potential marker for faulty situation awareness. They should never be brushed off as unimportant anomalies in the absence of evidence to support such a decision.

In many clinical situations there can be a significant pressure of time. Where this is not the case then no decision-making process should be concluded until the team is satisfied they have all the information and have considered all the options.

Where time is a pressure, a certain amount of pragmatism must be employed. There is plenty of evidence to confirm that practise and experience can mitigate some of the negative effects of abbreviating a decision-making process. Those making decisions under such circumstances need to remain aware of the short-cuts they have taken. They should be ready to receive feedback from their team, particularly if any member of the team has significant concerns about the proposed course of action.

Level 3 – having seen and understood we can now plan forward and communicate this with the team.

Team situation awareness

The individuals in the team may have a differing awareness of the situation depending on their previous experience, specialty, physical position, etc. The team's situation awareness will often be greater than any one individual's, however this can only be exploited if the individual elements are effectively communicated. The leader should actively encourage this.

3.9 Improving team and individual performance

In addition to effective communication, team working, situation awareness, leadership and followership skills, there are a number of other ways that team and individual performance can be further developed and improved.

Awareness of situations when errors are more likely

If we are aware that an error is more likely we can be more proactive in detecting them. Two common situations that make errors more likely are stress and fatigue. Stress is not only a source of error when we are overworked and overstimulated, but also, at the other end of the spectrum, when we are understimulated we become inattentive.

The acronym HALT has been used to describe situations when error is more likely:

H – Hungry
A – Angry
L – Late
T – Tired

IMSAFE has been used as a checklist in the aviation industry, asking whether the individual may be affected by:

I – Illness
M – Medication
S – Stress
A – Alcohol
F – Fatigue
E – Emotion

Ideally, individuals who are potentially compromised need to be supported appropriately, allowed time to recover and the team made aware. How this can be achieved in the middle of a night shift can be problematic.

Awareness of error traps

A common trap that people fall into is only seeing or registering the information that fits in with their current mental model. This is known as a *confirmation bias*. When this occurs people favour information that confirms their preconceptions or hypotheses regardless of whether the information is true. This may be observed within the healthcare setting during the process of a referral or handover. An example of this might be a clinician receiving a phone call requesting them to attend the ward to review an acutely deteriorating patient. The clinician is advised that the patient is a known asthmatic. On their way to the ward the clinician builds up a series of preconceived expectations around what they will find upon their arrival. They may even formulate a management plan whilst travelling to the scene, based upon their expectations. Once this mindset is established it can be difficult to shift.

On arrival, the clinician examines the systems affected by the presumed diagnosis. They seek to confirm their expectation by focusing on an auscultation of the chest at the expense of a thorough assessment. Upon hearing bilateral wheeze their preconceived ideas are confirmed and the remainder of the assessment is completed without due attention and more as a rehearsed exercise rather than an open-minded exploration. They fail to notice that the patient also has a soft stridor and is hypotensive. In this case the eventual diagnosis of anaphylaxis becomes at best a very late consideration, or at worst a situation that requires an objective newcomer to the team to point out the obvious.

Cognitive aids: checklists, guidelines and protocols

Cognitive aids such as guidelines are important because the human memory is not infallible. They also confer team understanding through the use of a standardised response. This reduces stress. This is especially true where an uncommon emergency event occurs. The team may be unfamiliar with one another and each member will be trying to remember what to do, what treatments are required and in what order. A good team leader will use the available cognitive aids as a prompt and the team's members can use it as a resource so that they can plan ahead. Safe practice is promoted through the use of these tools in an emergency rather than relying on memory.

Calling for help early

Trainee staff are often reluctant to call for senior help, partly due to not recognising the severity of the situation and partly due to concerns about wasting the time of seniors. With all emergency events, and in particular with paediatric emergencies, escalation and appropriate help should be summoned as soon as possible. Remember, help will not arrive instantly.

Using all available resources

Team resources include staff, observations, equipment, cognitive aids and the facilities in the local area. The team leader should continually consider the appropriateness of utilising available, un-tasked staff or equipment to optimise the patient's care and prevent a bottleneck in the treatment pathway.

Debriefing

Wherever possible a debriefing should be facilitated, even briefly, following clinical events. Ideally this should be normal procedure, rather than being reserved for catastrophic events. The aim of a debrief is to summarise any particular issues or problems that the team had, and reflect on how the team performed. Some organisations have set templates to facilitate this. It gives the opportunity for individuals, teams and organisations to continually develop.

3.10 Summary

In this chapter we have given a brief introduction to the human factors that can lead to poor team working, patient harm and adverse events. It is really important for you to use every opportunity to reflect and develop your own performance and influence the development of others and the team. Appropriate debriefing is included in the scenarios for the APLS course, which may be used to inform incorporation of this process into your own clinical practice.

PART 2
The seriously ill child

CHAPTER 4
Structured approach to the seriously ill child

Learning outcomes

After reading this chapter, you will be able to:
- Describe how to recognise the seriously ill child
- Describe a structured approach to the assessment of the seriously ill child
- Describe a structured approach to resuscitation and treatment of the seriously ill child

---

4.1 Introduction

As described in Chapter 1, the outcome for children following cardiac arrest is, in general, poor. Earlier recognition and management of potential respiratory, circulatory or central neurological failure will reduce mortality and secondary morbidity. Sections 4.2–4.5 outline the physical signs that should be checked during the rapid assessment of children. It is divided systematically into looking for signs of potential respiratory, circulatory and central neurological failure and constitutes the primary and secondary assessment.

The normal ranges are provided for reference in Table 4.1, these are referred to throughout the chapter.

4.2 Primary assessment of airway and breathing

Recognition of potential respiratory failure

The effort, efficacy and effect of breathing need to be assessed bearing in mind the effects of respiratory inadequacy on other organs in the child's body.

Effort of breathing

The degree of increase in the effort of breathing allows clinical assessment of the severity of respiratory disease. It is important to assess the following.

Respiratory rate

Normal resting respiratory rates at differing ages are shown in Table 4.1. Rates are higher in infancy, and fall with increasing age. Care should be taken in interpreting single measurements: infants can show rates of between 30 and 90 breaths per minute depending on their state of activity. The World Health Organisation (WHO) uses a cut-off of 60 breaths per minute for pneumonia in infants and young children. Most useful are trends in the measurement as an

---

Advanced Paediatric Life Support: A Practical Approach to Emergencies, Sixth Edition. Edited by Martin Samuels and Sue Wieteska.
© 2016 John Wiley & Sons, Ltd. Published 2016 by John Wiley & Sons, Ltd.

indicator of improvement or deterioration. At rest, tachypnoea indicates that increased ventilation is needed because of either lung or airway disease, or metabolic acidosis. A slow respiratory rate indicates fatigue, cerebral depression or a pre-terminal state.

Table 4.1 Normal ranges: respiratory rate (RR), heart rate (HR) and blood pressure (BP)

Age	Guide weight (kg) Boys	Guide weight (kg) Girls	RR At rest Breaths per minute 5th–95th centile	HR Beats per minute 5th–95th centile	BP Systolic 5th centile	BP Systolic 50th centile	BP Systolic 95th centile
Birth	3.5	3.5	25–50	120–170	65–75	80–90	105
1 month	4.5	4.5					
3 months	6.5	6	25–45	115–160			
6 months	8	7	20–40	110–160			
12 months	9.5	9			70–75	85–95	
18 months	11	10	20–35	100–155			
2 years	12	12	20–30	100–150	70–80	85–100	110
3 years	14	14		90–140			
4 years	16	16		80–135			
5 years	18	18			80–90	90–110	111–120
6 years	21	20		80–130			
7 years	23	22					
8 years	25	25	15–25	70–120			
9 years	28	28					
10 years	31	32					
11 years	35	35					
12 years	43	43	12–24	65–115	90–105	100–120	125–140
14 years	50	50		60–110			
Adult	70	70					

Recession

Intercostal, subcostal, sternal or suprasternal (tracheal tug) recession shows increased effort of breathing. This sign more readily develops in younger infants as they have a more compliant chest wall. Its presence in older children (i.e. over 6 or 7 years) suggests severe respiratory compromise. The degree of recession gives an indication of the severity of respiratory difficulty. In the child who has become exhausted through increased effort of breathing, recession decreases as they develop respiratory failure.

Inspiratory or expiratory noises

An inspiratory noise while breathing (stridor) is a sign of laryngeal or tracheal obstruction. In severe obstruction the stridor may also occur in expiration, but the inspiratory component is usually more pronounced. Wheezing indicates lower airway narrowing and is more pronounced in expiration. A prolonged expiratory phase also indicates lower airway narrowing. The volume of the noise is not an indicator of severity, as it may disappear in the pre-terminal state.

Grunting

Grunting is produced by exhalation against a partially closed glottis. It is an attempt to generate a positive end-expiratory pressure and prevent airway collapse at the end of expiration in children with 'stiff' lungs. This is a sign of severe respiratory distress and is characteristically seen in infants with pneumonia or pulmonary oedema. It may also be seen with raised intracranial pressure, abdominal distension or peritonism.

Accessory muscle use

As in adult life, the sternomastoid muscle may be used as an accessory respiratory muscle when the effort of breathing is increased. In infants, this is ineffectual and just causes the head to bob up and down with each breath.

Flaring of the nostrils

Flaring of the nostrils is seen especially in infants with respiratory distress.

Gasping

This is a sign of severe hypoxia and may be pre-terminal.

Exceptions

There may be absent or decreased evidence of increased effort of breathing in three circumstances:

1. In the infant or child who has had severe respiratory problems for some time, fatigue may occur and the signs of increased effort of breathing will decrease. Exhaustion is a pre-terminal sign.
2. Children with cerebral depression from raised intracranial pressure, poisoning or encephalopathy will have respiratory inadequacy without increased effort of breathing. The respiratory inadequacy in this case is caused by decreased respiratory drive.
3. Children who have neuromuscular disease (such as spinal muscular atrophy or muscular dystrophy) may present in respiratory failure without increased effort of breathing.

The diagnosis of respiratory failure in such children is made by observing the efficacy of breathing, and looking for other signs of respiratory inadequacy. These are discussed in the text.

Efficacy of breathing

Observations of the degree of chest expansion (or, in infants, abdominal excursion) provide an indication of the amount of air being inspired and expired. Similarly, important information is given by auscultation of the chest. Listen for reduced, asymmetrical or bronchial breath sounds. **A silent chest is an extremely worrying sign.**

Pulse oximetry can be used to measure the arterial oxygen saturation (SpO_2). A good plethysmographic (pulse) waveform is important to help confirm the accuracy of measurements. In severe shock and hypothermia, there may be poor or absent pulse detection. Measurements are also less accurate when the SpO_2 is less than 70%, with motion artefact, high levels of ambient light and in the presence of carboxyhaemoglobin. Oximetry in air gives a good indication of the efficacy of breathing, although to assess the adequacy of ventilation, some measure of carbon dioxide should be obtained. Any supplemental oxygen will mask problems with oxygenation due to ineffective breathing, unless the hypoxia is severe. Normal SpO_2 in an infant or child in air at sea level is 97–100%.

Effects of respiratory inadequacy on other organs

Heart rate

Hypoxia produces tachycardia in the older infant and child. Anxiety and a fever will also contribute to tachycardia, making this a non-specific sign. **Severe or prolonged hypoxia leads to bradycardia. This is a pre-terminal sign.**

Skin colour

Hypoxia (via catecholamine release) produces vasoconstriction and skin pallor. **Cyanosis is a late and pre-terminal sign of hypoxia** as it usually becomes apparent when SpO_2 falls to <70%, and only in the absence of anaemia. By the time central cyanosis is visible in acute respiratory disease, the patient is close to respiratory arrest. In the anaemic child, cyanosis may never be visible despite profound hypoxia. A few children will be cyanosed because of cyanotic heart disease, but may have adequate oxygen uptake within the lungs, and their cyanosis will be largely unchanged by oxygen therapy.

Mental status

The hypoxic or hypercapnic child will be agitated and/or drowsy. Gradually drowsiness increases and eventually consciousness is lost. These extremely useful and important signs are often more difficult to detect in small infants. The parents may say that the infant is just 'not himself'. The healthcare practitioner must assess the child's state of alertness by gaining eye contact and noting the response to voice and, if necessary, to painful stimuli. A generalised muscular hypotonia also accompanies hypoxic cerebral depression.

4.3 Primary assessment of the circulation

Recognition of potential circulatory failure

The cardiovascular status needs to be assessed bearing in mind the effects of circulatory inadequacy on other organs.

Cardiovascular status

Heart rate

Normal rates are shown in Table 4.1. The heart rate initially increases in shock due to catecholamine release and as compensation for decreased stroke volume. The rate, particularly in small infants, may be extremely high (up to 220 beats per minute).

An abnormally slow pulse rate, or bradycardia, is defined as less than 60 beats per minute or a rapidly falling heart rate associated with poor systemic perfusion. This is a pre-terminal sign.

Pulse volume

Although blood pressure is maintained until shock is severe, an indication of perfusion can be gained by comparative palpation of both peripheral and central pulses. Absent peripheral pulses and weak central pulses are serious signs of advanced shock, and indicate that hypotension is already present. Bounding pulses may be caused by an increased cardiac output (e.g. septicaemia), arteriovenous systemic shunt (e.g. patent arterial duct) or hypercapnia.

Capillary refill

Following cutaneous pressure on the centre of the sternum or on a digit for 5 seconds, capillary refill should occur within 2 seconds (Figure 4.1). A slower refill time than this can indicate poor skin perfusion, a sign which may be helpful in early septic shock, when the child may otherwise appear well, with warm peripheries.

The presence of fever does not affect the sensitivity of delayed capillary refill in children with hypovolaemia but a low ambient temperature reduces its specificity, so the sign should be used with caution in trauma patients who have been in a cold environment. Poor capillary refill and differential pulse volumes are neither sensitive nor specific indicators of shock in infants and children, but are useful clinical signs when used in conjunction with the other signs described. They should not be used as the only indicators of shock nor as quantitative measures of the response to treatment.

In children with pigmented skin, the sign is more difficult to assess. In these cases the nail beds are used and additionally the sole of the feet in young babies.

(a) (b)

(c) (d)

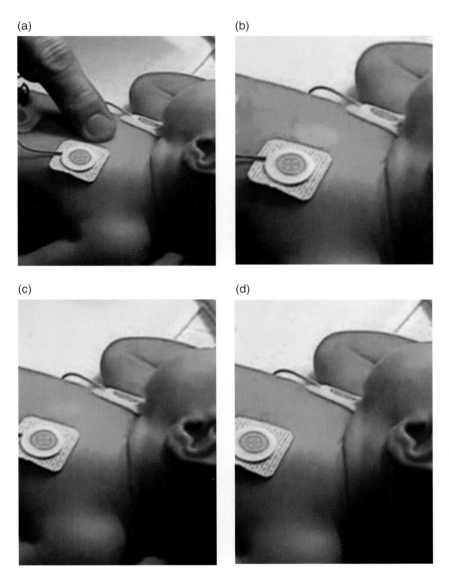

Figure 4.1 (a–d) Capillary refill assessment: apply pressure for 5 seconds and then release. Count in seconds how long it takes for the skin colour to return to normal

Blood pressure

Normal systolic pressures are shown in Table 4.1. In septic shock, target these normal values and respond to trends alongside the other indicators of shock. Use of the correct cuff size is crucial if an accurate blood pressure measurement is to be obtained. This caveat applies to both auscultatory and oscillometric devices. The width of the cuff should be more than 80% of the length of the upper arm and the bladder more than 40% of the arm's circumference.

If the blood pressure is less than the median systolic you should check for other signs of circulatory failure. **Hypotension (less than the 5th centile) is a late and pre-terminal sign of circulatory failure.** Once a child's blood pressure has fallen, cardiac arrest is imminent. Hypertension can be the cause or result of coma and raised intracranial pressure.

Effects of circulatory inadequacy on other organs

Respiratory system

A rapid respiration rate with an increased tidal volume, but without recession, may be caused by the metabolic acidosis resulting from circulatory failure.

Skin

Mottled, cold, pale skin peripherally indicates poor perfusion. A line of coldness may be felt to move centrally as circulatory failure progresses.

Mental status

Agitation and then drowsiness leading to unconsciousness are characteristic of circulatory failure. These signs are caused by poor cerebral perfusion. In an infant, parents may say that he is 'not himself'.

Urinary output

A urine output of less than 1 ml/kg/h in children and less than 2 ml/kg/h in infants indicates inadequate renal perfusion during shock. A history of reduced wet nappies or urine production should be sought.

Cardiac failure

The following features suggest a cardiac cause of respiratory inadequacy:

- Cyanosis, not correcting with oxygen therapy
- Tachycardia out of proportion to respiratory difficulty
- Raised jugular venous pressure
- Gallop rhythm/murmur
- Enlarged liver
- Absent femoral pulses

4.4 Primary assessment of disability

Recognition of potential central neurological failure

Neurological assessment should only be performed after airway (A), breathing (B) and circulation (C) have been assessed and treated. There are no neurological problems that take priority over ABC.

Both respiratory and circulatory failure will have central neurological effects. Conversely, some conditions with direct central neurological effects (such as meningitis, raised intracranial pressure from trauma, and status epilepticus) may also have respiratory and circulatory consequences.

Neurological function

Conscious level

A rapid assessment of conscious level can be made by assigning the patient to one of the categories shown in the box.

A	**A**lert
V	Responds to **V**oice
P	Responds only to **P**ain
U	**U**nresponsive to all stimuli

If the child does not respond to voice, it is important that response to pain is then assessed. A painful central stimulus can be delivered by sternal pressure, by supraorbital ridge pressure or squeezing the trapezius or Achilles tendon. Commonly, a child who is unresponsive or who only responds to pain has a significant degree of coma, equivalent to 8 or less on the Glasgow Coma Scale (GCS).

If the child responds to pain, it is best to note what the eyes and limbs did and what sounds or words were uttered, rather than simply categorising the child as 'P'. Simple descriptions that will form the basis of a subsequent formal GCS, such as 'opening eyes to pain' or 'localising to pain' are much more informative than 'P' alone. A child who does not open his eyes to pain, utters no sounds and extends his limbs has a GCS score of 4 and is likely to need prompt airway protection. A child who opens her eyes to pain, shouts recognisable words inappropriately and localises to the stimulus has a GCS of 10 and is at much less immediate risk. Both are classified as 'P'.

Posture

Many children who are suffering from a serious illness in any system are hypotonic. Stiff posturing such as that shown by decorticate (flexed arms, extended legs) or decerebrate (extended arms, extended legs) children is a sign of serious brain dysfunction (Figure 4.2). These postures can be mistaken for the tonic phase of a convulsion. Alternatively, a painful stimulus may be necessary to elicit these postures. Severe extension of the neck due to upper airway obstruction can mimic the opisthotonos that occurs with meningeal irritation. A stiff neck and full fontanelle in infants are signs which suggest meningitis.

(a)

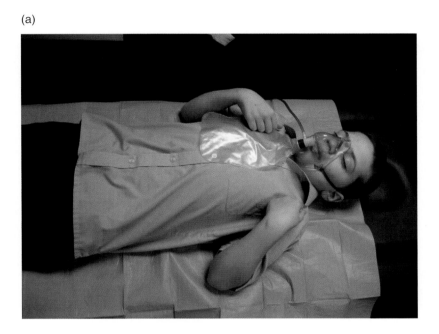

(b)

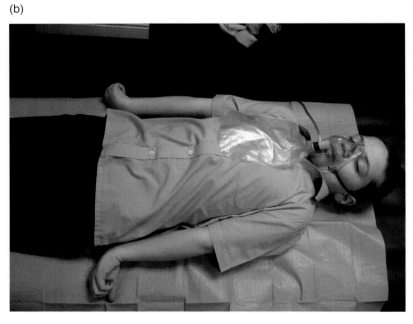

Figure 4.2 (a) Decorticate posturing, and (b) decerebrate posturing

Pupils

Many drugs and cerebral lesions have effects on pupil size and reactions. However, the most important pupillary signs to seek are dilatation, unreactivity and inequality, which indicate possible serious brain disorders.

Respiratory effects of central neurological failure

There are several recognisable breathing pattern abnormalities with raised intracranial pressure. However, they are often changeable and may vary from hyperventilation to Cheyne–Stokes breathing to apnoea. The presence of any abnormal respiratory pattern in a patient with coma suggests mid- or hind-brain dysfunction.

Circulatory effects of central neurological failure

Systemic hypertension with sinus bradycardia (Cushing's response) indicates compression of the medulla oblongata caused by herniation of the cerebellar tonsils through the foramen magnum. **This is a late and pre-terminal sign.**

4.5 Primary assessment of exposure

The examination of the seriously ill child will involve examination for markers of illness that will help provide specific emergency treatment.

Temperature

A fever suggests an infection as the cause of the illness, but may also be the result of prolonged convulsions or shivering. In young infants, infection may present with a low body temperature.

Rash and bruising

Examination is made for rashes, such as urticaria in allergic reactions, purpura, petechiae and bruising in septicaemia and child abuse, or maculopapular and erythematous rashes in allergic reactions and some forms of sepsis.

Reassessment

Single observations on respiratory and heart rates, degree of recession, blood pressure, conscious level, pupils, etc. are useful but much more information can be gained by frequent, repeated observations to detect a trend in the patient's condition. These are commonly now combined into a scoring system to provide an early warning of deterioration, e.g. the Paediatric Early Warning System (PEWS). There is no single validated tool, with different systems being used in different units.

Summary: the rapid clinical assessment of an infant or child

Airway and **B**reathing

- Effort of breathing
- Respiratory rate/rhythm
- Stridor/wheeze
- Auscultation
- Skin colour

Circulation

- Heart rate
- Pulse volume
- Capillary refill
- Skin temperature

Disability

- Mental status/conscious level
- Posture
- Pupils

Exposure

- Fever
- Rash and bruising

The whole assessment should take less than a minute.

Once airway (A), breathing (B) and circulation (C) are clearly recognised as being stable or have been stabilised, then definitive management of the underlying condition can proceed. During definitive management reassessment of ABCDE at frequent intervals will be necessary to assess progress and detect deterioration.

4.6 Structured approach to the seriously ill child

Treatment of a child in an emergency requires rapid assessment and urgent intervention. The structured approach includes:

- Primary assessment
- Resuscitation
- Secondary assessment and looking for key features
- Emergency treatment
- Stabilisation and transfer to definitive care

Primary assessment and resuscitation involve management of the vital ABC functions and assessment of disability (central nervous system function). This assessment and stabilisation occurs before any illness-specific diagnostic assessment or treatment takes place. Once the patient's vital functions are supported, secondary assessment and emergency treatment begins. Illness-specific pathophysiology is sought and emergency treatments are instituted. During the secondary assessment vital signs should be checked frequently to detect any change in the child's condition. If there is deterioration then primary assessment and resuscitation should be repeated.

Stabilisation and transfer to definitive care are covered in Chapter 25.

4.7 Primary assessment and resuscitation

In a severely ill child, a rapid examination of vital functions is required. The physical signs described in Sections 4.2–4.5 are checked in an ABC approach. This primary assessment and any necessary resuscitation must be completed before the more detailed secondary assessment is performed.

Airway

Primary assessment

- Assess patency by:
  - looking for chest and/or abdominal movement
  - listening for breath sounds
  - feeling for expired air
- Vocalisations, such as crying or talking, indicate ventilation and some degree of airway patency
- If there is obvious spontaneous ventilation, note other signs that may suggest upper airway obstruction:
  - the presence of stridor
  - evidence of recession
- If there is no evidence of air movement then chin lift or jaw thrust manoeuvres must be carried out. **Reassess the airway after any airway-opening manoeuvres**
- If there continues to be no evidence of air movement then airway patency can be assessed by performing an airway-opening manoeuvre while giving rescue breaths (see Chapter 19)

Resuscitation

- If the airway is not patent, then this can be secured by:
  - a chin lift or jaw thrust
  - the use of an airway adjunct
  - tracheal intubation

Breathing

Primary assessment

A patent airway does not ensure adequate ventilation. The latter requires an intact respiratory centre and adequate pulmonary function augmented by coordinated movement of the diaphragm and chest wall. The adequacy of breathing can be assessed as described in Section 4.2.

Resuscitation

- Give high-flow oxygen (flow rate 15 l/min) through a mask with a reservoir bag to any child with respiratory difficulty or hypoxia.
- In the child with inadequate respiratory effort, this should be supported either with bag–valve–mask ventilation or intubation and intermittent positive pressure ventilation.

Circulation

Primary assessment

The assessment of circulation has been described in Section 4.3. It is more difficult to assess than breathing and individual measurements must not be used on their own to diagnose circulatory failure.

Resuscitation

In every child with an inadequate circulation:

- Give high-flow oxygen through either a mask with a reservoir bag or an endotracheal tube if intubation has been necessary for airway control or inadequate breathing.
- Venous or intraosseous access should be gained and an immediate infusion of crystalloid (20 ml/kg) given. Urgent blood samples, especially blood glucose, may be taken at this point.

Disability (neurological evaluation)

Primary assessment

Both hypoxia and shock can cause a decrease in conscious level. Any problem with ABC must be addressed before assuming that a decrease in conscious level is due to a primary neurological problem. The rapid assessment of central neurological failure has been described in Section 4.4. In addition, any patient with a decreased conscious level or convulsions must have an initial glucose stick test performed.

Resuscitation

- Consider intubation to stabilise the airway in any child with a conscious level recorded as P or U (only responding to painful stimuli or unresponsive).
- If hypoglycaemia has been found, treat hypoglycaemia with a bolus of glucose (2 ml/kg of 10% glucose) followed by an IV infusion of glucose, after taking blood for glucose measurement in the laboratory and a sample for further studies.
- Intravenous lorazepam, buccal midazolam or rectal diazepam should be given for prolonged or recurrent fits (see Chapter 9 for further details).
- Manage raised intracranial pressure if present (see Chapter 8 for further details).

4.8 Secondary assessment and emergency treatment

The secondary assessment takes place once vital functions have been assessed and the treatment of life-threatening conditions has been instituted. It includes a medical history, a clinical examination and specific investigations. It differs from a standard medical history and examination in that it is designed to establish which emergency treatments are required to stabilise the child. Time is limited and a focused approach is essential. At the end of secondary assessment, the practitioner should have a better understanding of the illness affecting the child and may have formulated a differential diagnosis. Emergency treatments will be appropriate at this stage – either to treat specific conditions (such as asthma) or processes (such as raised intracranial pressure). The establishment of a definite diagnosis is part of definitive care.

The history often provides the vital clues that help the practitioner identify the disease process and hence be able to provide appropriate emergency care. In the case of children, the history is often obtained from an accompanying parent, although a history should be sought from the child if possible. Do not forget to ask pre-hospital staff about the child's initial condition and about treatments and response to treatments that have already been given.

Some children will present with an acute exacerbation of a known condition such as asthma or epilepsy. Such information is helpful in focusing attention on the appropriate system but the practitioner should be wary of dismissing new pathologies in such patients. The structured approach prevents this problem. Unlike trauma (which is dealt with later), illness affects systems rather than anatomical areas. The secondary assessment must reflect this and the history of the complaint should be sought with special attention to the presenting system or systems involved. After the presenting system has been dealt with, all other systems should be assessed and any additional emergency treatments commenced as appropriate.

The secondary assessment is not intended to complete the diagnostic process, but rather is intended to identify any problems that require emergency treatment.

The following gives an outline of a structured approach in the first hour of emergency management. It is not exhaustive but addresses the majority of emergency conditions that are amenable to specific emergency treatments in this time period. The symptoms, signs and treatments relevant to each emergency condition are elaborated in the relevant chapters that follow.

Respiratory

Secondary assessment

The following box gives common symptoms and signs that should be sought in the respiratory system. Emergency investigations are suggested.

Symptoms	**Signs**
Breathlessness	Cyanosis
Coryza	Tachypnoea
Cough	Recession
Noisy breathing – grunting, stridor, wheeze	Grunting
Drooling and inability to drink	Stridor
Abdominal pain	Wheeze
Chest pain	Chest wall crepitus
Apnoea	Tracheal shift
Feeding difficulties	Abnormal percussion note
Hoarseness	Crepitations on auscultation
	Acidotic breathing

Investigations
Oxygen saturation
Peak flow if asthma suspected
End-tidal/transcutaneous carbon dioxide if hypoventilation suspected
Blood culture if infection suspected
Chest X-ray (selective)
Arterial blood gases (selective)

Emergency treatment

- If 'bubbly' noises are heard, the airway is full of secretions, which may require clearance by suction.
- If there is a harsh stridor associated with a barking cough and severe respiratory distress, upper airway obstruction due to severe croup should be suspected and the child given nebulised adrenaline (400 micrograms/kg or 0.4 ml/kg of 1:1000 (maximum 5 ml) nebulised in oxygen).

- If there is a quiet stridor, drooling and a short history in a sick-looking child, consider epiglottitis or tracheitis. Intubation is likely to be urgently required, preferably by a senior anaesthetist. Do not jeopardise the airway by any unpleasant or frightening interventions. Give intravenous cefotaxime or ceftriaxone once the airway is secure.
- With a sudden onset and significant history of inhalation, consider a foreign body within the airway. If the 'choking child' procedure has been unsuccessful, the patient may require laryngoscopy. Do not jeopardise the airway by unpleasant or frightening interventions but contact a senior anaesthetist/ENT surgeon urgently. However, in extreme cases of life threat, immediate direct laryngoscopy to remove a visible foreign body with a Magill forceps may be necessary.
- Stridor following ingestion/injection of a known allergen suggests anaphylaxis. Children in whom this is likely should receive IM adrenaline (10 micrograms/kg or 150 micrograms (<6 years), 300 micrograms (6–12 years) or 500 micrograms (>12 years)).
- Children with a history of asthma or with wheeze and significant respiratory distress, decreased peak flow and/or hypoxia should receive oxygen therapy and inhaled β_2-agonists. Infants with wheeze and respiratory distress are likely to have bronchiolitis and require only oxygen if hypoxic.
- In acidotic breathing, take a blood sample for acid–base balance and blood sugar. Treat diabetic ketoacidosis with IV normal (physiological) saline and insulin.

Cardiovascular (circulation)

Secondary assessment

The box gives common symptoms and signs that should be sought in the cardiovascular system. Emergency investigations are suggested.

Symptoms	**Signs**
Breathlessness	Tachy- or bradycardia
Fever	Hypo- or hypertension
Palpitations	Abnormal pulse volume or rhythm
Feeding difficulties	Abnormal skin perfusion or colour
Drowsiness	Cyanosis/pallor
Pallor	Hepatomegaly
Fluid loss	Crepitations on auscultation
Poor urine output	Cardiac murmur
	Peripheral oedema
Investigations	Absent femoral pulses
Urea and electrolytes	Raised jugular venous pressure
Full blood count	Hypotonia
Arterial blood gas	Purpuric rash
Coagulation studies	
Blood culture	
Electrocardiogram	
Chest X-ray (selective)	

Emergency treatment

- Further boluses of fluid should be given to shocked children who have not had a sustained improvement to the first bolus given at resuscitation.
- Consider inotropes, intubation and central venous pressure monitoring with the third bolus.
- Consider IV cefotaxime/ceftriaxone in shocked children with no obvious fluid loss, as sepsis is likely.
- If a patient has a cardiac arrhythmia the appropriate protocol should be followed.
- If anaphylaxis is suspected, give IM adrenaline (10 micrograms/kg or 150 micrograms (<6 years), 300 micrograms (6–12 years) or 500 micrograms (>12 years)), in addition to fluid boluses.

- Give Prostin (alprostadil or dinoprostone) if duct-dependent congenital heart disease is suspected, e.g. in neonates with unresponsive hypoxia or shock.
- Surgical advice and intervention may be needed for gastrointestinal emergencies. The following symptoms and signs may suggest this.

Symptoms	Signs
Vomiting	Abdominal tenderness
Blood PR	Abdominal mass
Abdominal pain	Abdominal distension

Neurological (disability)

Secondary assessment

The following box gives common symptoms and signs that should be sought in the nervous system.

Symptoms	Signs
Headache	Altered conscious level
Convulsions	Convulsions
Change in behaviour	Altered pupil size and reactivity
Change in conscious level	Abnormal posture
Weakness	Abnormal oculocephalic reflexes
Visual disturbance	Meningism
Fever	Papilloedema or retinal haemorrhage
	Altered deep tendon reflexes
Investigations	Hypertension
Urea and electrolyte	Slow pulse
Blood sugar	Full and tense anterior fontanelle
Liver function tests	
Ammonia	
Blood culture	
Arterial blood gas	
Coagulation studies	
Blood and urine toxicology including carboxyhaemoglobin level	
Computed tomography brain scan	

Emergency treatment

- For convulsions follow the status epilepticus protocol (see Chapter 9).
- If there is evidence of raised intracranial pressure (decreasing conscious level, asymmetrical pupils, abnormal posturing and/or abnormal ocular motor reflexes) then the child should undergo:
  - Intubation and ventilation (to maintain a PCO_2 of 4.5–5.0 kPa (34–38 mmHg).
  - Nursing with head in-line and 20° head-up position (to help cerebral venous drainage).
  - IV infusion with IV hypertonic (2.7) 3% saline 3 ml/kg, or mannitol 250–500 mg/kg (1.25–2.5 ml of mannitol 20%) over 15 minutes, and repeated if needed, provided serum osmolality remains below 325 mOsm/l.
  - Consider dexamethasone (only for oedema surrounding a space-occupying lesion) 0.5 mg/kg 6-hourly.
- In a child with a depressed conscious level or convulsions, consider meningitis/encephalitis. Give cefotaxime/aciclovir.
- In drowsiness with sighing respirations, check blood sugar, acid–base balance and salicylate level. Treat diabetic ketoacidosis with IV normal saline and insulin.
- In unconscious children with pinpoint pupils, consider opiate poisoning. A trial of naloxone should be given.

External (exposure)

Secondary assessment

The box gives common symptoms and signs that should be sought externally.

Symptoms	Signs
Rash	Purpura
Swelling of lips/tongue	Urticaria
Fever	Angio-oedema

Emergency treatment

- In a child with circulatory or neurological symptoms and signs, a purpuric rash suggests septicaemia/meningitis. The patient should receive cefotaxime or ceftriaxone preceded by a blood culture.
- In a child with respiratory or circulatory difficulty, the presence of an urticarial rash or angio-oedema suggests anaphylaxis. Give IM adrenaline (10 micrograms/kg or 150 micrograms (<6 years), 300 micrograms (6–12 years) or 500 micrograms (>12 years)).

Further history

Developmental and social history

Particularly in a small child or infant, knowledge of the child's developmental progress and immunisation status may be useful. The family circumstances may also be helpful – it may be worth prompting parents to remember other details of the family's medical history.

Drugs and allergies

Any medication that the child is currently on or has been on should be recorded. If poisoning is a possibility, it is important to document any medication in the home that the child might have had access to, as even relatively benign over-the-counter medications for adults may cause serious toxicity in small children. A history of allergies should be sought.

4.9 Summary

The structured approach to the seriously ill child outlined here allows the practitioner to focus on the appropriate level of diagnosis and treatment during the first hour of care. Primary assessment and resuscitation are concerned with the maintenance of vital functions, while secondary assessment and emergency treatment allow more specific urgent therapies to be started. This latter phase of care requires a system-by-system approach and this minimises the chances of significant conditions being missed.

The following chapters and appendices discuss in more detail the recognition, resuscitation and emergency management of children with the following problems. In these chapters only components specific to the system being discussed will be covered and the generic approach discussed above will not be repeated, but should be used in all cases:

- Chapter 5: Breathing difficulties
- Chapter 6: Shock
- Chapter 7: Abnormalities of pulse rate or rhythm
- Chapter 8: Decreased conscious level
- Chapter 9: Convulsions
- Appendix E: Poisoning

CHAPTER 5
The child with breathing difficulties

Learning outcomes

After reading this chapter, you will be able to:
- Describe why infants and young children are susceptible to respiratory failure
- Describe how to assess children with breathing difficulties
- Describe how to resuscitate the child with life-threatening breathing difficulties

5.1 introduction

Most respiratory illnesses are self-limiting minor infections, but some present as potentially life-threatening emergencies, especially in children with underlying co-morbidity. Acute respiratory illnesses, such as pneumonia, are globally the largest single cause of death in children under five, accounting for 1.1 million of deaths per year (nearly 20%), with the majority of these occurring in the first 2 years of life. However, disorders outside the respiratory system may also cause apparent breathing difficulties, including cardiac disease, metabolic and neurological disorders and poisoning (Table 5.1). This chapter gives providers an approach to the assessment, resuscitation and emergency management of such children, as accurate diagnosis and prompt initiation of appropriate treatment are essential if unnecessary morbidity and mortality are to be avoided.

5.2 Susceptibility to respiratory failure

Severe respiratory illness may result in the development of respiratory failure, defined as an inability of physiological compensatory mechanisms to ensure adequate oxygenation and carbon dioxide clearance, resulting in arterial hypoxia with or without hypercapnia. Young children and infants develop respiratory failure more readily than older children and adults, reflecting important differences in the immune status, and the structure and function of the respiratory system of children and adults.

- Children, and particularly infants, are susceptible to infection with many viruses and bacteria to which adults have acquired immunity.
- The upper and lower airways in children are smaller and are more easily obstructed by mucosal swelling, secretions or a foreign body. Airway resistance is inversely proportional to the fourth power of the radius of the airway: a reduction in the radius by a half causes a 16-fold increase in airway resistance. Thus, 1 mm of mucosal oedema in an infant's trachea of 5 mm diameter results in a much greater increase in resistance than the same degree of oedema in a trachea of 10 mm diameter. From 2 months of age, airway resistance begins to decrease.
- The thoracic cage of young children is much more compliant than that of adults and thus provides less support for the maintenance of lung volume. When there is airways obstruction and increased inspiratory effort, this increased compliance results in marked chest wall recession and a reduction in the efficiency of breathing.

Advanced Paediatric Life Support: A Practical Approach to Emergencies, Sixth Edition. Edited by Martin Samuels and Sue Wieteska.
© 2016 John Wiley & Sons, Ltd. Published 2016 by John Wiley & Sons, Ltd.

Table 5.1 Causes of breathing difficulty in children, according to mechanism

Mechanism	Cause
Upper airway obstruction	Croup/epiglottitis Foreign body
Lower airway obstruction	Tracheitis Asthma/episodic viral wheeze Bronchiolitis
Disorders affecting lungs	Pneumonia Pulmonary oedema (e.g. in cardiac disease)
Disorders around the lungs	Pneumothorax Pleural effusion or empyema Rib fractures
Disorders of the respiratory muscles	Neuromuscular disorders
Disorders below the diaphragm	Peritonitis Abdominal distension
Increased respiratory drive	Diabetic ketoacidosis Shock Poisoning (e.g. salicylates) Anxiety attack and hyperventilation
Decreased respiratory drive	Coma Convulsions Raised intracranial pressure Poisoning

- The lung volume at end expiration is similar to the closing volume in infants, increasing the tendency to small airway closure and hypoxia. This may be exacerbated by an increased tendency to bronchoconstriction from alveolar or airway hypoxia.
- The number of alveoli is fewer in early childhood and this may increase the susceptibility to ventilation–perfusion mismatch.
- The respiratory muscles of young children are relatively inefficient. In infancy, the diaphragm is the principal respiratory muscle, and the intercostal and accessory muscles make relatively little contribution. Respiratory muscle fatigue can develop rapidly and result in respiratory failure and apnoea.
- The pulmonary vascular bed is relatively muscular in infancy, increasing the tendency with which pulmonary vasoconstriction occurs. In turn, this can lead to right to left shunting, ductal opening (in the early neonatal period), ventilation–perfusion mismatch and further hypoxia.
- In the first 1–2 months of life there may be a paradoxical inhibition of respiratory drive, with the result that infections can present with apnoea or hypoventilation, rather than the usual respiratory distress.
- Fetal haemoglobin is present in significant quantities until 4–6 months of age, and this results in the oxygen dissociation curve being shifted to the left, so that oxygen is given up less readily to the tissues; this makes infants more prone to tissue hypoxia and acidosis.

5.3 Clinical presentations of the child with breathing difficulty

Respiratory conditions can present with respiratory symptoms or symptoms within other systems:

Respiratory	Breathlessness Cough Noisy breathing (stridor or wheeze) Chest pain
Non-respiratory	Poor feeding Abdominal pain Meningism Changes in tone: hypotonia Change in colour or conscious level

Noisy breathing may be normal for the child or suggest pathology. Parents and carers commonly understand different meanings from those understood by doctors and nurses for the terms used to describe breathing noises, or may have their own terms. Useful historical features include relieving or aggravating factors (e.g. sleep, crying, feeding, position, exercise) and whether the voice or vocalisations are normal. Stridor is a high-pitched sound usually on inspiration from obstruction of the larynx or trachea and should be distinguished from stertor or snoring, which are lower pitched inspiratory noises suggestive of poor airway positioning or pharyngeal obstruction. Bubbly or gurgly noises suggest pharyngeal secretions, often seen in the child with neurodisability, who may have long-standing poor airway control and inability to spontaneously clear secretions. Wheeze is predominantly expiratory from lower airway obstruction, but may be called a variety of other names by parents. An expiratory grunt may suggest small airway closure or alveolar filling, such as found in pneumonia or pulmonary oedema.

Chest pain is an unusual symptom in children, and does not usually reflect cardiac disease, as it so often does in adults, and can suggest pneumonia. Similarly, pneumonia may present as abdominal pain.

While parents are usually alert to breathing difficulties in toddlers and older children, abnormal respiration may be more difficult for them to detect in infants. Infants with breathing difficulties may present with acute feeding problems. Feeding for an infant is one of the most strenuous activities, and its ease is often taken by parents as a gauge of their infant's well-being.

5.4 Primary assessment and resuscitation

This is dealt with in Chapter 4 and follows the ABCDE approach.

ABCDE features specific for breathing difficulties

> **Features suggesting cardiac cause of respiratory inadequacy**
>
> - Cyanosis, not correcting with oxygen therapy
> - Tachycardia out of proportion to respiratory difficulty
> - Raised jugular venous pressure
> - Gallop rhythm/murmur
> - Enlarged liver
> - Absent femoral pulses

Airway

- A patent airway is the first requisite. If the airway is not patent, an airway-opening manoeuvre should be used.
- The airway should then be secured with a pharyngeal airway device or by intubation with experienced senior help.

Breathing

- All children with breathing difficulties should receive high-flow oxygen through a face mask with oxygen as soon as the airway has been demonstrated to be adequate.
- Use a flow of 10–15 l/min via a face mask and reservoir bag to provide the patient with approaching 100% oxygen. If lower flows maintain adequate SpO_2 (94–98%), then nasal cannulae or nasopharyngeal catheters may be used for rates of <2 l/min.
- If the child is hypoventilating with a slow respiratory rate or weak effort, respiration should be supported with oxygen via a bag–valve–mask device and experienced senior help summoned.

Circulation

Fluid intake may have been reduced, particularly in infants presenting with breathing difficulties. Consider a fluid bolus (20 ml/kg of 0.9% saline) if there are signs of circulatory failure and particularly when intubation and positive pressure ventilation is initiated.

5.5 Secondary assessment and looking for key features

While the primary assessment and resuscitation are being carried out, a focused history of the child's health and activity over the previous 24 hours and any significant previous illness should be gained. All children with breathing difficulties will have varying degrees of respiratory distress and cough, so these are not useful diagnostic discriminators.

Certain key features, which will be identified clinically in the above assessment and from the focused history, can point the clinician to the likeliest working diagnosis for emergency treatment.

- Inspiratory noises, i.e. stridor, point to upper airway obstruction   Section 5.6
- Expiratory noises, i.e. wheeze, point to lower airway obstruction   Section 5.7
- Fever without stridor suggests pneumonia   Section 5.8
- Signs of heart failure point to congenital or acquired heart disease   Section 5.9
- Short history, exposure to allergen and urticarial rash point to anaphylaxis   Sections 6.6 and 6.9
- Suspicion of ingestion and absence of cardiorespiratory pathology point to poisoning   Section 5.11

5.6 Approach to the child with stridor

Obstruction of the upper airway (larynx and trachea) is potentially life threatening. The small cross-sectional area of the upper airway renders the young child particularly vulnerable to obstruction by oedema, secretions or an inhaled foreign body (Table 5.2).

Table 5.2 Causes of stridor

Incidence (UK)	Diagnosis	Clinical features
Very common	Croup – viral laryngo-tracheo-bronchitis	Coryzal, barking cough, mild fever, hoarse voice
Uncommon	Foreign body aspiration	Sudden onset, history of choking
Rare	Epiglottitis	Drooling, muffled voice, septic appearance, absent cough
	Bacterial tracheitis	Harsh cough, chest pain, septic appearance
	Trauma	Neck swelling, crepitus, bruising
	Retropharyngeal abscess or peritonsillar abscess	Drooling, septic appearance
	Inhalation of hot gases	Facial burns, peri-oral soot
	Infectious mononucleosis	Sore throat, tonsillar enlargement
	Angioneurotic oedema	Itching, facial swelling, urticarial rash
	Diphtheria	Travel to endemic area, unimmunised

Reassess airway

Is the airway partially obstructed or narrowed and what is the likely cause? Note the presence of inspiratory noises.

- If 'bubbly' noises are heard, the airway is full of secretions requiring clearance and suggests that the child is very fatigued, or has a depressed conscious level and is unable to clear the secretions with their own cough.
- If stertorous (snoring) respiratory noises are heard, consider partial obstruction of the airway due to a depressed conscious level.
- If there is a harsh stridor associated with a barking cough, upper airway obstruction due to croup should be suspected.
- If a quiet stridor in a sick-looking child without cough, consider epiglottitis.
- If stridor was of sudden onset, with no prodromal symptoms or a history suggestive of inhalation, consider a foreign body aspiration.

Reassess breathing

What degree of effort is needed for breathing and what is its efficacy and effect? The answer to this question will inform the clinician as to the severity of the upper airway obstruction. A pulse oximeter should be put in place and the oxygen saturation noted both on breathing air and high-flow oxygen.

Airway emergency treatment

In the child with a compromised but functioning airway, an important principle in all cases is to avoid worsening the situation by upsetting the child. Crying and struggling may quickly convert a partially obstructed airway into a completely obstructed one. Administration of oxygen, nebulised adrenaline or the performance of a radiograph may all require skill. Parents' help should be enlisted.

Partial obstruction from secretions or a depressed conscious level

- Use suction to clear an airway partially obstructed by secretions as long as there is no stridor.
- Support the airway with the chin lift or jaw thrust manoeuvre in a child with stertorous breathing due to a depressed conscious level or extreme fatigue and seek senior airway support.
- Further maintenance of the airway can be accomplished with an oro- or nasopharyngeal airway, but the child may require intubation.
- Whilst help is summoned, continuous positive airway pressure can be given to patients with a reduced conscious level using a face mask, oxygen flow and breathing circuit, e.g. an anaesthetic breathing circuit (Ayre's T-piece), if familiar with using such circuits.

Croup

- Give nebulised adrenaline (400 micrograms/kg or 0.4 ml/kg of 1:1000 (maximum 5 ml)) with oxygen through a face mask to patients with severe respiratory distress in association with harsh stridor and a barking cough, provided it does not unduly upset the child. This will produce a transient improvement beginning within 10–30 minutes and lasting for up to 2 hours. It may need to be repeated, and if so, additional measures should be taken to ensure the airway is managed by senior staff.
- Children who require adrenaline for the emergency treatment of croup should also receive oral or nebulised steroids, such as oral dexamethasone or prednisolone (see later in chapter).
- Adrenaline reduces the clinical severity of obstruction, although the effect is short lived, but is usually of sufficient duration for the corticosteroids to take effect. Patients should be observed closely with continuous ECG and oxygen saturation monitoring, as they may still deteriorate and require tracheal intubation. Adrenaline may contribute to a tachycardia, but other side effects are uncommon. This treatment is best used to 'buy time' in which to assemble an experienced team to treat a child with severe croup. Failure to respond to nebulised adrenaline should question the diagnosis of croup – consider bacterial tracheitis, epiglottitis or foreign body.
- Give humidified oxygen through a face mask, and monitor the oxygen saturation. Hypoxia is a late sign of croup and reflects alveolar hypoventilation secondary to airways obstruction and ventilation–perfusion mismatch. Whilst the respiratory rate and the degree of sternal recession are valuable clinical indicators of severity and response to treatment, the degree of hypoxia is the best assessment. However, hypoventilation may be masked when the child is receiving high ambient oxygen. The oxygen saturation with the child breathing air should be checked intermittently.

Foreign body aspiration

- Foreign body aspiration must be suspected for any witnessed choking episodes. Although a history of inhalation may be elicited from the parent, foreign body aspiration cannot be excluded on either normal physical examination or chest radiograph. Laryngo-bronchoscopy is needed for all children with a history suggestive of foreign body aspiration.
- Do not jeopardise the airway by unpleasant or frightening interventions, but contact a senior anaesthetist/ENT surgeon urgently.
- In extreme cases of life threat, immediate direct laryngoscopy with Magills forceps to remove a visible foreign body (Figure 5.1) may be necessary.

Epiglottitis

The diagnosis of acute epiglottitis is made from the characteristic history and clinical findings, as described in Table 5.2.

- Intubation is likely to be required. Contact a senior anaesthetist urgently, who will perform a gaseous induction of anaesthesia. When deeply anaesthetised, the child can be laid on his back to allow laryngoscopy and intubation. Tracheal intubation may be difficult because of the intense swelling and inflammation of the epiglottis ('cherry red epiglottis') (Figure 5.2). A smaller tube than the one usually required for the child's size will be necessary. An ENT surgeon capable of performing a tracheotomy should be present.

(a)

(b)

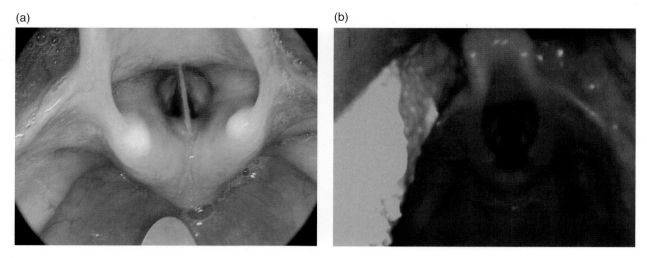

Figure 5.1 (a) Larynx with foreign body obstruction, and (b) normal larynx

(a)

(b)

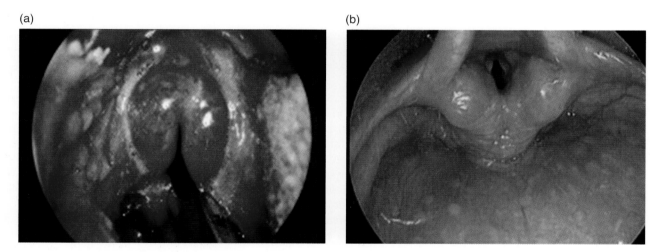

Figure 5.2 (a) Larynx epiglottitis, and (b) normal larynx

- Do not jeopardise the airway by unpleasant or frightening interventions. Do not lie the child down if he or she prefers sitting up.
- Interventions, such as lateral radiographs of the neck and venepuncture, must be avoided as they disturb the child and have precipitated fatal total airway obstruction.
- Nebulised medications such as adrenaline or steroids are of uncertain benefit, and if used, upset to the child should be avoided.

Anaphylaxis

See Section 6.9 for details of the emergency treatment of anaphylaxis.

Specific upper airway conditions

Most cases of upper airway obstruction in children are the result of infection, but inhalation of a foreign body or hot gases (house fires), angioneurotic oedema and trauma can all result in obstruction. The normal airway may also become obstructed in the unconscious, supine patient.

Croup

Background

Croup (acute laryngo-tracheo-bronchitis) is defined as an acute clinical syndrome with inspiratory stridor, a barking cough, hoarseness and variable degrees of respiratory distress. Parainfluenza viruses are the commonest pathogens but others include respiratory syncytial virus, influenza and adenoviruses. The peak incidence of croup is in the second year of life and most hospital admissions are in children aged between 6 months and 5 years. Between 1% and 5% of children are admitted with croup.

The typical features of a barking cough, harsh stridor and hoarseness are often preceded by fever and coryza for 1–3 days. The symptoms often start, and are worse, at night. Many children have stridor and a mild fever (<38.5°C), with little or no respiratory difficulty. If tracheal narrowing is minor, stridor will be present only when the child hyperventilates or is upset. As the narrowing progresses, the stridor becomes both inspiratory and expiratory, and is present even when the child is at rest. Some children, and particularly those below the age of 3 years, develop the features of increasing obstruction with marked sternal and subcostal recession, tachycardia, tachypnoea and hypoxia leading to agitation. If the infection extends distally to the bronchi, wheeze may also be audible. Some children have repeated episodes of croup.

Treatment

Steroids modify the natural history of croup: they give rise to clinical improvement within 30 minutes, and decrease the need for hospitalisation, the duration of hospitalisation and the need for intubation. Current treatments include:

- Oral dexamethasone 150 micrograms/kg or prednisolone 0.5–1.0 mg/kg
- Inhaled nebulised budesonide 2 mg

Oral steroids are the treatment of choice, but if the child will not take oral medication or is vomiting, then inhaled budesonide should be used. Both can be repeated after 12 hours if clinically indicated.

A very small proportion of children admitted to hospital with croup require tracheal intubation. The decision to intubate is a clinical one based on increasing tachycardia, tachypnoea and chest retraction, or the appearance of cyanosis, exhaustion or confusion. Ideally, the procedure should be performed under general anaesthetic by an experienced paediatric anaesthetist, unless there has been a respiratory arrest. A tracheal tube of smaller gauge than usual is often required. If there is doubt about the diagnosis, or difficulty in intubation is anticipated, it is recommended that an ENT surgeon capable of performing a tracheotomy is present.

Bacterial tracheitis

Bacterial tracheitis, or pseudomembranous croup, is an uncommon but life-threatening form of upper airway infection. Infection of the tracheal mucosa with *Staphyloccocus aureus*, streptococci or *Haemophilus influenzae* B (Hib) results in copious, purulent secretions and mucosal necrosis. The child appears toxic, with a high fever and the signs of progressive upper airway obstruction. The croupy cough, absence of drooling and a longer history help distinguish this condition from epiglottitis. Over 80% of children with this illness need intubation and ventilatory support to maintain an adequate airway, as well as intravenous antibiotics (cefotaxime or ceftriaxone plus flucloxacillin).

Epiglottitis

Background

Acute epiglottitis shares some clinical features with croup but it is a quite distinct entity. Although much less common than croup, its importance is that unless the diagnosis is made rapidly and appropriate treatment commenced, total obstruction and death may ensue. This is far less commonly seen in countries where Hib immunisation is routine, but may still occur in cases of vaccine failure and in unimmunised children.

Infection with Hib causes intense swelling of the epiglottis and the surrounding tissues and obstruction of the larynx. Epiglottitis is most common in children aged 2–6 years, but it can occur in infants and in adults. The onset of the illness is usually acute with high fever, lethargy, a soft inspiratory stridor and rapidly increasing respiratory difficulty over 3–6 hours.

In contrast to croup, cough is minimal or absent. Typically, the child sits immobile, with the chin slightly raised and the mouth open, drooling saliva. The patient appears very toxic and pale, and has poor peripheral circulation (most are septicaemic). There is usually a high fever (>39°C). Because the throat is so painful, the child is reluctant to speak and unable to swallow drinks or saliva.

> Disturbance of the child, and particularly attempts to lie the child down, to examine the throat with a spatula, or to insert an intravenous cannula, can precipitate total obstruction and must be avoided.

Treatment

After securing the airway, blood should be sent for culture and treatment with intravenous cefotaxime or ceftriaxone commenced. With appropriate treatment, most children can be extubated after 24–36 hours and they recover fully within 3–5 days. Complications such as hypoxic cerebral damage, pulmonary oedema and other serious *Haemophilus* infections are rare. In countries where the Hib vaccine is in use, there should be an investigation into vaccine failure.

Foreign body aspiration

Background

Foreign body aspiration is commonest in infants less than 3 years of age – a history of a witnessed choking event is very suggestive as the child is often too young to give a history. Infants have a smaller airway than adults and their larynx is in a relatively high position with the epiglottis close to the root of the tongue, increasing the risk of aspiration. Incisors bite through food while molars are necessary to masticate food in preparation for swallowing. Molars erupt approximately 6 months after incisors, thus infants are unable to pulp their food and the bite-sized food they generate is the ideal shape to obstruct an airway if aspirated. Infants often run around and talk while chewing, may put non-organic foreign bodies in their mouth while playing and may be inattentive and easily distractible. Foodstuffs (nuts, grapes, sweets, meat) are the commonest foreign bodies. In contrast to croup there is usually no history of prodromal viral upper respiratory tract infection or pyrexia.

All suspected foreign body aspiration should have a chest radiograph. Flat objects such as coins tend to align in the sagittal plane in the trachea whereas objects in the oesophagus tend to align in the anterior plain. The majority of foreign bodies are radio-lucent and therefore not visible on plain chest radiographs, but there may be secondary evidence of localised gas trapping, atelectasis or mediastinal shift. In approximately 20% of foreign body aspirations, the chest radiograph is normal.

Treatment

Removal through a bronchoscope under general anaesthetic should be performed as soon as possible because there is a risk that coughing will move the object into the trachea and cause life-threatening obstruction. In the case of a stridulous child with a relatively stable airway and a strong suspicion of foreign body inhalation, careful gaseous induction of anaesthesia should be induced by an experienced anaesthetist, with the presence of an ENT surgeon to perform a tracheotomy in case of deterioration. The foreign body can then be removed under controlled conditions.

Anaphylaxis

Background

Anaphylaxis is a potentially life-threatening, immunologically mediated reaction with respiratory or circulatory effects that develop over minutes, often associated with skin or mucosal changes. Laryngeal oedema causing upper airway obstruction is one manifestation. Food, especially nuts, drugs (including contrast media and anaesthetic drugs) and venom are the commonest causes of this. Prodromal symptoms of flushing, itching, facial swelling and urticaria usually precede stridor. Abdominal pain, diarrhoea, wheeze and shock may be additional or alternative manifestations of anaphylaxis (see Section 6.9 for further details).

A severe episode of anaphylaxis can be predicted in patients with a previous severe episode or a history of increasingly severe reaction, a history of asthma or treatment with β-blockers. Measurement of blood levels of mast cell tryptase at presentation can be helpful in confirming the diagnosis.

Treatment

See Section 6.9 for the treatment of anaphylaxis.

Other causes of upper airways obstruction

Although croup accounts for the large majority of cases of acute upper airway obstruction, several other uncommon conditions need to be considered in the differential diagnosis. Diphtheria is seen only in children who have not been immunised against the disease. Always ask about immunisations in any child with fever and signs of upper airway obstruction, particularly if they have been to endemic areas recently. Specific treatment of diphtheric croup includes penicillin, steroids and antitoxin.

Marked tonsillar swelling in infectious mononucleosis or acute tonsillitis can occasionally compromise the upper airway. The passage of a nasopharyngeal tube may give instant relief and steroids are often helpful.

Retropharyngeal abscess or peritonsillar abscess are uncommon, but both can present with fever and the features of upper airway obstruction together with feeding difficulties. Treatment is by surgical drainage and intravenous antibiotics.

5.7 Approach to the child with wheeze

The two common causes of lower respiratory obstruction are:

1. Acute severe asthma or episodic viral wheeze.
2. Bronchiolitis.

Bronchiolitis is mostly confined to the under 1-year-olds and asthma is much more commonly diagnosed in the over 1-year-olds.

Acute severe asthma

It can be difficult to assess the severity of an acute exacerbation of asthma. Clinical signs correlate poorly with the severity of airway obstruction. Some children with acute severe asthma do not appear distressed, and young children with severe asthma are especially difficult to assess.

Historical features associated with more severe or life-threatening airway obstruction include:

- A long duration of symptoms and symptoms of regular nocturnal awakening
- Poor response to treatment already given in this episode
- A severe course of previous attacks, including the use of intravenous therapy, and those who have required admission to an intensive care unit

After resuscitation and before progressing to specific treatment for acute asthma in any setting, it is essential to assess accurately the severity of the child's condition. The following clinical signs should be recorded regularly, e.g. every 30–60 minutes, or before and after each dose of bronchodilator:

- Pulse rate
- Respiratory rate and degree of recession
- Use of accessory muscles of respiration
- Degree of agitation and conscious level
- SpO_2
- Peak flow (if possible in over 6–7-year-olds)

Two degrees of severity are described to indicate the appearance of asthmatic children at the most severe end of the spectrum. These are severe and life-threatening asthma (Table 5.3).

Table 5.3 Symptoms of severe and life-threatening asthma

Acute severe asthma	Life-threatening asthma
Too breathless to feed or talk	Exhaustion
Respiratory rate:	Poor respiratory effort
>30/min (>5 years)	Silent chest
>50/min (2–5 years)	Hypotension
Pulse rate:	Conscious level depressed/agitated
>120 beats/min (>5 years)	Consider whether this could be anaphylaxis (see Section 6.9 for
>130 beats/min (2–5 years)	further details)

Arterial oxygen saturation by a pulse oximeter (SpO_2) is useful in assessing severity, monitoring progress and predicting outcome in acute asthma. More intensive in-patient treatment is likely to be needed for children with $SpO_2 < 92\%$ in air after initial bronchodilator treatment.

The peak expiratory flow (PEF) can be a valuable measure of severity, but children under 6 years old and those who are very dyspnoeic are usually unable to produce reliable readings.

Examination features that are poor signs of severity include the degree of wheeze, respiratory rate and pulsus paradoxus. A chest radiograph is indicated only if there is severe dyspnoea, uncertainty about the diagnosis, asymmetry of chest signs or signs of severe infection.

Asthma emergency treatment

- Assess ABC.
- Give high-flow oxygen via a face mask with a reservoir bag.
- Attach pulse oximeter and aim to keep SpO_2 at 94–98%.
- Give a β_2-agonist, such as salbutamol:
  - In those with mild to moderate asthma and maintaining $SpO_2 > 92\%$ in air, use a pressurised aerosol 1000 micrograms (10 sprays) via a valved holding chamber (spacer) with/without a face mask. Children with mild to moderate asthma are less likely to have tachycardia and hypoxia if given β_2-agonists via a pressurised aerosol and spacer. Children aged <3 years are likely to require a face mask connected to the mouthpiece of a spacer for successful drug delivery. Inhalers should be sprayed into the spacer in individual puffs and inhaled immediately by tidal breathing.
  - In those with severe or life-threatening asthma, or when oxygen is needed, use nebulised salbutamol 2.5 mg (<5 years) or 5 mg (>5 years) (with ipratropium bromide) with oxygen at a flow of 6–8 l/min in order to provide small enough particle sizes. Higher flows may be used, but more of the nebulised drug may be lost from the face mask. This can be repeated every 20-30 minutes.
- Give oral prednisolone 1 mg/kg or, if vomiting, IV hydrocortisone 4 mg/kg.
- If receiving nebulised salbutamol, mix with ipratropium bromide 250 micrograms (<2 years: 125 micrograms) driven with oxygen. This may be given every 20–30 minutes initially, reducing the dose as improvement occurs. In severe asthma, the nebulisers can be continuous as breaks between them can lead to a rebound of symptoms.
- If an infant or child is clearly in respiratory failure with poor respiratory effort, a depressed conscious level and poor saturation despite maximum oxygen therapy, attempt to support ventilation with a bag–valve–mask and arrange for urgent intubation. Give an IV bronchodilator such as salbutamol infusion (e.g. a bolus of 15 micrograms/kg; <2 years: 5 micrograms/kg).

Reassess ABC and monitor the response to treatment carefully. Assessment is based on physical signs and oxygen saturation measurements performed immediately before and 15–30 minutes after inhaled treatment. This should be accompanied by improved peak flow measurement.

If not responding, or deteriorating condition

- For severe or life-threatening asthma, intravenous bronchodilators are effective: consider IV aminophylline, magnesium sulphate or salbutamol. There is no clear evidence that one intravenous therapy is superior to another.
- Give magnesium sulphate 40 mg/kg over 20 minutes.
- Give IV salbutamol 15 micrograms/kg over 10 minutes in patients aged 2 years and older (<2 years: 5 micrograms/kg). The latter may be followed by IV infusion of 1–5 micrograms/kg/min, whilst monitoring ECG and serum potassium regularly to allow for the detection and treatment of hypokalaemia. Note the loading dose is equivalent to 1.5 micrograms/kg/min.
- Contact the paediatric intensive care unit (PICU) or the retrieval service and senior anaesthetic support.
- Consider intubation for mechanical ventilation: either rapid sequence induction with IV ketamine or inhalational anaesthesia may help bronchodilatation (see box).
- If the child is not on oral theophylline or other methylxanthines, give a loading dose of IV aminophylline 5 mg/kg over 20 minutes, monitoring the ECG for arrhythmias, followed by an infusion of 1 mg/kg/h.
- If respiratory effort is poor or deteriorating, or conscious level is depressed, or SpO_2 is low and falling despite maximum oxygen therapy, attempt to support ventilation with a bag–valve–mask, or with a mask, T-piece and bag with high-flow oxygen, whilst arranging for urgent intubation. Use a slow inflation rate (<12 inflations/min) as marked hyperinflation prolongs expiration.

Indications for intubation

- Increasing exhaustion
- Progressive deterioration in:
  - clinical condition
  - SpO_2 – decreasing and/or oxygen requirement increasing
  - PCO_2 – increasing

Mechanical ventilation is rarely required. There are no absolute criteria, as the decision to intubate is usually based on the clinical condition of the child and response to previous treatment. In cases of acute severe asthma that respond to treatment, there is usually little value to be gained from routine blood gas measurement. However, in those responding poorly, a blood gas with raised CO_2 should expedite the decision to intubate. Children with acute asthma who require mechanical ventilation need transfer to the PICU. The prognosis is good, but complications such as air leak and lobar collapse are common. All intubated children must have frequent or continuous CO_2 monitoring.

If responding and improving

- If there has been improvement (SpO_2 >92% in air, minimal recession, PEF >50% of normal value), it may be possible to consider discontinuing intravenous treatment.
- When oxygen is no longer needed, change from a nebulised bronchodilator to the use of 8–10 aerosol sprays of a β_2-agonist inhaler, giving one spray at a time during tidal breathing through a spacer with mouthpiece or mask.
- Reduce the frequency of inhaled therapy from half-hourly to 4-hourly, reducing frequency as improvement occurs.

Inhaler technique should be checked and an asthma action plan provided. The child's maintenance treatment should be reviewed and altered if inadequate. Ensure that the child has appropriate medical follow-up.

Other measures

- Reassure the child and avoid upset
- Monitor the ECG and SpO_2
- Ensure that there is avoidance of any identifiable trigger
- Intravenous fluids: restrict to two-thirds of the normal requirements
- Antibiotics: do not give routinely, as most asthma attacks are triggered by viral infections

Drug treatment

The drug treatments available for severe acute asthma are given in Table 5.4.

Table 5.4 Drug treatment of severe acute asthma	
Oxygen	High flow
Nebulised β_2-bronchodilator	Salbutamol 2.5–5 mg as required according to severity and response
	Terbutaline 2.5–10 mg
Nebulised ipratropium bromide	250 mcg (<2 years 125 mcg) every 20–30 minutes

Prednisolone	1 mg/kg/day for 3 days (max. dose/day 40 mg)
	Or intravenous hydrocortisone succinate:
	  loading dose 4 mg/kg
	  continuous infusion 1 mg/kg/h

Intravenous salbutamol	Loading dose 15 mcg/kg in children aged over 2 years Continuous infusion 1–5 mcg/kg/min
IV magnesium	40 mg/kg over 20 minutes
Aminophylline	Loading dose 5 mg/kg IV over 20 minutes* Continuous infusion 1 mg/kg/h

*Omit if the child has received oral theophylline in the previous 12 hours.

- Corticosteroids expedite recovery from acute asthma. Although a single dose of oral prednisolone is effective, many paediatricians use a 3–5-day course. There is no need to taper off the dose for courses lasting up to 10–14 days, unless the child is on maintenance treatment with oral or high-dose inhaled steroids. Unless the child is vomiting, there is no advantage in giving steroids parenterally.
- Intravenous aminophylline also has a role in the child who fails to respond adequately. A loading dose is given over 20 minutes, followed by a continuous infusion. Seizures, severe vomiting and fatal cardiac arrhythmias may follow rapid infusion. Continuous ECG monitoring should therefore be undertaken during infusion of the loading dose. If the child has received slow-release theophylline in the previous 12 hours the loading dose should be omitted.
- Intravenous magnesium sulphate is a safe treatment for acute asthma. Doses of 40 mg/kg/day (maximum 2 g) by slow infusion have been used. Studies of efficacy for severe childhood asthma unresponsive to more conventional therapies have shown evidence of benefit.
- Intravenous salbutamol has been shown to offer an advantage over inhaled delivery. Although inhaled drugs should be given first as they are accessible and more acceptable to the child, intravenous salbutamol has a place in severe or life-threatening episodes that do not respond promptly to inhaled therapy. Important side effects include sinus tachycardia and hypokalaemia: serum potassium levels should be checked 12-hourly, and supplementation may be needed.
- The order of use, dosages and combinations of aminophylline, magnesium and intravenous salbutamol remain a matter of uncertainty.
- Nebulised magnesium sulphate (150 mg added to nebulised salbutamol and ipratropium) may be useful in severe asthma with SpO_2 <92% in air.
- There is no evidence to support the routine use of inhaled steroids or heliox for the treatment of acute asthma in childhood.

Background information on asthma

Acute exacerbation of asthma is the commonest reason for a child to be admitted to hospital in the UK. In 2011, asthma caused 18 deaths in under 15-year-olds; reviews of such cases often identify preventable factors in both the recognition and management of the condition.

The classic features of acute asthma are cough, wheeze and breathlessness. In young children, they may have no triggers other than viral infections and no interval symptoms. Such cases are often termed viral-induced wheeze or episodic viral wheeze, but should be treated as acute asthma. An increase in symptoms and decreasing response to bronchodilator, along with difficulty in walking, talking or sleeping, all indicate worsening asthma.

Upper respiratory tract infections (URTIs) are the commonest precipitant of symptoms of asthma in the pre-school child. Viruses cause 90% of these infections. Exercise-induced symptoms are more frequent in the older child. Emotional upset, laughing or excitement may also precipitate acute exacerbations. It is hard to assess the importance of allergen exposure to the onset of acute symptoms in an individual with asthma, partly because of the ubiquitous nature of the common allergens (house dust mite, grass pollens, moulds) and partly because delay in the allergic response makes a cause and effect relationship difficult to recognise. A rapid fall in air temperature, exposure to a smoky atmosphere and other chemical irritants such as paints and domestic aerosols may trigger an acute attack.

Bronchiolitis emergency treatment

Management is primarily supportive – fluid replacement, gentle suctioning of nasal secretions, prone position (if in hospital), oxygen therapy and respiratory support if necessary.

- Assess ABC.
- Ensure that the airway is patent and clear: use of a Yankauer suction catheter applied to the nares can help to ensure that the nose and nasopharynx are cleared, which can have a significant impact on an infant's respiratory distress.
- Give a high concentration of oxygen via a mask with reservoir bag. Monitor the SpO_2 and keep at 94–98%. Milder and improving cases may use oxygen via nasal cannulae at <2 l/min.
- Consider using humidity, prone positioning and high-flow, humidified systems (flows of 1–2 l/kg/min).
- Maintain hydration and nutrition. In infants with significant respiratory distress, maintain hydration by feeding via a nasogastric tube, or intravenously at two-thirds the usual maintenance. Remember, nasogastric tubes may partially occlude the airway. Breastfeeding may be too stressful, in which case breast milk should be expressed and given via a gastric tube.
- Monitor for apnoea/hypoventilation in those under 2 months old:
  - SpO_2,
  - respiratory frequency/apnoea monitor, and
  - PCO_2 – transcutaneous, capillary or end-tidal.
- Heated, humidified, high-flow nasal cannulae (HHHFNC) therapy and continuous positive airway pressure (CPAP) are both believed to improve the work of breathing by preventing dynamic airway collapse during the expiration thereby reducing air trapping and improving gas exchange. CPAP results in decreased respiratory rate and PCO_2, and clinical practice suggests that CPAP decreases the need for mechanical ventilation with greatest benefit if instituted early. Indications for CPAP include severe respiratory distress, a requirement for FiO_2 >0.5 or infants with apnoeas.
- Mechanical ventilation is required in 2% of infants admitted to hospital. In severe cases, infants with the following may need intubation and mechanical ventilation:
  - recurrent apnoea,
  - exhaustion, or
  - severe hypercapnia and hypoxia.
- All intubated infants must have continuous SpO_2 and CO_2 monitoring.
- Both nebulised 3% saline and nebulised adrenaline with corticosteroids have been subjected to trials, but without showing substantial benefit.
- Bronchodilators, steroids, antibiotics and physiotherapy are not useful.

Background information on bronchiolitis

Bronchiolitis is the most common serious respiratory infection of childhood: 10% of infants are affected and 2–3% are admitted to hospital with the disease in their first year of life. Ninety per cent of patients are aged 1–9 months; it is unusual after 1 year of age. There is an annual winter epidemic. Respiratory syncitial virus (RSV) is the pathogen in 60–70% of cases, the remainder being caused by other respiratory viruses, such as parainfluenza, influenza, human metapneumovirus and adenoviruses. Acute bronchiolitis is not a primary bacterial infection, and secondary bacterial involvement is uncommon.

Fever and a clear nasal discharge precede a dry cough and increasing breathlessness. Wheezing may be present with crackles audible on auscultation. Feeding difficulties associated with increasing dyspnoea are often the reason for admission to hospital. Recurrent apnoea is a serious and potentially fatal complication, and is seen particularly in infants born prematurely. Infants with co-morbidities including premature birth, immunodeficiency, left to right shunt congenital heart disease or interstitial lung diseases are more prone to develop severe disease. The findings on examination are characteristic (Table 5.5).

Table 5.5 Bronchiolitis: characteristic findings on examination

Sign	Findings
Tachypnoea	>50 breaths/min
Recession	Subcostal and intercostal
Cough	Sharp, dry
Hyperinflation of the chest	Sternum prominent, liver depressed
Tachycardia	>140 beats/min Consider arrhythmia if >220 beats/min
Crackles	Fine end-inspiratory
Wheezes	High-pitched expiratory > inspiratory
Colour	Cyanosis or pallor
Breathing pattern	Irregular breathing/recurrent apnoea

Risk factors for severity in bronchiolitis

- Age under 6 weeks
- Premature birth
- Chronic lung disease
- Congenital heart disease
- Immunodeficiency

Infants with bronchiolitis rarely need a chest radiograph. If performed it usually shows hyperinflation and often evidence of collapse or consolidation, particularly in the upper lobes (Figure 5.3). RSV and other viruses can be identified on nasopharyngeal secretions. Blood gas analysis, which is required in only the most severe cases, shows lowered oxygen and raised CO_2 levels.

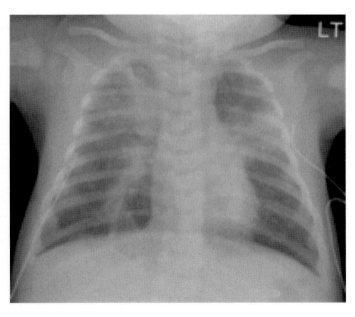

Figure 5.3 Chest X-ray of bronchiolitis

Bronchiolitis may trigger heart failure in an infant with a previously undiagnosed cardiac lesion. Distinguishing features are listed in Table 5.6.

Table 5.6 Features that help distinguish heart failure from bronchiolitis	
Heart failure	**Bronchiolitis**
Feeding difficulty with growth failure	
Restlessness, sweating	
Tachycardia and tachypnoea	Coryzal and harsh cough
Pallor, sweating and cool peripheries	
Large heart with displaced apex beat	Normal or apparently small heart
Large liver	Liver lower than normal
Gallop rhythm	
Murmur	No murmur
Chest X-ray shows pulmonary congestion and large heart	Hyperinflation on chest X-ray

The natural history of bronchiolitis is of a self-limiting disease that usually lasts 3–7 days.

Although many causes of breathing difficulties are associated with infection, a high fever is usually associated only with pneumonia, epiglottitis and bacterial tracheitis. Although many cases of asthma are precipitated by an URTI, the asthmatic child is rarely febrile and a low-grade fever is characteristic of bronchiolitis. Therefore, in the absence of stridor and wheeze, breathing difficulties in association with a significant fever are likely to be due to pneumonia.

5.8 Approach to the child with fever

Pneumonia emergency treatment

- Assess ABC.
- Provide a high concentration of oxygen via a face mask with reservoir bag. Attach a pulse oximeter; if a low flow maintains SpO_2 at 94–98%, then nasal cannulae may be used with a flow <2 l/min.
- It is not possible to differentiate reliably between bacterial and viral infection on clinical, haematological or radiological grounds, so children diagnosed as having significant pneumonia should receive antibiotics. The choice of antibiotic is usually according to local policy, but for infants and older children amoxicillin is effective against most bacteria. For young infants or if there is a septic component, cefotaxime would be considered. Other options include the use of:
  - flucloxacillin – if *Staphylococcus aureus* is suspected, or
  - macrolide antibiotic – if atypical pneumonia or pertussis (unimmunised infant) is suspected.
- Maintain hydration: extra fluid may be needed to compensate for loss from fever, and restriction may be needed because of inappropriate antidiuretic hormone (ADH) secretion. Fluid overload can contribute to worsening breathlessness.
- Clinical examination and the chest radiograph may reveal a pleural effusion (Figure 5.4). This should be confirmed with ultrasound and, if large, it should be drained to relieve breathlessness, aid diagnosis and allow the instillation of intrapleural fibrinolytic agents. Ultrasound may guide the positioning of an intrapleural drain. Details of the procedure can be found in Chapter 23.
- Airway and breathing support may especially be needed in children with neurodisability or neuromuscular weakness, who may have poor airway control and weak respiratory muscles even when well.

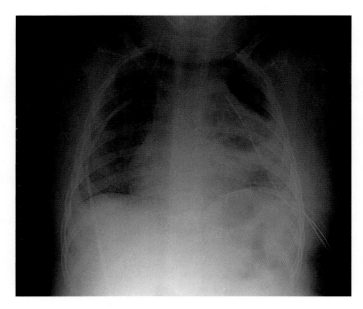

Figure 5.4 Chest X-ray of pneumonia

Background to pneumonia

Pneumonia in childhood was responsible globally for 13% of deaths of children aged under 5 years in 2013 (WHO data). Infants, and children with congenital abnormalities or chronic illnesses, are at particular risk. A wide spectrum of pathogens causes pneumonia in childhood, and different organisms are important in different age groups. The incidence of viral infections decreases with increasing age, while the incidence of bacterial infections remains stable across all ages. Viral infections typically peak during the autumn and winter season, whereas bacterial pneumonia exhibits less marked seasonal fluctuation.

In the newborn, organisms from the mother's genital tract, such as *Escherichia coli* and other Gram-negative bacilli, group B β-haemolytic *Streptococcus* and *Chlamydia trachomatis* are the most common pathogens. In infancy, respiratory viruses are the most frequent cause, but *Streptococcus pneumoniae*, *Haemophilus* and, less commonly, *Staphylococcus aureus* are also important. In school-aged children, viruses become less frequent pathogens and bacterial infection, especially *Mycoplasma pneumoniae*, *S. pneumoniae* and *Chlamydia pneumoniae*, are important. *Bordetella pertussis* can present with pneumonia as well as with classic whooping cough, even in children who have been fully immunised. It can cause a severe pneumonitis, leading to respiratory failure in unimmunised infants.

Fever, cough, breathlessness and chest recession in the younger child and lethargy are the usual presenting symptoms. The cough is often dry initially but then becomes loose. Older children may produce purulent sputum but in those below the age of 5 years it is usually swallowed. Pleuritic chest pain, neck stiffness and abdominal pain may be present if there is pleural inflammation. Classic signs of consolidation such as decreased percussion, decreased breath sounds and bronchial breathing are often absent, particularly in infants, and a chest radiograph is needed. This may show lobar consolidation, widespread bronchopneumonia or, rarely, cavitation of the lung. Pleural effusions may occur, particularly in bacterial pneumonia and this may organise to empyema. An ultrasound of the chest will delineate the size and nature of pleural collection and if needed will guide placing of a chest drain. Blood cultures, swabs for viral isolation and a full blood count should also be performed. It can be useful to save an acute serum for further microbiological diagnosis.

All children diagnosed as having significant pneumonia should receive antibiotics. Oral antibiotics are sufficient in most cases, unless there is vomiting or severe respiratory distress. The initial choice of antibiotics depends on the age of the child and local policy. Newborns and young infants should receive broad-spectrum intravenous antibiotics such as cetotaxime or ceftriaxone. For older infants and preschool children, oral amoxicillin is suitable. For school-aged children, a macrolide such as clarithromycin is suitable. Check for any antibiotic allergy. Antibiotics should be given for 7–10 days, although complicated pneumonias, e.g. with empyema, may require several weeks' duration.

In children with no respiratory difficulty, treatment will occur at home with a penicillin or macrolide. Infants, and children who look toxic, have definite dyspnoea, an SpO_2 below 93%, grunting or signs of dehydration should be admitted and usually require intravenous treatment initially. Oxygen (if SpO_2 < 93%) and an adequate fluid intake (70% maintenance, because of possible inappropriate ADH secretion) are also required. Secretion management techniques are not beneficial in previously healthy children with community-acquired pneumonia, but may help children with neurodisability or neuromuscular weakness.

Mechanical ventilation is rarely required unless there is a serious underlying condition. Transfer to the PICU should be considered with the following: an FiO_2 >0.6 to keep the SpO_2 at 94–98%, shock, exhaustion, rising CO_2, apnoea or irregular breathing. If a child has recurrent or persistent pneumonia, they should be referred to a respiratory specialist so further investigation may be undertaken.

5.9 Approach to the child with heart failure

Infants and children with serious cardiac pathology may present with breathlessness, cyanosis or cardiogenic shock. The immediate management of shock is described in Chapter 6.

Causes of heart failure that may present as breathing difficulties

Left ventricular volume overload or excessive pulmonary blood flow:

Ventricular septal defect	Atrioventricular septal defect
Common arterial trunk	Persistent arterial duct

Left heart obstruction:

Hypertrophic cardiomyopathy	Critical aortic stenosis
Aortic coarctation	Hypoplastic left heart syndrome

Primary 'pump' failure:

Myocarditis	Cardiomyopathy

Dysrhythmia:

Supraventricular tachycardia	Complete heart block

Heart failure emergency treatment

Reassess ABC

- If there are signs of shock – poor pulse volume or low blood pressure with extreme pallor and depressed conscious level – treat the child for cardiogenic shock (see Chapter 6).
- If circulation is adequate and oxygen saturation is normal or improves significantly with oxygen by face mask but there are signs of heart failure, then the breathing difficulty is due to pulmonary congestion secondary to a large left to right shunt. The shunt may be through a ventricular septal defect (VSD), atrioventricular septal defect (AVSD), patent ductus arteriosus (PDA) or, more rarely, an aortopulmonary window or truncus arteriosus. In many cases a heart murmur will be heard. A chest X-ray will usually provide supportive evidence in the form of cardiomegaly and increased pulmonary vascular markings. Give:
  - high-flow oxygen by face mask with a reservoir, and
  - diuretics should be commenced. In most cases, oral diuretics are adequate and a combination of loop diuretics (frusemide (furosemide)) with a potassium-sparing diuretic (amiloride or spironolactone) in twice or thrice daily doses should be commenced. Electrolytes should be checked prior to commencing diuretics. In severe cases, the first dose of frusemide may need to be given intravenously.
- Babies in the first few days of life who present with breathlessness and increasing cyanosis largely unresponsive to oxygen supplementation are likely to have duct-dependent congenital heart disease such as tricuspid or pulmonary atresia. See Section 6.10 for further details and treatment.
- Children of all ages who present with breathlessness from heart failure may have myocarditis. This is characterised by a marked sinus tachycardia and the absence of signs of structural abnormality. The patients should be treated with oxygen and diuretics.

A full blood count and measurements of serum urea and electrolytes, calcium, glucose and arterial blood gases should be performed on all patients in heart failure. A routine infection screen including blood cultures is recommended, especially in infants. A full 12-lead ECG and a chest radiograph are essential. All patients suspected of having heart disease should be discussed with a paediatric cardiologist, as transfer to a tertiary centre will usually be required. Echocardiography will establish the diagnosis in most cases.

Background to heart failure in infancy and childhood

In infancy, heart failure is usually secondary to structural heart disease, and medical management is directed at improving the clinical condition prior to definitive surgery. There are some complex congenital heart defects in which the presence of a PDA is essential to maintain pulmonary or systemic flow. The normal PDA closes functionally in the first 24 hours of life. Infants with duct-dependent right or left heart lesions present in the first few days of life as the ductus arteriosus starts closing in response to transition from fetal to postnatal life. With modern obstetric management, many infants are now diagnosed antenatally so that they may be delivered within cardiac units. Newborns also more commonly undergo newborn oximetry screening, which also allows earlier detection of cases. This has resulted in fewer infants with serious congenital heart disease, including those with duct-dependent disease, presenting to paediatric or emergency departments. See Section 6.10 for further details.

In the older child, myocarditis and cardiomyopathy are the usual causes of the acute onset of heart failure and remain rare. Presenting features include fatigue, effort intolerance, anorexia, abdominal pain and cough. The presence of chest pain and arrhythmia should also be included as clues towards a diagnosis of myocarditis. On examination, a marked sinus tachycardia, hepatomegaly and raised jugular venous pressure are found with inspiratory crackles on auscultation. ECG and cardiac enzymes may be helpful in diagnosis.

5.10 Approach to the child with anaphylaxis

This is covered in detail in Section 6.9.

5.11 Approach to the child with metabolic and poisoning problems

Diabetes

As hyperventilation is a feature of the severe acidosis produced by diabetes, occasionally a child may present with a primary breathing difficulty. The correct diagnosis is usually easy to establish and management is described in Appendix B.

Poisoning

There may be apparent breathing difficulties following the ingestion of a number of poisons. The respiratory rate may be increased by poisoning with:

- Salicylates
- Ethylene glycol (antifreeze)
- Methanol
- Cyanide

However, usually only poisoning with salicylates causes any diagnostic dilemma. Poisoning with drugs that cause a depression of ventilation will present as a diminished conscious level. The management of the poisoned child is dealt with in Appendix E.

5.12 Summary

You should use the structured approach in the assessment and management of the child with breathing difficulties:

- Primary assessment
- Resuscitation
- Secondary assessment and looking for key features
- Emergency treatment
- Stabilisation and transfer to definitive care

CHAPTER 6
The child in shock

Learning outcomes

After reading this chapter, you will be able to:
- Identify the causes of shock in infants and children
- Describe the pathophysiology of shock
- Describe how to assess children with shock
- Describe how to resuscitate the child with life-threatening shock
- Describe the emergency treatment of the different causes of shock
- Identify the properties of different resuscitation fluids

6.1 Introduction

Shock is an acute, life-threatening syndrome of circulatory dysfunction resulting in inadequate delivery of oxygen and other nutrients to meet tissue metabolic demands. The final pathway is a failure of both substrate delivery and removal of metabolites leading to a state of acute cellular oxygen deficiency irrespective of the initial insult triggering shock, which can be any severe disease or injury. This in turn leads to anaerobic metabolism and cellular acidosis, culminating in loss of normal cellular function, cell death, organ dysfunction and eventually death, if not recognised and appropriately treated.

Maintenance of adequate tissue perfusion and oxygen supply depends on blood volume, cardiac output and arterial oxygen content. Cardiac output is the product of heart rate and stroke volume, and is directly proportional to preload (venous return), afterload (systemic vascular resistance) and cardiac contractility. Oxygen-carrying capacity is defined by haemoglobin content and arterial oxygenation. Therefore, an insult affecting any of these can lead to a shock state.

Inadequate tissue perfusion resulting in impaired cellular respiration (i.e. shock) may result from defects of the heart pump (cardiogenic), loss of fluid (hypovolaemic), abnormalities of vessels (distributive), flow restriction (obstructive) or inadequate oxygen-releasing capacity of blood (dissociative). In many causes of shock, several mechanisms may coexist, therefore the clinician must consider which of several alternative emergency treatments will be effective for any individual patient.

6.2 Pathophysiology of shock

Shock results from an acute failure of circulatory function. Inadequate amounts of nutrients, especially oxygen, are delivered to body tissues and there is inadequate removal of tissue waste products. Other than underlying illnesses, age-dependent maturation of different organ systems and the body's defence mechanisms define the response to shock.

Shock is a progressive state which can be divided into three phases: compensated, uncompensated and irreversible. Although artificial, this division is useful because each phase has characteristic clinico-pathological manifestations and outcome.

Advanced Paediatric Life Support: A Practical Approach to Emergencies, Sixth Edition. Edited by Martin Samuels and Sue Wieteska.
© 2016 John Wiley & Sons, Ltd. Published 2016 by John Wiley & Sons, Ltd.

Compensated shock

In this early phase, physiological neuro-hormonal compensatory mechanisms maintain vital (i.e. brain, heart and kidneys) organ perfusion. Sympathetic nervous system reflexes increase systemic arterial resistance, divert blood away from non-essential tissues, constrict the venous reservoir and increase the heart rate to maintain cardiac output. The systolic blood pressure remains normal, whereas the diastolic pressure may be elevated due to the increased systemic arterial resistance. Increased secretion of angiotensin and vasopressin allows the kidneys to conserve water and salt, while reduced renal perfusion leads to reduced urine output, and intestinal fluid is reabsorbed from the digestive tract. The clinical signs characteristic of this stage are mild agitation or confusion, skin pallor, increased heart rate, cold peripheral skin with decreased capillary return and reduced urine output. Early recognition is crucial as appropriate therapeutic interventions at this stage can completely reverse shock. In older patients, raised cardiac output with decreased systemic resistance may give rise to warm extremities and wide pulse pressure.

Uncompensated shock

If shock is unrecognised or untreated in the early stage, it progresses further and the compensatory mechanisms fail to support the circulatory system. Poorly perfused tissue beds can no longer sustain aerobic metabolism and comparatively inefficient anaerobic metabolism becomes their major source of energy production. Anaerobic metabolism produces lactate; the acidosis is further compounded by intracellular carbonic acid formed because of the inability of the circulation to remove carbon dioxide. Acidosis reduces myocardial contractility and impairs the response to circulating catecholamines.

A further result of anaerobic metabolism is the failure of the energy-dependent sodium–potassium pump, which maintains the normal homeostatic environment for optimal cellular function. Lysosomal, mitochondrial and membrane functions deteriorate without this homeostasis. Sluggish blood flow and chemical changes in small vessels lead to platelet adhesion and may produce damaging chain reactions in the kinin and coagulation systems, heralding the onset of disseminated intravascular coagulation (DIC).

If recognised in this stage, shock may still be reversible if appropriately treated. Clinical manifestations of this stage are a normal or falling blood pressure, tachycardia, prolonged capillary refill, cold peripheries, acidotic breathing, depressed cerebral state and severely reduced or absent urine output. Blood gases reveal metabolic acidosis and blood lactate is increased.

Irreversible shock

If the shock goes untreated, it progresses to an irreversible stage where the cellular damage cannot be reversed even if cardiovascular function is restored to adequate levels. Despite haemodynamic correction, multiple organ failure occurs. This underlies the clinical observation that during shock progression a point is reached where death of the patient becomes inevitable, despite appropriate therapeutic intervention. Hence early recognition and appropriate treatment is vital.

6.3 Classification of the causes of shock

The causes of shock are listed in Table 6.1, with the more common in bold. It can be seen that the most common cause in paediatric patients is hypovolaemia from a number of different conditions. The cause of shock is often multifactorial. For example, in septic shock, hypovolaemia, cardiac dysfunction, abnormal vascular tone and dissociative shock due to impaired mitochondrial function may occur simultaneously.

6.4 Approach to the child in shock

Early recognition of shock is crucial and requires a high index of suspicion and knowledge of the conditions that predispose children of different ages and co-morbidities to shock. For example, it is important to know a history of congenital heart disease, immunodeficiency, trauma, surgery, toxin ingestion or allergies.

The child may present with fever, rash, pallor, poor feeding, drowsiness, history of trauma or poisoning. Other than certain obvious causes of shock like external haemorrhage, signs and symptoms of early compensated shock can be easily missed.

Table 6.1 Causes of shock

Causes of shock		Chapter
Hypovolaemic	**Haemorrhage**	11
	Gastroenteritis, stomal losses	6
	Intussusception, volvulus	6
	Burns	16
	Peritonitis	
Distributive	**Septicaemia**	6
	Anaphylaxis	6
	Vasodilating drugs	
	Spinal cord injury	15
Cardiogenic	Arrhythmias	7
	Heart failure (cardiomyopathy, myocarditis)	5–7
	Valvular disease	
	Myocardial contusion	12
Obstructive	Congenital cardiac (coarctation, hypoplastic left heart, aortic stenosis)	7
	Tension/haemopneumothorax	12
	Flail chest	12
	Cardiac tamponade	12
	Pulmonary embolism	
Dissociative	Profound anaemia	6
	Carbon monoxide poisoning	Appendix E
	Methaemoglobinaemia	

6.5 Primary assessment and resuscitation

ABCDE features specific for shock

- There is often tachypnoea (acidotic breathing).
- Monitor the heart rate/rhythm, blood pressure, capillary refill time, toe–core temperature difference and urine output.
- If the heart rate is above 200 beats/min in an infant or above 150 beats/min in a child, or if the rhythm is abnormal, perform a 12-lead ECG.
- It is important to check the blood for glucose, lactate, base excess and gas exchange, preferably not a cold peripheral capillary sample.
- Mental status/conscious level (AVPU; see Chapter 4): agitation at first evolving to obtundation and coma.
- Posture: children in shock are usually hypotonic.
- Rash is often a key clinical indicator for the cause of shock. Haemorrhagic purpura, although characteristic of meningococcal sepsis, may be seen in severe sepsis of other aetiologies particularly pneumococcal sepsis. Generalised erythema, conjunctivitis and mucositis may indicate toxic shock syndrome.
- Fever suggests an infective cause.

Airway

- Ensure airway is open: consider airway-opening manoeuvres, airway adjuncts or urgent induction of anaesthesia and intubation to secure the airway.

Breathing

- Adequate airway: give high-flow oxygen through a face mask with a reservoir, or, if needed and available, high-flow nasal cannula oxygen.
- Hypoventilating: support with oxygen via a bag–valve–mask device and seek experienced, senior help for early tracheal intubation and mechanical ventilation.

Circulation

- Gain intravenous (IV) or intraosseous (IO) access:
  - Insert two wide-bore IV cannulae if possible, immediately proceed to IO access if peripheral venous access is difficult.
  - Femoral venous access can be used in situations where peripheral or IO access is impossible and experienced help is available.
- Take blood for blood gas (including lactate, haemoglobin and ionised calcium), glucose stick test and laboratory tests including full blood count, electrolytes, renal and liver function tests, C-reactive protein (CRP) or procalcitonin (if available), blood culture, meningococcal/streptococcal polymerase chain reaction (PCR), cross-match and coagulation studies.

In the industrialised world with access to inotropes and mechanical ventilation, initial resuscitation of hypovolemic shock begins with boluses of up to 20 ml/kg crystalloid over 5–10 minutes, titrated to reversing hypotension, increasing urine output (>1 ml/kg/h), and attaining normal capillary refill, peripheral pulses and level of consciousness. Reassess the patient after each fluid bolus to look for signs of improvement. Albumin may be considered in the child requiring repeated fluid boluses, however there is insufficient evidence to recommend its routine use.

- Be cautious in those with primary cardiogenic shock and in those with signs of raised intracranial pressure (ICP): the first group may still benefit from a judicious fluid bolus (5–10 ml/kg) to optimise preload. It is important to seek the urgent advice of a paediatric cardiologist for further treatment. In patients with signs suggestive of raised ICP (i.e. relative bradycardia and hypertension, posturing or seizures), hypotension is detrimental for cerebral perfusion, but excessive fluids carry the theoretical risk of worsening cerebral oedema; hence fluids should be given cautiously in 10 ml/kg aliquots with careful reassessment of clinical signs after each fluid bolus.
- In non-hypotensive children with severe haemolytic anaemia (severe malaria or sickle cell crises), blood transfusion is considered superior to crystalloid boluses.
- Give inotropes if hypotension does not respond to initial fluid resuscitation or if hepatomegaly or new respiratory crackles develop. For improved circulation, peripheral IV or IO access can be used for inotrope infusion when a central line is not available.
- Expert advice regarding intubation and ventilation should be sought in patients who have received more than 40 ml/kg fluid with signs of ongoing shock. Mechanical ventilation decreases the energy requirements of the heart and respiratory muscles, allows delivery of adequate concentrations of oxygen and helps reduce the risk of development of pulmonary oedema. It also facilitates the placement of indwelling catheters for arterial and central venous access.
- Renal perfusion should be monitored with a urinary catheter and hourly urine output measurement as it is an important marker of renal perfusion.
- Give an antibiotic such as ceftriaxone or cefotaxime for those with an obvious or suspected diagnosis of septicaemia, e.g. in the presence of a purpuric rash, or in those where the aetiology is unknown. Blood cultures should be obtained before administering antibiotics when possible but this should not delay administration of antibiotics.
- In patients with trauma, haemorrhage must be looked for and controlled for effective management of shock. If uncontrolled bleeding is external, it can be controlled by direct pressure, but if internal, control may not be possible until surgery. This has led to a much more cautious fluid regime: pre-hospital paramedics are now likely to be using repeated boluses of fluid of 5 ml/kg. In hospital it is recommended that if there is no response to the initial bolus of 5–10 ml/kg, the massive haemorrhage protocol should be considered with urgent surgical assessment and appropriate management. In some instances, the benefits of hypotensive resuscitation should be balanced against other factors: head injury, for example, might be worsened by hypotension. If head injury is present or suspected, blood pressure should be kept at normal levels to maintain cerebral perfusion.
- If a tachyarrhythmia is identified as the cause of shock, up to three synchronous electric shocks at 1.0, 2.0 and 2.0 J/kg should be given (see Chapter 7):
  - If the arrhythmia is broad-complex and synchronous shocks are not activated by the defibrillator then attempt an asynchronous shock.
  - A conscious child should be anaesthetised first.

- If the tachyarrhythmia is supraventricular tachycardia (SVT) then this can be treated with IV/IO adenosine as this can often be administered more quickly than a synchronous electric shock.
- If anaphylaxis is obvious give adrenaline 10 micrograms/kg IM or 150 micrograms (<6 years), 300 micrograms (6–12 years) or 500 micrograms (>12 years).

Disability

If there is coexistent evidence of raised intracranial pressure, manage as in Chapter 8.

'Don't ever forget glucose' (DEFG)

Hypoglycaemia may give a similar clinical picture to that of compensated shock. This must always be excluded by an urgent glucose bedside test and blood glucose estimation. Shock and hypoglycaemia may coexist due to limited glycogen reserves and the fact that ill children may not have had adequate nutritional intake.

6.6 Key features of the child in shock

While the primary assessment and resuscitation are being carried out, a focused history of the child's health and activity over the previous 24 hours and any significant previous illness should be gained. Certain key features that will be identified from this – and the initial blood test results – can point the clinician to the likeliest working diagnosis for emergency treatment.

• A history of vomiting and/or diarrhoea points to fluid loss either externally (e.g. gastroenteritis) or into the abdomen (e.g. volvulus, intussusception, ruptured appendix)	Section 6.7
• The presence of fever and/or rash points to septicaemia	Section 6.8
• The presence of urticaria, angioneurotic oedema or history of allergen exposure points to anaphylaxis	Section 6.9
• The presence of cyanosis unresponsive to oxygen or a grey colour with signs of heart failure in a baby under 4–6 weeks points to duct-dependent congenital heart disease	Section 6.10
• The presence of heart failure in an older infant or child points to cardiomyopathy or myocarditis	Section 6.11
• A history of sickle cell disease or a recent diarrhoeal illness and a very low haemoglobin points to acute haemolysis. A history of sickle cell disease, abdominal pain and enlarged spleen points to acute splenic sequestration	Sections 6.12 and 6.13
• An immediate history of major trauma points to blood loss and, more rarely, tension pneumothorax, haemothorax, cardiac tamponade or spinal cord transection	Part 3
• The presence of severe tachycardia and an abnormal rhythm on the ECG points to a cardiac cause for shock	Chapter 7
• A history of polyuria and the presence of acidotic breathing and a very high blood glucose points to diabetes ketoacidosis	Appendix B
• A history of drug ingestion points to poisoning	Appendix E

6.7 Approach to the child with non-haemorrhagic fluid loss

Infants are more likely than older children to present with shock due to sudden and rapid fluid losses due to gastroenteritis or with concealed fluid loss secondary to a 'surgical abdomen' such as a volvulus. This is due both to the infant's low physiological reserve and increased susceptibility to these conditions.

In infants, gastroenteritis may occasionally present as circulatory collapse with little or no significant history of vomiting or diarrhoea. This is due to sudden massive loss of fluid from the bowel wall into the gut lumen, causing a depletion of intravascular volume. The infecting organism can be any of the usual diarrhoeal pathogens, of which viruses are the most common.

Having completed the primary assessment and resuscitation and identified by means of the key features that fluid loss is the most likely diagnosis, the child is reassessed to identify the response to the first fluid bolus.

Emergency treatment of hypovolaemic shock due to non-haemorrhagic fluid loss

Reassess ABC

- The child has had one fluid bolus of 20 ml/kg IV crystalloids.
- If signs of shock persist after the first bolus, give a second fluid bolus of crystalloid or colloid:
  - In gastroenteritis, one to two boluses usually restore circulating volume.
  - In gastroenteritis, immediately initiate oral or nasogastric rehydration with oral rehydration solution (see Appendix B) and restart normal feeding within 4–6 hours.
- Recheck acid–base status and electrolytes:
  - Acidosis will usually be corrected by treatment of shock; bicarbonate losses need to be corrected only in patients who have proven large bicarbonate losses in the stool.
  - Sodium imbalance may occur, this may cause convulsions (see Appendix B). If convulsions are present rapidly increase hyponatraemia (NaCl 3% 4 ml/kg in 15 minutes) to a serum Na of 125 mmol/l or, if earlier, until the convulsion terminates. Once the seizure has stopped, or if there is asymptomatic hyponatraemia, slowly correct serum Na (maximum 8–12 mmol/l/day).
- Consider diagnostic possibilities:
  - Abdominal X-ray or ultrasound scan to detect distended bowel, intra-abdominal air or fluid.
  - Consider urgent surgical referral especially if bile-stained vomiting or abdominal guarding is present. Ensure that the patient has had antibiotics as sepsis or toxic shock syndrome may mimic an acute abdomen.
  - Consider sepsis (secondary to the surgical abdomen) and give appropriate IV antibiotics.
- Consider tracheal intubation and mechanical ventilation, particularly if more than 40 ml/kg of fluid are required with signs of ongoing shock.
- Consider a third fluid bolus if still shocked; at this stage also consider the need for inotropes and monitoring of central venous pressure (CVP).
- The child's bladder should have been catheterised in order to accurately assess the urinary output.

6.8 Approach to the child with septic shock

The incidence of septic shock varies with age and is highest in infants. It carries significant mortality and morbidity. Septic shock is the classic example of a combination of several factors contributing to the shock. These include hypovolaemia (fever, often associated diarrhoea, vomiting and anorexia, together with alterations in capillary permeability leading to capillary leakage), cardiogenic (impaired cardiac function due to hypovolaemia and direct myocardial suppressive factors from infecting organisms and the host inflammatory response), distributive (alterations in vascular tone with vasoconstriction in some vascular beds and vasodilatation in others) and dissociative (there is a non-specific sepsis-induced mitochondrial dysfunction impairing cellular oxygen utilisation) elements. Septic shock is defined as sepsis with cardiovascular end-organ dysfunction.

Infection with *Neisseria meningitidis* (the meningococcus) is the commonest cause of community-acquired septicaemia in infants and children. In countries where a vaccine against meningococcus C has been introduced, there has been a significant fall in the number of cases of infection due to this organism. Other causes of septicaemia in children include group B streptococcal infection in young infants, Gram-negative sepsis in relation to underlying urinary tract or gut problems and group A streptococcal sepsis. In children with underlying co-morbidities, respiratory or neurological infection is important, and infection of long-term indwelling devices (such as venous catheters) is becoming increasingly prevalent.

The cardinal sign of meningococcal septicaemia is a purpuric rash in an ill child. At the onset, however, the rash may be absent, or mistaken for viral exanthems and a careful search should be made for purpura in any unwell child. In about 15% of patients with meningococcal septicaemia, a blanching erythematous rash replaces or precedes a purpuric one, and in 7% of cases no rash occurs.

In toxic shock syndrome the initial clinical picture includes a high fever, diffuse erythema, headache, confusion, conjunctival and mucosal hyperaemia (strawberry tongue), scarlatiniform rash, subcutaneous oedema, vomiting and watery diarrhoea. Findings may also include a trivial injury such as an infected wound, cut, scratch, minor burn or scald, surgical wound infection or coexistent deep-seated infection such as pneumonia or bone/joint infection. Early administration of anti-staphylococcal/streptococcal antibiotics, concurrent with initial resuscitation, is vital. Intravenous immunoglobulin should be considered along with urgent drainage of any localised pus.

Early adequate fluid resuscitation is the key to survival in children with septic shock; however, indiscriminate or overaggressive fluid resuscitation can be harmful. Choice of fluid is still debated (see Section 6.15).

Having completed the primary assessment and resuscitation and identified by means of the key features that septicaemia is the most likely diagnosis, the child is reassessed.

Emergency treatment of septic shock

Reassess ABC

- Give a fluid bolus of crystalloids and reassess for signs of improvement. Subsequent boluses could be either crystalloids or colloids. Children often require repeated boluses of fluid to achieve relative stability (up to 200 ml/kg in the first 24 hours has been used to treat severe shock, i.e. 2.5 times the blood volume).
- Ensure that an antibiotic has been given as soon as possible, preferably after doing a blood culture. A third-generation cephalosporin, such as cefotaxime or ceftriaxone, is usually used, but an antistaphylococcal antibiotic (e.g. clindamycin) should be considered if there is possible toxic shock syndrome. There are some specific considerations:
  - Under 3 months old: add amoxicillin to cover *Listeria*.
  - Use cefotaxime (not ceftriaxone) in premature or jaundiced infants, in hypoalbuminaemia and if a calcium infusion is being used.
  - If hospital acquired or neutropenic, consider tazobactam.
  - If previous culture of resistant organism, give appropriate antibiotic (e.g. methicillin-resistant *Staphylococcus aureus* (MRSA): add vancomycin; extended-spectrum β-lactamases (ESBL): meropenem).
  - If vascular access device has been used for more than 48 hours add vancomycin.
- Expert advice regarding intubation and ventilation should be sought in patients who have received more than 40 ml/kg fluid with signs of ongoing shock. Positive pressure ventilation decreases energy requirements of the heart and respiratory muscles, allows delivery of adequate concentrations of oxygen and helps reduce the risk of development of pulmonary oedema. It also facilitates placement of indwelling catheters for arterial and central venous access. All intubated children must have continuous SpO_2 and capnography, with frequent blood gas monitoring.
- At this point it is necessary to consider inotropes and ideally to monitor CVP. Central venous access should be achieved using a multilumen catheter via the femoral or internal jugular vein. Optimising CVP may improve cardiac output with less risk of inducing heart failure. Cardiac failure may be induced by excessive IV fluids, especially if severe anaemia, malnutrition or a primary cardiac disorder is present.
- When a third fluid bolus is required, start inotropes; in children with hypodynamic shock with a high systemic vascular resistance (SVR) (cold extremities), dopamine or adrenaline (if rapidly deteriorating) are recommended. Dopamine is prepared as an IV solution (e.g. 30 mg/kg made up to 50 ml with NaCl 0.9%: 1 ml/h = 0.1 micrograms/kg/min); start at a dose of 10 micrograms/kg/min and increase to 15 or 20 micrograms/kg/min if there is a poor response. Adrenaline has both inotropic and chronotropic activity and greater β_2 effects in peripheral vasculature allowing vasodilatation. Start at a dose of 0.05 micrograms/kg/min and increase to 2 micrograms/kg/min if necessary. In hyperdynamic shock with low SVR (warm shock), noradrenaline might be the first choice (use the same dose as adrenaline). Because of an increase in mortality with delay in time to inotrope use, it is now recommended that peripheral inotropes can be used whilst central access (or IO) is being attained. The peripheral access site must be closely monitored. (Nor)adrenaline solutions should be 10 times diluted.
- In refractory shock with suspected or definite adrenal insufficiency, take blood for cortisol level and give hydrocortisone at 50 mg/kg/day as a continuous infusion.

> It is difficult to manage a seriously ill patient requiring mechanical ventilation and inotropic support without intensive care facilities and invasive monitoring. If these treatments are required, a PICU must be involved early to give advice and to retrieve the patient.

Further investigations

In addition to the blood tests taken during resuscitation, the following blood tests are needed in the septic child: calcium, magnesium, phosphate, coagulation screen, meningo-/streptococcal PCR and arterial blood gas. Electrolyte and acid–base abnormalities can have a deleterious effect on myocardial function. They should be sought and corrected early (see Appendix A). **Do not give bicarbonate to correct metabolic acidosis due to hypovolaemia.**

Source control

Urgently look for possible source of infection and remove; for example necrotising fasciitis requires surgical debridement, line infection requires removal of the line as soon as other access is obtained, and an abscess should be drained.

Reassess disability

Meningitis may accompany septicaemia. Assess neurological status (conscious level, using the Glasgow Coma Score, pupillary size and reaction, and posture), particularly looking for signs of raised ICP. If, despite effective treatment of shock, there is decreasing conscious level or abnormal posturing or focal neurological signs, treat for raised ICP.

Treatment of disability in shock

The priority in patients with a mixed picture of shock and meningitis is management of shock, as adequate brain perfusion is dependent on adequate cardiac output. If signs of raised ICP persist, tracheal intubation and mechanical ventilation should be initiated urgently.

- Support ventilation (maintain a PCO_2 of 4.5–5.5 kPa (34–41 mmHg).
- Nurse with the head in-line in a 20° head-up position (to help cerebral venous drainage).
- Insert a urinary catheter early, and monitor urine output.
- Maintenance of a normal blood pressure to ensure an adequate cerebral perfusion pressure is mandatory. Treatment of the shocked state takes priority over treatment of increased ICP. An adequate blood pressure is necessary to maintain cerebral perfusion.
- Lumbar puncture must be avoided as its performance may cause death through coning of the brain stem through the foramen magnum.
- Paediatric intensive care skills and monitoring are paramount in these patients. Seek advice early.

6.9 Approach to the child with anaphylaxis

Anaphylaxis is a potentially life-threatening, immunologically mediated reaction to ingested, inhaled or topical substances, which may present as either shock or respiratory distress. Common triggers include certain foods, especially nuts, egg and shellfish, and drugs such as penicillin, anaesthetic agents and radiographic contrast media. The life-threatening features include breathing difficulties with stridor or wheeze, or shock, due to acute vasodilatation and fluid loss from the intravascular space caused by increased capillary permeability. Any of these may lead to collapse and respiratory or cardiac arrest.

Prodromal symptoms of flushing, itching, facial swelling, urticaria, abdominal pain, vomiting and diarrhoea, wheeze and stridor may precede shock or may be the only manifestations of anaphylaxis. The presence of these additional symptoms confirms anaphylaxis as the cause of breathlessness and/or shock in a child. Most patients will have a history of previous, less severe allergic reactions; some may have a 'medic-alert' bracelet or carry their own adrenaline. Confirmation of the diagnosis may be aided by measurement of blood mast cell tryptase levels.

Key points in the history may point to a severe reaction:

- Previous severe reaction
- History of increasingly severe reactions
- History of asthma
- Treatment with β-blockers

Symptoms and signs vary according to the body's response to the allergen. These are shown in Table 6.2.

Table 6.2 Symptoms and signs in allergic reaction

	Symptoms	Signs
Allergic reactions	Burning sensation in mouth, itching of lips, mouth and throat, coughing, feeling of warmth, nausea, abdominal pain, loose bowel motions, sweating	Urticarial rash, angio-oedema, conjunctivitis
Anaphylaxis	Difficulty breathing, noisy breathing, cyanosis, agitation, collapse	Wheeze, stridor, tachycardia with hypotension, poor pulse volume and pallor, respiratory arrest or cardiac arrest

Emergency treatment of anaphylaxis (Figure 6.1)

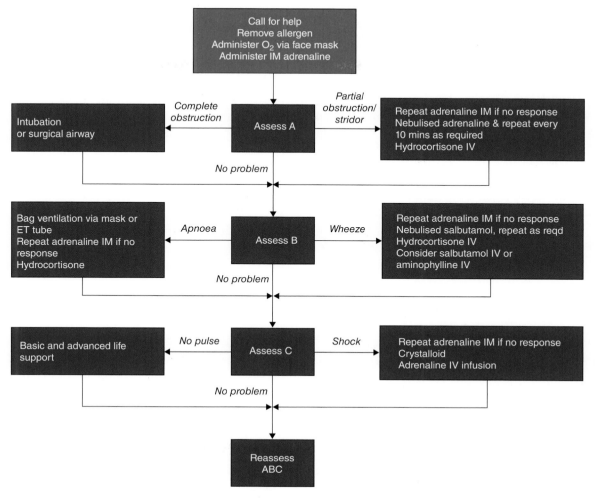

Drugs in anaphylaxis	Dosage by age			
	Less than 6 months	**6 months to 6 years**	**6–12 years**	**More than 12 years**
Adrenaline IM – pre-hospital practitioners	150 micrograms (0.15 ml of 1:1000)		300 micrograms (0.3 ml of 1:1000)	500 micrograms (0.5 ml of 1:1000)
Adrenaline IM – in-hospital practitioners	10 micrograms/kg *0. 1ml/kg of 1:10 000 (infants and young children) OR 0.01 ml/kg of 1:1000 (older children)[1]*			
Adrenaline IV	Titrate 1 microgram/kg*			
Crystalloid	20 ml/kg			
Hydrocortisone (IM or slow IV)	25 mg	50 mg	100 mg	200 mg

*1 microgram/kg given over 1 minute (range 30 seconds to 10 minutes), e.g. according to local protocol, one of these adrenaline doses can be diluted in saline to a volume of 10 ml, giving a solution of 1mcg/kg/ml.

[1]The strength of IM adrenaline is not intended to be prescriptive, 1:1000 or 1:10 000 could be used depending on what is practicable. The problem with sticking solely to 1:1000 is that when used in infants and small children, you are then drawing up very small volumes.

Figure 6.1 Emergency treatment of anaphylaxis. [ET, endotracheal]

Specific treatment includes:

- High-flow oxygen
- Intramuscular adrenaline: either 10 micrograms/kg or 150 micrograms (<6 years), 300 micrograms (6–12 years) or 500 micrograms (>12 years)
- Nebulised adrenaline for stridor 400 micrograms/kg or 0.4 ml/kg of 1:1000 (maximum 5 ml), as for croup
- Nebulised bronchodilator for wheeze

The management of anaphylactic shock requires airway management and ventilation, administration of adrenaline and aggressive fluid resuscitation. Intubation will be required for severe cases. Note that the IM route is the preferred route for the delivery of adrenaline. IV/IO adrenaline should be reserved for children with life-threatening shock or airway obstruction, for whom an IM injection has had to be given in repeated doses or been ineffective or for those in cardiac arrest. The patient must be carefully monitored.

Having completed the primary assessment and resuscitation and identified by means of the key features that anaphylaxis is the most likely diagnosis, the child is reassessed.

Further emergency management of anaphylaxis

For ongoing shock, and shock resistant to treatment, continue with boluses of crystalloid or colloid and ventilatory support and give further doses of IM adrenaline every 5 minutes if the symptoms are not reversed. Additional inotropes will not be needed because the adrenaline used for the treatment of anaphylaxis is a powerful inotrope. However, in the face of shock resistant to IM adrenaline and one or two boluses of fluid, an infusion of IV adrenaline may be life saving. The dose is 0.1–5.0 micrograms/kg/min and the patient should be closely monitored for pulse and blood pressure.

In addition to the above treatment, it is also customary to give patients with anaphylaxis an antihistamine and corticosteroids. The role these drugs play in management is limited, as their onset of action is too delayed to be of much benefit in the first hour.

6.10 Approach to the infant with a duct-dependent congenital heart disease

Features suggesting a cardiac cause of circulatory inadequacy

- Cyanosis, not correcting with oxygen therapy
- Tachycardia out of proportion to respiratory difficulty
- Raised jugular venous pressure
- Gallop rhythm, murmur
- Enlarged heart on chest X-ray
- Enlarged liver
- Absent femoral pulses

The ductus arteriosus connects the systemic and pulmonary circulations in fetal life. Infants with duct-dependent right or left heart lesions present in the first few days of life as the ductus arteriosus starts closing in response to transition from fetal to postnatal life.

Neonates with duct-dependent pulmonary circulation (e.g. pulmonary atresia, critical pulmonary stenosis, tricuspid atresia, tetralogy of Fallot) present in the first few days of life with increasing cyanosis unresponsive to supplemental oxygen and signs of severe hypoxaemia with little respiratory distress before collapsing with cardiogenic shock. A high index of suspicion is required to diagnose these conditions, as frequently there is no audible murmur. Patients may have tachycardia, tachypnoea and an enlarged liver.

Neonates with duct-dependent systemic circulation (e.g. coarctation of the aorta, critical aortic stenosis, hypoplastic left heart syndrome, interrupted aortic arch) usually present in the first few days of life with inability to feed, breathlessness, a grey appearance and collapse with poor peripheral circulation and cardiogenic shock. These infants are severely ill with signs of poor organ perfusion with severe metabolic acidosis, poor urine output and decreased conscious level. Pulses can be difficult to feel in these patients because of left-sided obstruction to cardiac output and a difference may be noticed in the upper and lower limb pulses and blood pressure depending on the site of the lesion.

Children with transposition of the great arteries are duct dependent for both circulations (systemic and pulmonary).

Having completed the primary assessment and resuscitation and identified by means of the key features that duct-dependent congenital heart disease is the most likely diagnosis, the child is reassessed.

Emergency treatment of duct-dependent congenital heart disease

Reassess ABC

- Oxygen therapy will often provide limited benefit. Since it may accelerate duct closure, use oxygen judiciously or discontinue if there is no effect. Keep a low threshold for tracheal intubation and mechanical ventilation in patients with cardiogenic shock. This decreases metabolic demands of the body and assists cardiac function.

> The most experienced personnel should be summoned for support in these situations as use of anaesthetic-induction agents can worsen the situation. Frequent discussion with a paediatric cardiologist and intensivist is mandatory.

- Give an IV infusion of dinoprostone (prostaglandin E2 (PGE2)), this will usually reopen and keep the arterial duct patent, which will help in stabilising the patient before definitive surgical intervention.
- Cyanotic baby or one with poorly palpable pulses who is otherwise well and non-acidotic: start at 10–15 nanograms/kg/min.
- Acidotic or unwell baby with suspected duct-dependent lesion: start at 20 nanograms/kg/min. If no response within first hour, increase to up to 50 nanograms/kg/min.
- In suspected left-sided obstruction: aim for palpable pulses, normal pH and normal lactate. In suspected right-sided obstruction: aim for SpO_2 75–85% and normal lactate. If there is suspected or known transposition of the great arteries or hypoplastic left or right heart syndrome with SpO_2 <70% or worsening lactates liaise urgently with cardiology and/or intensive care as rapid assessment and atrial septostomy may be necessary. Prostaglandins can cause apnoea in some infants; frequent assessment is necessary to identify those who need ventilatory support. Prostaglandins can also cause vasodilatation and subsequent drop in blood pressure. Such patients may benefit from a fluid bolus to optimise preload.

Investigations

- Chest X-ray
- ECG
- Full blood count, arterial blood gases, urea and electrolytes (including calcium), glucose and lactate
- Blood cultures since differential diagnosis with sepsis might be difficult

Discuss with and transfer to a paediatric cardiology unit. Monitor pre- and post-ductal saturations.

6.11 Approach to the child with shock due to cardiomyopathy

Cardiomyopathy/myocarditis is uncommon, but may rarely be found in an infant or child presenting with shock, arrhythmias and signs of heart failure with no history of congenital heart disease. It may be difficult to differentiate these patients from septic patients and treatment is dictated by the management of shock. If such a patient were in the first few weeks of life, a trial of prostaglandin (PGE1 or 2) would be appropriate and would be beneficial for duct-dependent circulations as discussed.

Having completed the primary assessment and resuscitation and having identified by means of the key features that cardiomyopathy/myocarditis is the most likely diagnosis, the child is reassessed.

Emergency treatment of cardiomyopathy/myocarditis

The section on emergency treatment can be revised with management depending on whether the child presents with cardiac failure or shock. Those presenting in heart failure need to be managed as per American Heart Association guidance for heart failure, including use of angiotensin-converting enzyme inhibitors. In those presenting in shock and suspected to have myocarditis or cardiomyopathy, aggressive fluid resuscitation needs to be avoided and inotropes need to be used on advice of the intensive care team. Adrenaline is usually the preferred inotrope and can be used both centrally and peripherally. The role of the extracorporeal membrane oxygenation and ventricular assist devices needs to be recognised with the focus on the child being stabilised and transferred urgently to the right centre.

Reassess ABC

- Give high-flow oxygen
- Give a cautious fluid bolus of 5–10 ml/kg. Children may be fluid depleted and have cardiac dysfunction, so judicious use of fluid would not be harmful. Aggressive fluid resuscitation needs to be avoided and inotropes (e.g. adrenaline and/or dobutamine) need to be used only on advice of the paediatric intensive care team or paediatric cardiologist. Careful assessment and consideration is required of the cardiac haemodynamics, namely preload, contractility and afterload.
- Treatment then needs to be titrated according to the clinical picture. Consider a diuretic, if the child is not shocked, to offload the heart, such as IV frusemide 0.5–1 mg/kg.

Investigations

- Chest X-ray
- ECG
- Full blood count, arterial blood gases, urea and electrolytes including calcium, glucose and lactate
- Blood cultures

> Urgent cardiology advice should be sought. Echocardiography should establish the diagnosis in almost all cases. Consider early liaison and transfer to a paediatric cardiac centre as these children can be extremely difficult to manage.

6.12 Approach to the child with profound anaemia

Severe anaemia exists if the haemoglobin level is less than 50 g/l. If acute haemolysis is the cause of anaemia, urine will usually be dark brown in colour, the child will be lethargic with their palms and soles near white, and there may be signs of heart failure. The most usual situation in which a child develops sudden severe haemolysis is in the case of septicaemia associated with sickle cell disease or haemolytic uraemic syndrome (HUS). In children returning from endemic areas, severe malaria may present with severe anaemia, with or without haemolysis.

Emergency treatment of profound anaemia

- Transfusion should in general be considered when the haemoglobin level is less than 50 g/l.
- The presence of heart failure affects the decision to transfuse; diuretics will be required or an exchange transfusion may be safer. Fluid overload may exacerbate or lead to cardiogenic shock and pulmonary oedema.
- Treatment may also be required as for sepsis with volume support, intubation and inotropes.
- Fresh blood should be used where possible, if not available use packed cells.
- Management of these children includes early paediatric intensive care advice and transfer.

6.13 Approach to the child with sickle cell crisis

Sickle cell disease is characterised by episodic clinical events called 'crises'. Vaso-occlusive crisis is the most common and occurs when abnormal red cells clog small vessels, causing tissue ischaemia. The other crises are acute chest syndrome, sequestration crisis (severe anaemia and hypotension, resulting from pooling of blood in the spleen and liver), aplastic crisis and hyper-haemolytic crisis. Factors that precipitate or modulate the occurrence of sickle cell crises are not fully understood, but infections, hypoxia, dehydration, acidosis, stress and cold are believed to play some role.

Oxygen therapy, rehydration, antibiotics and analgesia are considered standard treatment in sickle cell crises. Parenteral morphine is also considered essential for relieving pain in severe vaso-occlusive crises and acute chest syndrome.

6.14 After resuscitation and emergency treatment of shock

Following successful restoration of adequate circulation, varying degrees of organ dysfunction may remain, and should be actively sought and managed. The problems are similar but of a lesser degree than those expected following resuscitation from cardiac arrest. Thus after the initial resuscitation and emergency treatment, the patient should have a review of ABC, as well as a full systems review to ensure stabilisation for safe and effective transfer (see Chapter 25).

6.15 Use of fluids in resuscitation

Which fluid?

Crystalloid and colloid fluids are available for volume replacement. Dextrose infusions are not appropriate fluids for resuscitation and can be dangerous, for example, by lowering serum sodium and predisposing to hyponatraemic seizures. For further details of the composition of different fluids, see Appendix B.

- Compared with colloids, crystalloid fluids diffuse more readily into the interstitial space.
- Compared with colloids, crystalloid fluids may be associated with more peripheral oedema.
- Where a capillary leak exists, crystalloid fluids allow more water to enter the interstitial space because of a lower osmotic pressure.
- Crystalloid fluids need greater volumes than colloids to expand the vascular space.

There has been a long-standing debate about whether crystalloid or colloid solutions should be used in resuscitation. No definitive answer can be given still. Where small volumes of fluid are needed, the choice of fluid is probably less important.

In acute collapse, a smaller volume of colloid fluid is needed than crystalloid to produce a given increase in intravascular volume, and so a more rapid correction of haemodynamic derangement may be possible with colloid solutions if these are readily available.

When larger volumes of fluid are used, the choice of fluid becomes more important. As the circulating volume of a child is approximately 80 ml/kg, if more than 40 ml/kg of fluid is used for resuscitation, one-half of the child's circulating volume will have been given. If much more fluid resuscitation is needed, significant haemodilution may result, and consideration should be given to using blood for fluid resuscitation with measurements of the CVP (effectively cardiac preload) to guide fluid resuscitation and the haematocrit to guide the need for blood transfusion. Where large volumes are used, colloids could be preferred in paediatric practice. 'Normal' saline (0.9% NaCl solution), and colloids suspended in normal saline, are often infused because they are easily available, and are isotonic with plasma. Their non-physiological levels of chloride and lack of buffer, however, cause metabolic acidosis. In cases where large amounts of crystalloids are used, a more balanced solution such as Ringers lactate is now the preferred choice.

If blood is needed, a full cross-match should be undertaken, which takes about 1 hour to perform. For urgent need, type-specific non-cross-matched blood (which is ABO Rhesus compatible but has a higher incidence of transfusion reactions) takes about 15 minutes to prepare. In dire emergencies O-negative blood must be given.

How much fluid?

The volume of fluid needed will depend on clinical assessment. However, the clinical situation may dictate the rapidity with which repeat boluses are given. For example, in a retrospective review of children with septic shock, early administration of large volumes of fluid (>40 ml/kg in the first hour) was associated with better outcome than smaller volume resuscitation, encouraging an aggressive approach in septicaemia. In contrast, where shock is caused by penetrating trauma requiring definitive surgical management, maximal fluid resuscitation may be best delayed until surgery, as improving perfusion without improving oxygen-carrying capacity results in a worse outcome.

If large volumes are needed, resuscitation is best guided by measurement of the CVP, invasive blood pressure and urine output. Patients requiring large-volume resuscitation need early involvement from and transfer to a paediatric intensive care unit. When large volumes are used, fluids should be warmed.

In conclusion, there is no definitive evidence demonstrating which fluid is best for resuscitation. Other important questions – how much and when should fluids be used – also remain to be answered. Clinical trials will be needed to answer these questions, although they are likely to be difficult to perform. At present, optimal management should be guided by knowledge of the pathophysiology underlying the disease, and of the different roles of the different fluids.

6.16 Summary

You should use the structured approach in the assessment and management of the child with shock:

- Primary assessment
- Resuscitation
- Secondary assessment and looking for key features
- Emergency treatment
- Stabilisation and transfer to definitive care

CHAPTER 7
The child with an abnormal pulse rate or rhythm

Learning outcomes

After reading this chapter, you will be able to:

- Describe how to assess children with an abnormal pulse rate or rhythm
- Describe how to resuscitate the child with life-threatening brady- or tachyarrhythmia

---

7.1 Introduction

In tachyarrhythmias in children, the rate is fast but the rhythm is largely regular. Causes include the following.

Causes of tachyarrhythmias in children

- Re-entrant congenital conduction pathway abnormality (common)
- Poisoning
- Metabolic disturbance
- After cardiac surgery
- Cardiomyopathy
- Long QT syndrome

In bradyarrhythmias in children, the rate is slow and the rhythm usually irregular. Causes include the following.

Causes of bradyarrhythmias in children

- Pre-terminal event in hypoxia or shock
- Raised intracranial pressure
- Conduction pathway damage following cardiac surgery
- Congenital heart block (rare)
- Long QT syndrome

Presentations include the following.

Presentations of arrhythmias in children

- History of palpitations (verbal child)
- Poor feeding (pre-verbal child)
- Heart failure or shock

Advanced Paediatric Life Support: A Practical Approach to Emergencies, Sixth Edition. Edited by Martin Samuels and Sue Wieteska.
© 2016 John Wiley & Sons, Ltd. Published 2016 by John Wiley & Sons, Ltd.

7.2 Primary assessment and resuscitation

ABCDE features specific for abnormal rate/rhythm

Airway

- Ensure the airway is open – consider airway-opening manoeuvres, airway adjuncts or urgent induction of anaesthesia and intubation to secure the airway.

Breathing

- Breathing: high-flow oxygen through a face mask with reservoir.
- Hypoventilating or bradycardia: support with a bag–valve–mask device and consider intubation and ventilation.

Circulation

- Heart rate: this is the defining observation for this presentation. An abnormal pulse rate is defined as one falling outside the normal range given in Chapter 1.
- Most serious disease or injury states are associated with a sinus tachycardia. In infants this may be as high as up to 220 beats per minute (bpm) and in children up to 180 bpm. Rates over these figures are highly likely to be tachyarrhythmias, but in any case of significant tachycardia, i.e. 200 bpm in an infant and 150 bpm in a child, an ECG rhythm strip should be examined and, if in doubt, a full 12-lead ECG performed. Very high rates may be impossible to count manually and the pulse oximeter will often be unreliable. Again, a rhythm strip is advised.
- An abnormally slow pulse rate is defined as one less than 60 bpm or a rapidly falling heart rate associated with poor systemic perfusion. This will almost always be in a child who requires major resuscitation.

Monitor the ECG:

1. Is the rate:
   too fast?
   too slow?
2. Is the rhythm:
   regular?
   irregular?
3. Are the QRS complexes:
   narrow?
   broad?

Bradycardia

- Bradycardia is usually a pre-terminal rhythm. It is seen as the final response to profound hypoxia and ischaemia and its presence is ominous.
- Bradycardia is precipitated by vagal stimulation as occurs in tracheal intubation and suctioning and may be found in postoperative cardiac patients. The rhythm is usually irregular.
- Bradycardia may be seen in patients with raised intracranial pressure. These patients may have presented with coma and their management can be found in Chapters 8 and 14.
- Bradycardia can be a side effect of poisoning with digoxin or β-blockers and the management can be found in Appendix E.

Tachyarrhythmia

- Tachyarrhythmia with absent P-waves and a narrow QRS complex on the ECG is supraventricular tachycardia. The rhythm is usually regular.
- Tachyarrhythmia with a wide QRS complex on the ECG is ventricular tachycardia; this can be provoked by:
  - hyperkalaemia, or
  - poisoning with tricyclic antidepressants. Additional details on the management of the poisoned child with ventricular tachycardia can be found in Appendix E.

Resuscitation

- Heart rate <60 beats/min: with shock, start chest compressions, obtain vascular access and give a bolus of 20 ml/kg crystalloid.
- Ventricular tachycardia (VT): with shock, treat with synchronised DC cardioversion starting at 2 J/kg. This can be repeated and the dose can be increased if needed.
  - The child who is responsive to pain should be anaesthetised or sedated first.
  - If the synchronous shocks for VT are ineffectual (because the defibrillator cannot recognise the abnormally shaped QRS complex), then the shocks may have to be given asynchronously, recognising that this is a more risky procedure. Without conversion, however, the rhythm may deteriorate to ventricular fibrillation (VF) or asystole.
  - Synchronisation relies on the ability of the defibrillator to recognise the QRST complex, and is designed to avoid shock delivery at a point in the cardiac cycle likely to precipitate VF.
- Supraventricular tachycardia (SVT): give IV/IO adenosine 100 micrograms/kg to a maximum single dose of 500 micrograms/kg (300 micrograms/kg if the baby is aged under 1 month) if this can be administered more quickly than a synchronous electric shock.
- Bloods: full blood count, renal function and glucose.

7.3 Approach to the child with bradycardia

In paediatric practice bradycardia is almost always a pre-terminal finding in patients with respiratory or circulatory insufficiency. Airway, breathing and circulation should always be assessed and treated if needed before pharmacological management of bradycardia (Figure 7.1). Incidental bradycardia in a clinically well child may be seen in athletic and sporty children and does not require any treatment.

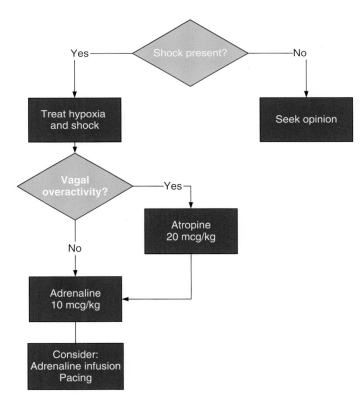

Figure 7.1 Algorithm for the management of bradycardia

Reassess ABC

- If there is hypoxia and shock, treat with:
  - High concentration oxygen, bag–mask ventilation, intubation and intermittent positive pressure ventilation.
  - Volume expansion (20 ml/kg of crystalloid repeated as recommended in the treatment of shock).
  - If the above is ineffective titrate slowly adrenaline 10 micrograms/kg IV.
  - If the above is ineffective, infuse adrenaline 0.05–2 micrograms/kg/min IV.

- If there has been vagal stimulation:
  - Treat with adequate ventilation.
  - Give atropine 20 micrograms/kg IV/IO (minimum dose 100 micrograms; maximum dose 600 micrograms).
  - The dose may be repeated after 5 minutes (maximum total dose of 1 mg in a child and 2 mg in an adolescent).
- If there has been poisoning, seek expert toxicology help.

7.4 Approach to the child with supraventricular tachycardia

Supraventricular tachycardia is the most common non-arrest arrhythmia during childhood and is the most common arrhythmia that produces cardiovascular instability during infancy. SVT in infants generally produces a heart rate >220 bpm, and often 250–300 bpm. Lower heart rates occur in children during SVT. The QRS complex is narrow, making differentiation between marked sinus tachycardia due to shock and SVT difficult, particularly because SVT may also be associated with poor systemic perfusion.

The following characteristics may help to distinguish between sinus tachycardia and SVT (Figures 7.2 and 7.3).

- Sinus tachycardia is typically characterised by a heart rate less than 200 bpm in infants and children, whereas infants with SVT typically have a heart rate greater than 220 bpm.
- P-waves may be difficult to identify in both sinus tachycardia and SVT once the ventricular rate exceeds 200 bpm. If P-waves are identifiable, they are usually upright in leads I and AVF in sinus tachycardia while they are negative in leads II, III and AVF in SVT. In SVT, P-wave morphology is likely to be variable depending on substrate.
- In sinus tachycardia, the heart rate varies from beat to beat and is often responsive to stimulation, but there is no beat to beat variability in SVT.
- Termination of SVT is abrupt, whereas the heart rate slows gradually in sinus tachycardia in response to treatment.
- A history consistent with shock (e.g. gastroenteritis or septicaemia) is usually present with sinus tachycardia.

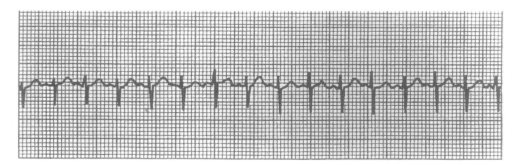

Figure 7.2 Sinus tachycardia

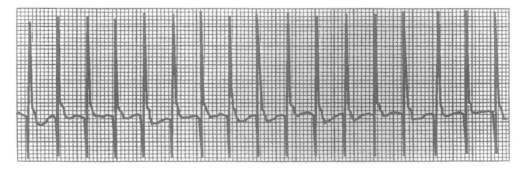

Figure 7.3 Supraventricular tachycardia

Cardiopulmonary stability during episodes of SVT is affected by the child's age, duration of SVT and prior ventricular function and ventricular rate. Older children usually complain of light-headedness, dizziness or chest discomfort or they note the fast heart rate. Very rapid rates may be undetected for long periods in young infants until they develop a low cardiac output state and shock. This deterioration in cardiac function occurs because of increased myocardial oxygen demand and limitation in myocardial oxygen delivery during the short diastolic phase associated with very rapid heart rates. If baseline myocardial function is impaired (e.g. in a child with a cardiomyopathy), SVT can produce signs of shock in a relatively short time.

Follow the algorithm for SVT (Figure 7.4).

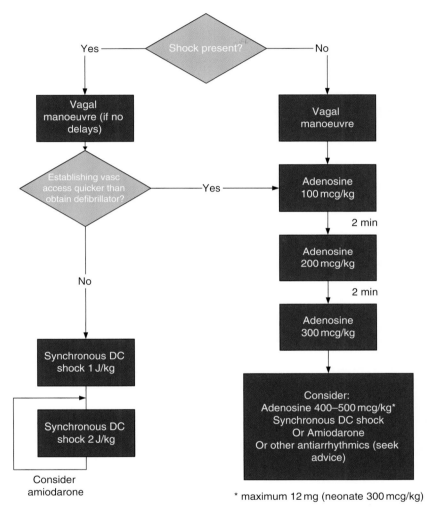

Figure 7.4 Algorithm for the management of supraventricular tachycardia

Reassess ABC

- Try vagal stimulation while continuing ECG monitoring. The following techniques can be used:
  - Elicit the 'diving reflex', which produces an increase in vagal tone, slows atrioventricular conduction and interrupts the tachycardia. This can be done by the application of a rubber glove filled with iced water over the face, or if this is ineffectual, wrapping the infant in a towel and immersing the face in iced water for 5 seconds.
  - One-sided carotid sinus massage.
  - Older children can try a Valsalva manoeuvre. Some children know that a certain position or action will usually effect a return to sinus rhythm. Blowing hard through a straw may be effective for some children.
  - Do not use ocular pressure in an infant or child, because ocular damage may result.
- If these manoeuvres are unsuccessful, give:
  - Intravenous adenosine: start with a rapid intravenous bolus of 100 micrograms/kg, and if success is not achieved, then after 2 minutes use 200 micrograms/kg. The next dose should be 300 micrograms/kg. The maximum single dose that

should be given is 500 micrograms/kg (300 micrograms/kg in a child under 1 month) up to a maximum of 12 mg. Continuous ECG monitoring, preferably with a paper ECG recording, should be done during adenosine administration so that the effect of the drug can be clearly demonstrated. Adenosine acts very rapidly with a half-life of less than 10 seconds. This means that side effects of flushing, nausea, dyspnoea and chest tightness are short-lived. It also means, however, that the effect may be short lasting and the SVT may recur.

- If the drug is given through a small peripheral vein, an insufficiently high concentration may reach the heart and therefore a larger dose may need to be given. Preferably, the drug should be injected into a large peripheral vein and followed rapidly by a saline flush. In older children a vein in the cubital fossa is preferred because of proximity to the heart. Adenosine is the drug of choice for SVT because of its efficacy and safety record.
- If the stable SVT of a child has not been converted to a normal rhythm with intravenous adenosine, it is essential to seek the advice of a paediatric cardiologist before further treatment. One of the following may be suggested:
  - Propranolol can be given by mouth in a dose of 250–500 micrograms/kg 3–4 times daily.
  - Propranolol (25–50 micrograms/kg slowly intravenously): as asystole may occur, IV propranolol is not a preferable option where there are not the facilities to undertake pacing. A paediatric cardiologist may advise a small dose to be given with cardiac monitoring. **Do not give propranolol if the patient has been given verapamil.**
  - Flecainide (2 mg/kg over at least 10 minutes): this is a membrane stabiliser but can be proarrhythmic and has a negative inotropic effect. It is good at terminating SVT and can be used by slow IV infusion (1–2 mg/kg) over 10–20 minutes, with continuous ECG monitoring.
  - Amiodarone: this drug can be used in refractory atrial tachycardia. The dose is 5 mg/kg over 30 minutes. Subsequent infusion may be required at a variable rate.
  - DC cardioversion under general anaesthetic is preferable, but if used only one drug should be given and further cardiological advice sought.
  - Digoxin: dosage schedules vary with age and underlying condition. This is no longer considered the preferred option and should only be given on the advice of a cardiologist.
  - Verapamil: the dose is 100–300 micrograms/kg, to a maximum of 5 mg. This should not be used in children under 1 year of age, as it has been associated with irreversible hypotension and asystole at this age. The drug should be terminated when sinus rhythm is seen, even if the calculated dose has not been given. Do not use if a patient has received β-blockers, flecainide or amiodarone.

7.5 Approach to the child with ventricular tachycardia

In the haemodynamically stable child with ventricular tachycardia, a history should be carefully obtained to identify an underlying cause for the tachycardia because this will often determine ancillary therapy.

- Consider the following underlying causes:
  - Congenital heart disease and surgery.
  - Myocarditis or cardiomyopathy.
  - Poisoning with tricyclic antidepressants, procainamide or quinidine.
  - Renal disease or another cause of hyperkalaemia.
  - Channelopathies (long QT syndromes, catecholaminergic polymorphic VT).
- Look for characteristics of the ECG indicative of torsade de pointes: polymorphic VT with QRS complexes that change in amplitude and polarity so that they appear to rotate around an isoelectric line. This is seen in conditions characterised by a long QT interval or drug poisoning, such as with quinine, quinidine, disopyramide, amiodarone, tricyclic antidepressants or digoxin.
- Check serum potassium, magnesium and calcium levels.
- Analysis of the ECG should be done in consultation with a paediatric cardiologist, who should be sent a copy urgently.

Follow the algorithm for ventricular tachycardia (Figure 7.5).

Reassess ABC

- In the haemodynamically unstable child, the treatment is synchronised DC cardioversion starting at 2 J/kg. It can be repeated and the dose can be increased if needed.
- The treatment of the haemodynamically stable child with VT should always include early consultation with a paediatric cardiologist. They may suggest:

- amiodarone (5 mg/kg over 20 minutes; 30 minutes in neonates), or
- intravenous procainamide (15 mg/kg over 30–60 minutes, monitor ECG and blood pressure).
- Both can cause hypotension, which should be treated with volume expansion.
- Rare specific VT types may respond to IV verapamil.
- In cases where the ventricular arrhythmia has been caused by drug toxicity, sedation/anaesthesia and DC shock may be the safest approach. Use synchronous shocks initially, as these are less likely to produce ventricular fibrillation than an asynchronous shock. If synchronous shocks are ineffectual, subsequent attempts will have to be asynchronous if the child is in shock.
- The treatment of torsade de pointes VT is emergency defibrillation followed by magnesium sulphate in a rapid IV infusion (several minutes) of 25–50 mg/kg (up to 2 g) and possibly lidocaine. Intravenous β-blockers may help calm the adrenergic storm.

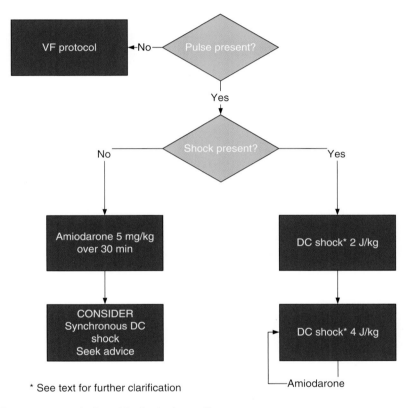

Figure 7.5 Algorithm for the management of ventricular tachycardia

It is important not to delay a safe therapeutic intervention for longer than necessary in VT as the rhythm often deteriorates quite quickly into pulseless VT or VF. Sometimes wide-complex tachycardia can be SVT with bundle branch block and aberrant conduction. This can be very difficult to differentiate from VT by a non-specialist. A safer approach is to treat it as VT. A dose of adenosine may help identify the underlying aetiology of the arrhythmia, but should be used with extreme caution in haemodynamically stable children with wide-complex tachycardia because acceleration of the tachycardia and significant hypotension are known risks and should not delay definitive treatment in children with shock. Seek advice.

7.6 Summary

You should use the structured approach in the assessment and management of the child with an abnormal pulse rate or rhythm:

- Primary assessment
- Resuscitation
- Secondary assessment and looking for key features
- Emergency treatment
- Stabilisation and transfer to definitive care

CHAPTER 8
The child with a decreased conscious level

Learning outcomes

- After reading this chapter, you will be able to:
- Recognise the causes of decreased conscious level in infants and children
- Describe the pathophysiology of raised intracranial pressure
- Describe how to assess children with a decreased conscious level
- Describe how to resuscitate the child with a decreased conscious level

---

8.1 Introduction

The conscious level may be altered by disease, injury or intoxication. The level of awareness decreases as a child passes through stages from drowsiness (mild reduction in alertness and increase in hours of sleep) to unconsciousness (unrousable, unresponsive). Because of variability in the definition of words describing the degree of coma, the Glasgow Coma Scale (GCS) and the Children's Glasgow Coma Scale (Table 8.1) have been developed as semiquantitative measures and, more importantly, as an aid to communication between carers. The GCS was developed and validated for use in the head-injured patient but has come to be used as an unvalidated tool for the description of conscious states from all pathologies.

In children, coma is caused by a diffuse metabolic insult (including cerebral hypoxia and ischaemia) in 95% of cases, and by structural lesions in the remaining 5%. Metabolic disturbances can produce diffuse, incomplete and asymmetrical neurological signs falsely suggestive of a localised lesion. Early signs of metabolic encephalopathy may be subtle, with reduced attention and blunted affect. The conscious level in metabolic encephalopathies is often quite variable from minute to minute. The most common causes of coma are summarised in the following box.

Disorders causing coma in children (*Continued overleaf*)

- Hypoxic ischaemic brain injury following respiratory or circulatory failure
- Epileptic seizures
- Trauma:
  - intracranial haemorrhage
  - brain swelling
- Infections:
  - meningitis
  - encephalitis
  - cerebral and extracerebral abscesses
  - malaria

Advanced Paediatric Life Support: A Practical Approach to Emergencies, Sixth Edition. Edited by Martin Samuels and Sue Wieteska.
© 2016 John Wiley & Sons, Ltd. Published 2016 by John Wiley & Sons, Ltd.

- Intoxication
- Metabolic:
  - renal or hepatic failure
  - hypo- or hypernatraemia
  - hypoglycaemia
  - hypothermia
  - hypercapnia
  - inherited metabolic disease
- Cerebrovascular event, secondary to arteriovascular malformation or tumour
- Cerebral tumour
- Hydrocephalus, including blocked intraventricular shunts

Table 8.1 Glasgow Coma Scale and Children's Glasgow Coma Scale

Glasgow Coma Scale (4–15 years)		Children's Glasgow Coma Scale (<4 years)	
Response	Score	Response	Score
Eye opening		Eye opening	
Spontaneously	4	Spontaneously	4
To verbal stimuli	3	To verbal stimuli	3
To pain	2	To pain	2
No response to pain	1	No response to pain	1
Best motor response		Best motor response	
Obeys verbal command	6	Spontaneous or obeys verbal command	6
Localises to pain	5	Localises to pain or withdraws to touch	5
Withdraws from pain	4	Withdraws from pain	4
Abnormal flexion to pain (decorticate)	3	Abnormal flexion to pain (decorticate)	3
Abnormal extension to pain (decerebrate)	2	Abnormal extension to pain (decerebrate)	2
No response to pain	1	No response to pain	1
Best verbal response		Best verbal response	
Orientated and converses	5	Alert; babbles, coos words to usual ability	5
Disorientated and converses	4	Less than usual words, spontaneous irritable cry	4
Inappropriate words	3	Cries only to pain	3
Incomprehensible sounds	2	Moans to pain	2
No response to pain	1	No response to pain	1

Children with a decreased conscious level are usually presented by parents who are very aware of the seriousness of the symptom. They may also have noted other features such as fever, headache or exposure to poisoning, which may aid the clinician in making a presumptive diagnosis.

8.2 Pathophysiology of raised intracranial pressure

In very young children, before the cranial sutures are closed, considerable intracranial volume expansion may occur if the process is slow (i.e. hydrocephalus). However, if the process is rapid and in children with a fixed volume cranium, increase in volume due to brain swelling, haematoma or cerebrospinal fluid (CSF) blockage will cause raised intracranial pressure (ICP). Initially, CSF and venous blood within the cranium decrease in volume. Soon, this compensating mechanism fails and as the ICP continues to rise the cerebral perfusion pressure (CPP) falls and cerebral arterial blood flow is reduced. CPP is defined as mean arterial pressure (MAP) minus ICP:

$$CPP = MAP - ICP$$

Reduced CPP reduces cerebral blood flow (CBF). Normal CBF is over 50 ml/100 g brain tissue/min. If the CBF falls below 20 ml/100 g brain tissue/min, the brain suffers ischaemia. The aim is to keep CPP above 40–60 mmHg; there may be age-specific thresholds with infants at the lower end and adolescents at the upper end of this range.

Increasing ICP will push brain tissue against more rigid intracranial structures. Two clinical syndromes are recognisable by the site of localised brain compression (Figure 8.1).

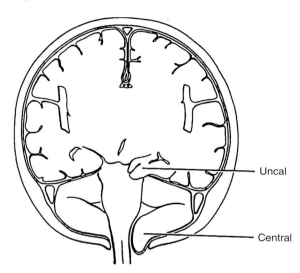

Figure 8.1 Herniations of the brain

Central syndrome

The whole brain is pressed down towards the foramen magnum and the cerebellar tonsils herniate through it ('coning'). Neck stiffness may be noted. A slow pulse, raised blood pressure and irregular respiration leading to apnoea are seen terminally, usually preceded by significant tachycardia.

Uncal syndrome

The intracranial volume increase is mainly in the supratentorial part of the intracranial space. The uncus, which is part of the hippocampal gyrus, is forced through the tentorial opening and compressed against the fixed free edge of the tentorium. If the pressure is unilateral (e.g. from a subdural or extradural haematoma), this leads to third nerve compression and an ipsilateral dilated pupil. Next, an external oculomotor palsy appears, so the eye cannot move laterally. Hemiplegia may then develop on either or both sides of the body, depending on the progression of the herniation.

8.3 Primary assessment and resuscitation

ABCDE

The first steps in the management of the patient with a decreased conscious level are to assess and if necessary support airway, breathing and circulation. This will ensure that the diminished conscious level is not secondary to hypoxia and/or ischaemia and that whatever the cerebral pathology it will not be worsened by a lack of oxygenated blood supply to the brain.

Follow the algorithm for coma (Figure 8.2).

Features specific for child with decreased conscious level
Airway

- Ensure the airway is open – consider airway-opening manoeuvres, airway adjuncts or intubation to secure the airway.
- If the child has an AVPU score of 'P' or 'U', or the gag or cough reflex is absent, the airway is at risk. It should be maintained by an airway manoeuvre or adjunct and senior help requested to secure it.

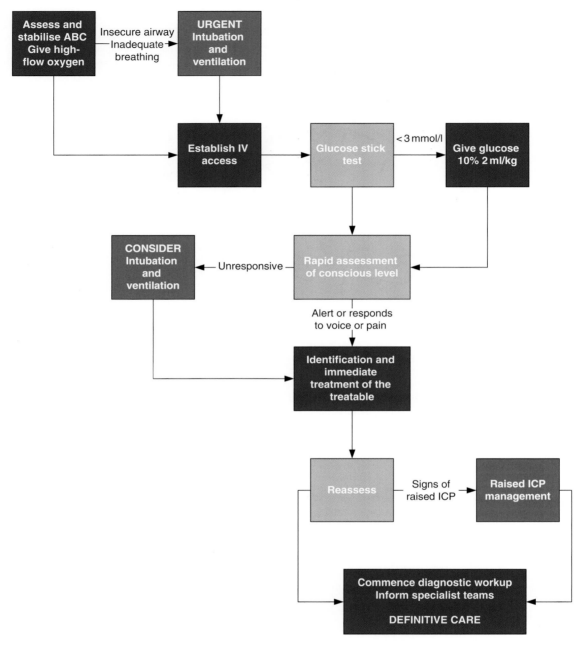

Figure 8.2 Algorithm for the initial management of coma. [ICP, intracranial pressure]

Breathing

- Effects on breathing: acidotic sighing respirations may suggest metabolic acidosis from diabetes, an inborn error of metabolism or salicylate/ethylene glycol poisoning as a cause for the coma.

Resuscitation

- All children with a decreased conscious level should receive high-flow oxygen through a face mask with a reservoir.
- If the child is hypoventilating, respiration should be supported with oxygen via a bag–valve–mask device and consideration given to intubation and ventilation. Inadequate breathing in coma can lead to a rise in arterial PCO_2, which can cause a dangerous rise in ICP.

Circulation

- Heart rate: the presence of an inappropriate bradycardia will suggest raised ICP.
- Blood pressure: significant hypertension could indicate a possible cause for the coma or may be a result of it.

Resuscitation

Circulation needs to be optimised; if ICP is high, then cerebral perfusion will be compromised. However, overenthusiastic fluid administration should be avoided.

- Establish IV/IO access quickly.
- Check blood glucose – DEFG: 'Don't ever forget glucose'.
- Take blood for a rapid bedside and laboratory test for glucose. If in doubt or the test is unavailable, it is safer to treat as if hypoglycaemia is present (<3 mmol/l): give a bolus of 10% glucose IV 2 ml/kg, followed by 5% glucose solutions (10% in infants). Without the follow-on infusion, there is a risk of rebound hypoglycaemia, which may also occur with larger bolus doses of glucose.
- If hypoglycaemia is a new condition for the patient take 5 ml of lithium heparin blood before giving the glucose and send it to the laboratory for the plasma to be frozen. This will allow later investigation of the cause of the hypoglycaemic state.
- Take blood samples for blood culture, full blood count, renal and liver function tests, plasma ammonia (send rapidly to the laboratory ideally on ice), blood group and save/cross-match, and blood gas analysis.
- Give a broad-spectrum antibiotic such as cefotaxime or ceftriaxone to any child in whom sepsis or meningitis/encephalitis is suspected. Also consider early administration of aciclovir if herpes encephalitis cannot be excluded quickly.
- Give a 20 ml/kg rapid bolus of crystalloid to any patient with signs of shock unless there is evidence of trauma, when a bolus of 10 ml/kg should be used. Reassess the need for repeated boluses with persistent shock.

Disability

- Posture: decorticate or decerebrate posturing in a previously normal child should suggest raised ICP.
- Look for neck stiffness in a child and a full or tense fontanelle in an infant, which suggest meningitis.
- The presence of convulsive movements should be sought: these may be subtle.
- If a rash is present, ascertain if it is purpuric as an indicator of meningococcal/streptococcal disease or non-accidental injury.
- Fever is suggestive evidence of an infectious cause (but its absence does not exclude it) or poisoning with ecstasy, cocaine or salicylates. Hypothermia suggests poisoning with barbiturates or ethanol.
- Look for evidence of poisoning: history or characteristic smell (see Appendix E).

There should be a specific assessment for intracranial hypertension. There are very few absolute signs of raised ICP, these being papilloedema, a bulging fontanelle and the absence of venous pulsation in retinal vessels. All three signs are often absent in acutely raised ICP. In a previously well, unconscious child (GCS <9) who is not in a postictal state, the signs in the box are suggestive of raised ICP.

Signs of raised intracranial pressure

1. Abnormal oculocephalic reflexes (avoid in patients with neck injuries):
   - When the head is turned to the left or right a normal response is for the eyes to move away from the head movement; an abnormal response is no (or random) movement
   - When the head is flexed, a normal response is deviation of the eyes upward; a loss of conjugate upward gaze is a sign suggestive of raised ICP
2. Abnormal posture (see Figure 4.2):
   - Decorticate (flexed arms, extended legs)
   - Decerebrate (extended arms, extended legs)
   Posturing may need to be elicited by a painful stimulus
3. Abnormal pupillary responses: unilateral or bilateral dilatation suggests raised ICP
4. Abnormal breathing patterns: there are several recognisable breathing pattern abnormalities in raised ICP. However, they are often changeable and may vary from hyperventilation to Cheyne–Stokes breathing to apnoea
5. Cushing's triad: slow pulse, raised blood pressure and breathing pattern abnormalities are a late sign of raised ICP

Resuscitation

Undertake appropriate medical management of raised ICP, if noted.

- Intubate and support ventilation (maintain a PCO_2 of 4.5–5.5 kPa or 34–41 mmHg).
- Nurse with the head in-line in a 20° head-up position (to help cerebral venous drainage).
- Give hypertonic (3%) saline 3 ml/kg followed by a continuous infusion of 0.1–1.0 ml/kg/h of the same solution. Serum osmolality should be maintained <360 mOsm/l. Mannitol can be used as an alternative (250–500 mg/kg; i.e. 1.25–2.5 ml of 20% solution IV over 15 minutes), and give 2-hourly as required, provided serum osmolality is not greater than 325 mOsm/l).
- Consider dexamethasone (only for oedema surrounding a space-occupying lesion) 0.5 mg/kg 6-hourly.

Lumbar puncture

> Lumbar puncture should not be performed in a child in coma.

The purpose of a lumbar puncture is to confirm the diagnosis of meningitis/encephalitis and to identify the organism and its antibiotic sensitivity. There is a risk of coning and death if a lumbar puncture is performed in a child with significantly raised ICP. Normal fundi or a normal CT scan do not exclude acutely, severely raised ICP. The lumbar puncture can be performed some days later when the child's condition allows, to confirm or refute the diagnosis of meningitis/encephalitis if antibiotic treatment or aciclovir, respectively, has been started. In addition, the results of blood cultures and PCR are therefore important.

The relative contraindications to a lumbar puncture are shown in the box.

Relative contraindications to lumbar puncture

- Prolonged or focal seizures
- Focal neurological signs, e.g. asymmetry of limb movement and reflexes, ocular palsies
- A widespread purpuric rash in an ill child. In this case IV cefotaxime/ceftriaxone should be given immediately, preferably after a blood culture
- Glasgow Coma Scale score of less than 13
- Pupillary dilatation
- Impaired oculocephalic reflexes (doll's eye reflexes)
- Abnormal posture or movement, decerebrate or decorticate posturing, or cycling movements of the limbs
- Inappropriately low pulse, elevated blood pressure and irregular respirations (i.e. signs of impending brain herniation)
- Thrombocytopenia or coagulation disorder
- Papilloedema
- Hypertension

8.4 Secondary assessment and looking for key features

While the primary assessment and resuscitation are being carried out, a focused history of the child's health and activity over the previous 24 hours and any significant previous illness should be gained. In a patient in coma, it is often impossible to be certain of the diagnosis in the first hour. The main immediate aims are therefore to maintain homeostasis and 'treat the treatable'.

Specific points for history taking include:

- Recent trauma
- Pre-existing neurological disability
- History of epilepsy
- Poison ingestion: specifically enquire about medicine/agents that the child might have been exposed to.
- Known chronic condition (e.g. renal disease, cardiac abnormality, diabetes)
- Last meal
- Known metabolic disorder or family history of one
- Previous episodes of encephalopathy with illness.
- Recent trips abroad.

Specific additional neurological examination includes:

- Eye examination:
  - pupil size and reactivity (Table 8.2)
  - fundal changes: haemorrhage and papilloedema (trauma, hypertension)
  - ophthalmoplegia: lateral or vertical deviation
- Reassess posture and tone: look for lateralisation
- Assess deep tendon reflexes and plantar responses: look for lateralisation

Lateralisation suggests a localised rather than a generalised lesion, but this is often a false indicator in childhood. The child will almost certainly need a CT or magnetic resonance imaging (MRI) scan.

Table 8.2 Summary of pupillary changes

Pupil size and reactivity	Cause
Small reactive pupils	Metabolic disorders
	Medullary lesion
Pinpoint pupils	Metabolic disorders
	Narcotic/organophosphate ingestions
Fixed midsize pupils	Midbrain lesion
Fixed dilated pupils	Hypothermia
	Severe hypoxia
	Barbiturates (late sign)
	During and post seizure
	Anticholinergic drugs
Unilateral dilated pupil	Rapidly expanding ipsilateral lesion
	Tentorial herniation
	Third nerve lesion
	Epileptic seizures

A general physical examination may add clues to point to a working diagnosis. Specific findings include the following:

- Skin: rash, haemorrhage, trauma and evidence of neurocutaneous syndromes
- Scalp: evidence of trauma
- Ears and nose:
  - bloody or clear discharge: base of skull fracture (see Chapter 14)
  - evidence of otitis media or mastoiditis: may accompany meningitis
- Neck tenderness or rigidity: meningitis or cerebrovascular accident
- Odour: alcohol intoxication, ketones in diabetic ketoacidosis or metabolic disorders
- Abdomen: enlarged liver (in conjunction with hypoglycaemia, inherited metabolic disease)

The key features, which will be identified clinically, from the history, examination and the initial blood test results, can point the clinician to the likeliest working diagnosis for emergency treatment.

- Coma that develops over several hours, associated with irritability and/or fever and a rash points to meningitis/encephalitis   Section 8.6
- A history of opiate ingestion and/or pinpoint pupils points to poisoning with opiates   Section 8.8
- Coma occurring in the setting of, or just after, a minor illness presenting with vomiting, hepatomegaly and hypoglycaemia points to metabolic encephalopathy   Section 8.8
- A history of travel abroad might point to malaria   Section 8.9
- Coma associated with significant hypertension points to hypertensive encephalopathy   Section 9.7

- A history of onset of coma over an hour or so in an otherwise well child is suggestive of poisoning
- A vague and inconsistent history and/or suspicious bruising in an infant are suggestive of non-accidental head injury; the presence of retinal haemorrhage is supportive evidence of this
- Hyperglycaemia points to diabetes
- A history of very sudden onset of coma, sometimes with a preceding headache points to a cerebrovascular accident

Appendix E

Chapter 14

Appendix B

In addition, unless meningitis can be excluded by the clear identification of another cause for coma, it should be assumed present as the consequence of missed diagnosis is catastrophic and the risk of unnecessary treatment with antibiotics small. This also applies to meningoencephalitis from *Mycoplasma* and herpes, and the use of erythromycin and aciclovir, respectively. Early initiation of treatment is important because these have a worse prognosis when treatment is seriously delayed. Senior advice should be sought.

8.5 Further general treatment of coma

- Give normal fluid maintenance, avoid hypoglycaemia and maintain electrolyte balance, unless there is evidence of raised ICP or increased antidiuretic hormone secretion.
- Maintain normoglycaemic state:
  - use 5% glucose solutions (10% in young infants), increasing as needed, and
  - be cautious of administering insulin to hyperglycaemic patients, as this may be stress induced.
- Assess and maintain electrolyte balance:
  - if possible keep serum sodium in the normal range, 135–145 mmol/l, and
  - avoid hyponatraemia by using crystalloid or adding extra sodium in the maintenance fluids.
- Treat seizures if present and give prophylactic anticonvulsants if the child has repeated seizures.
- Insert a gastric tube to aspirate stomach contents. Perform gastric lavage in appropriate circumstances (see Appendix E).
- Regulate temperature, ensuring hyperthermia above 37.5°C is avoided.
- Undertake appropriate medical management of raised ICP, if noted, as discussed.
- Maintain skin care to prevent bedsores, and eye padding to avoid xerophthalmia.

8.6 Approach to the child with meningitis/encephalitis

After the neonatal period, the commonest cause of bacterial meningitis is *Neisseria meningitidis* (meningococcus). There is still a mortality rate of around 5% and a similar rate of permanent serious sequelae. Infection with *Streptococcus pneumoniae* is less common and may follow an upper respiratory infection with or without otitis media. Long-term morbidity and mortality occur in up to 30% of cases. Widespread Hib vaccination has reduced the incidence of *Haemophilus influenzae* infection. A wide range of infections may also cause encephalitis.

Diagnosis of bacterial meningitis

In the 3-year-old child and under

Bacterial meningitis is difficult to diagnose in its early stages in this age group. The classic signs of neck rigidity, photophobia, headache and vomiting are often absent. A bulging fontanelle is a sign of advanced meningitis in an infant, but even this serious and late sign will be masked if the baby is dehydrated from fever and vomiting. Almost all children with meningitis have some degree of raised ICP, so that, in fact, the signs and symptoms of meningitis are primarily those of raised ICP. The following are signs of possible meningitis in infants and young children:

- Coma
- Drowsiness (often shown by lack of eye contact with parents or doctor)
- High-pitched cry or irritability that cannot be easily soothed by parent
- Poor feeding
- Unexplained pyrexia
- Convulsions with or without fever
- Apnoeic or cyanotic attacks
- Purpuric rash

In older children of 4 years and over

These children are more likely to have the classic signs of headache, vomiting, pyrexia, neck stiffness and photophobia. Some present with coma or convulsions. In all unwell children, and children with an unexplained pyrexia, a careful search should be made for neck stiffness and for a purpuric rash. The finding of such a rash in an ill child is almost pathognomic of meningococcal infection, for which immediate treatment is required (see Section 6.8).

Emergency treatment of meningitis

Reassess ABCD

- Specific assessment should be made of the severity of raised ICP, as many of the clinical signs of meningitis arise from this.
- After the above assessment, give intravenous cefotaxime or another suitable antibiotic if meningitis is suspected and this has not yet been given. Treat a child with possible raised ICP and meningitis without performing a lumbar puncture. Ensure blood cultures and PCR have been taken, as these may help in the diagnosis.
- Treat with aciclovir and a macrolide in a febrile, comatose child for the rare respective possibilities of herpes simplex virus and *Mycoplasma* encephalitis.
- Give dexamethasone (150 micrograms/kg, max. 10 mg, four times a day) in suspected or confirmed bacterial meningitis, aiming to start within 4 hours of antibiotics (not later than 12 hours). Do not use in infants younger than 3 months, but in older infants and children corticosteroids can reduce the rate of severe hearing loss and possibly other long-term neurological sequelae.

8.7 Approach to the child poisoned with opiates

These children are usually toddlers who have drunk the green liquid form of methadone. The sedative effect of the drug may reduce the conscious level sufficiently to put the airway at risk and cause hypoventilation.

Emergency treatment of opiate poisoning

Reassess ABC

Following stabilisation of airway, breathing and circulation, the specific antidote is naloxone. An initial bolus dose of 10 micrograms/kg is used but some children need doses as high as 100 micrograms/kg, up to a maximum of 2 mg. Naloxone has a short half-life, relapse often occurring after 20 minutes. Further boluses, or an infusion of 10–20 micrograms/kg/min, may be required.

It is important to normalise carbon dioxide before the naloxone is given because adverse events such as ventricular arrhythmias, acute pulmonary oedema, asystole or seizures may otherwise occur. This is because the opioid system and the adrenergic system are inter-related. Opioid antagonists and hypercapnia stimulate sympathetic nervous system activity. Therefore, if ventilation is not provided to normalise carbon dioxide prior to naloxone administration, the sudden rise in adrenaline concentration can cause arrhythmias.

8.8 Approach to the child with metabolic coma

The most common metabolic disorders that can result in encephalopathy are hypoglycaemia and diabetic ketoacidosis (see Appendix B). Nevertheless, metabolic coma can arise from a variety of conditions, including a number of rare, inborn errors of metabolism. These illnesses often present with a rapidly progressive encephalopathy, vomiting, drowsiness and convulsions or coma. There may be associated hepatomegaly (from fatty change), hypoglycaemia, abnormal liver enzymes or hyperammonaemia. In a case of otherwise unexplained coma with a GCS of <12, a key urgent investigation is a plasma ammonia. Interpretation of the concentration can be difficult, as can specific treatment of the hyperammonaemia. In this event seek advice from a specialist in inherited metabolic disease and the paediatric intensive care unit.

8.9 Approach to the child with malaria

Plasmodium falciparum causes 95% of deaths and most severe complications. It is transmitted by the bite of an infected *Anopheles* mosquito, and less commonly by infected blood transfusion, needle stick injuries or by the transplacental route.

The clinical features of severe disease include reduced conscious level, convulsions, metabolic acidosis, hypoglycaemia and severe normocytic anaemia. Cerebral malaria may produce encephalopathy, rapid-onset coma and raised intracranial pressure. Diagnosis requires microscopy of a thick film (quick diagnosis) and thin film (species identification). Obtain a complete history for the laboratory, including the likely country or region of origination.

Specific emergency treatment of cerebral malaria

Reassess ABCDE

- IV/IO artesunate (2.4 mg/kg on admission, then at 12 and 24 hours, then once a day) is the recommended treatment for severe *P. falciparum* malaria. Quinine is an acceptable alternative if artesunate is not available (loading dose 20 mg/kg over 4 hours. in glucose 5% then 10 mg/kg every 8 hours). Give with ECG monitoring.
- Consider antibiotics, e.g. IV cefotaxime since the risk of concomitant bacterial (Gram-negative) infections is high in children.
- Monitor and treat hypoglycaemia as needed.
- If there is evidence of life-threatening anaemia (haemoglobin <5 g/dl) consider transfusion, especially if there are signs of heart failure. Be cautious with fluid administration!

8.10 Approach to the child with systemic hypertensive crisis

See Sections 9.6 and 9.7.

8.11 Stabilisation and transfer to definitive care

After the child has been stabilised and conditions such as hypoglycaemia, meningitis and opiate poisoning have been treated as indicated, some children will remain undiagnosed. These children and those in whom there is any suggestion of lateralisation or intracranial hypertension should have an urgent CT scan. Children who remain very ill and those in whom the cause of coma is as yet unidentified will require transfer to a paediatric intensive care unit and the involvement of other specialists such as from neurology, inherited metabolic diseases or endocrinology as indicated. With any evidence of intracranial bleeds, time-critical transfer/review is required.

Patients will almost certainly need intubation and ventilation for safe transfer by the retrieval team (see Chapter 25). In such patients neurological assessment cannot be continued, and there should therefore be clear documentation of neurological signs, including their progression before transfer is commenced.

8.12 Summary

You should use the structured approach in the assessment and management of the child with a decreased conscious level:

- Primary assessment
- Resuscitation
- Secondary assessment and looking for key features
- Emergency treatment
- Stabilisation and transfer to definitive care

CHAPTER 9
The convulsing child

9.1 Introduction

Generalised convulsive status epilepticus (CSE) is currently defined as a generalised convulsion lasting 30 minutes or longer, or when successive convulsions occur so frequently over a 30-minute period that the patient does not recover consciousness between them. Although the outcome of CSE is mainly determined by its cause, the duration of the convulsion is also important. In addition, the longer the duration of the convulsions, the more difficult it is to terminate it. In general, convulsions that persist beyond 5 minutes may not stop spontaneously, so it is usual practice to institute anticonvulsive treatment after it has lasted 5 or more minutes.

Common causes of convulsions in children include fever (<6 years), meningitis/encephalitis, epilepsy, hypoxia and metabolic abnormalities. Status epilepticus occurs in approximately 1–5% of patients with epilepsy. Up to 5% of children with febrile seizures will present with CSE.

Status epilepticus can be fatal, but mortality is lower in children than in adults – at about 4–6%. Death may be due to complications of the convulsion, including obstruction of the airway, hypoxia and aspiration of vomit, to overmedication, cardiac arrhythmias or to the underlying disease process. Complications of prolonged convulsions include cardiac arrhythmias, hypertension, pulmonary oedema, hyperthermia, disseminated intravascular coagulation and myoglobinuria. Adverse neurological outcomes (persistent epilepsy, motor deficits, learning and behavioural difficulties) are age dependent, occurring in 6% of those over 3 years but 29% of those under 1 year.

9.2 Pathophysiology of prolonged convulsions

A generalised convulsion increases the cerebral metabolic rate at least three-fold. Initially, there is an increased sympathetic activity with the release of catecholamines, which lead to peripheral vasoconstriction and increased systemic blood pressure. There is also a loss of cerebral arterial regulation and, following the increase in systemic blood pressure, there is a resulting increase in cerebral blood flow to provide the necessary oxygen and energy. If convulsions continue, the systemic blood pressure falls and this is followed by a fall in cerebral blood flow. Lactic acid rapidly accumulates and there is subsequently cell death, oedema and raised intracerebral pressure resulting in further worsening of cerebral perfusion.

Advanced Paediatric Life Support: A Practical Approach to Emergencies, Sixth Edition. Edited by Martin Samuels and Sue Wieteska.
© 2016 John Wiley & Sons, Ltd. Published 2016 by John Wiley & Sons, Ltd.

9.3 Primary assessment and resuscitation

ABCDE

The first steps in the management of the convulsing patient are to assess and, if necessary, support airway, breathing and circulation. This will ensure that the convulsion is not secondary to hypoxia and/or ischaemia and that whatever the cerebral pathology, it will not be worsened by lack of oxygenated blood supply to the brain. An important early step is to identify and treat any hypoglycaemia.

Features specific for the convulsing child

Airway

- Ensure the airway is open – consider airway-opening manoeuvres or airway adjuncts.
- If the child is breathing satisfactorily, the recovery position should be adopted to minimise the risk of aspiration of vomit.

Breathing

- Look for stridor or grunting. Grunting may be caused by the convulsion or raised intracranial pressure and may not be a sign of respiratory distress in this instance.

Resuscitation

- Give high-flow oxygen through a face mask with reservoir.
- If respiratory effort is inadequate, support with a bag–valve–mask device and consider intubation and ventilation.

Circulation

- Heart rate: the presence of an inappropriate bradycardia will suggest raised intracranial pressure.
- Blood pressure: significant hypertension could indicate a possible cause for the convulsion but more likely is a result of it.
- Look for a rash: if present, ascertain if it is purpuric as an indicator of meningococcal/streptococcal disease or non-accidental injury.
- Fever is suggestive evidence of an infectious cause (but its absence does not suggest the opposite) or poisoning with ecstasy, cocaine or salicylates. Hypothermia suggests poisoning with barbiturates or ethanol.
- Consider the evidence for poisoning: history or characteristic smell (see Appendix E).

Resuscitation

- Gain intravenous or intraosseous access.
- Take blood for a rapid bedside and laboratory test for glucose. If in doubt or a test is unavailable, it is safer to treat as if hypoglycaemia is present (<3 mmol/l): give a bolus IV of 2 ml/kg 10% glucose, followed by 5% glucose solutions (10% in infants). Without the follow-on infusion there is a risk of rebound hypoglycaemia, which may also occur with larger bolus doses of glucose.
- If hypoglycaemia is a new condition for the patient take 5 ml of lithium heparin blood before giving the glucose and send to the laboratory for the plasma to be frozen. This will allow later investigation of the cause of the hypoglycaemic state.
- Give a 20 ml/kg rapid bolus of crystalloid to any patient with signs of shock and reassess need for repeated boluses.
- Give an antibiotic such as cefotaxime or ceftriaxone if a diagnosis of septicaemia is considered or made obvious by the presence of a purpuric rash, preferably after blood has been taken for culture.
- Give an antibiotic such as cefotaxime or ceftriaxone to any child in whom a diagnosis of meningitis is considered with signs that may include a stiff neck or bulging fontanelle, preferably after blood has been taken for culture. Do not delay to perform a lumbar puncture. Also consider early administration of aciclovir if herpes encephalitis cannot be excluded quickly.

Disability

- Assess mental status/conscious level (AVPU).
- Pupillary size and reaction (see Table 8.2).
- Posture: decorticate or decerebrate posturing in a previously normal child should suggest raised intracranial pressure. These postures can be mistaken for the tonic phase of a convulsion. Consider also the possibility of a drug-induced dystonic reaction or a psychogenic, pseudo-epileptic attack. All these movement disorders are distinguishable from tonic–clonic status epilepticus as long as they are considered.
- Look for neck stiffness in a child and a full or tense fontanelle in an infant, which suggest meningitis.

9.4 Secondary assessment and looking for key features

While the primary assessment and resuscitation are being carried out, a focused history of the child's health and activity over the previous 24 hours and any significant previous illness should be gained.

Specific points for history taking include:

- Current febrile illness
- Recent trauma
- History of epilepsy
- Poison ingestion
- Last meal
- Known illnesses, specifically diabetes and adrenal insufficiency

9.5 Emergency treatment of the convulsion

The immediate emergency treatment requirement, after ABC stabilisation and exclusion or treatment of hypoglycaemia, is to stop the convulsion.

Reassess ABC

This evidence-based consensus guideline is not intended to cover all circumstances. There are patients with recurrent convulsive status whose physicians recognise that they respond to certain drugs and not to others and for these children an individual protocol is more appropriate. In addition, seizures in neonates are managed differently to those of infants and children.

The protocol is suitable for the majority of children with CSE who present acutely on wards or in an emergency department (Figure 9.1). It is not applicable to non-convulsive status epilepticus. It is important to respect the time intervals between the steps.

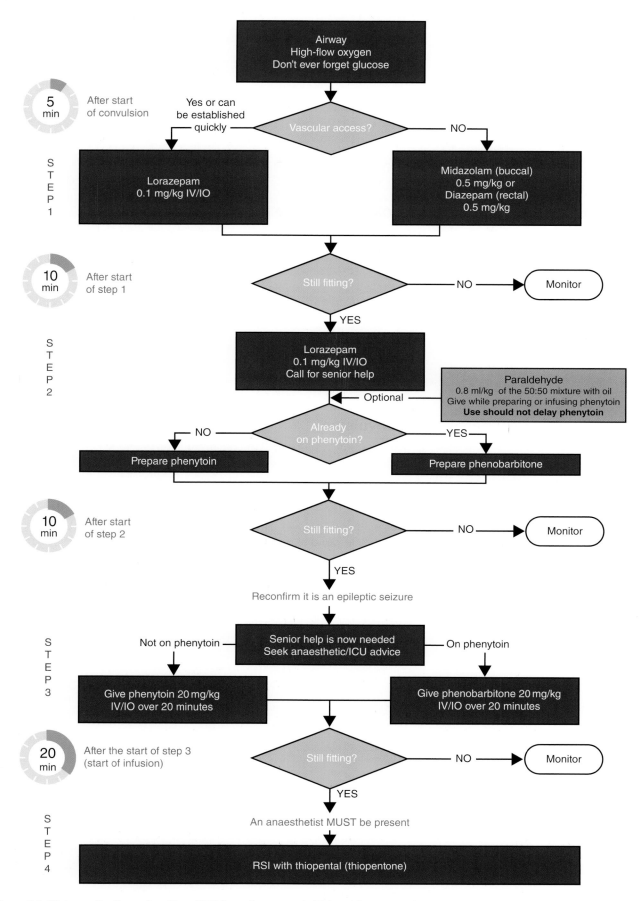

Figure 9.1 Status epilepticus algorithm. [ICU, intensive care unit; RSI, rapid sequence induction]

Step 1 is undertaken 5 minutes after the seizure has started. If this has started in the pre-hospital environment it may be more than 5 minutes after the seizure started before the child arrives in the department – you would therefore move immediately to step 1 on arrival.

STEP 1
- Many children may have already undergone step 1 before arrival in hospital. In that case proceed to step 2
- If in a pre-hospital setting or when IV/IO access is not established and if the seizure has lasted longer than 5 minutes, give buccal midazolam 0.5 mg/kg (max. 10 mg) or rectal diazepam 0.5 mg/kg
- If IV/IO access is already established or can be established quickly, give IV/IO lorazepam 0.1 mg/kg

STEP 2
- *If the convulsion continues for 10 minutes after start of step 1* and in the hospital setting, give a second dose of benzodiazepine, and call for senior help
- If the child has received buccal midazolam or rectal diazepam before or in hospital, and is still convulsing, obtain IV access to give one dose of IV lorazepam (0.1 mg/kg, max. 4 mg). Do not give more than two doses of benzodiazepine, including any pre-hospital medication. If IV access still has not been achieved, obtain IO access
- Start to prepare phenytoin for step 3
- Reconfirm it is an epileptic seizure

In the majority of children, treatment in steps 1 to 2 will be effective

STEP 3
- At this stage senior help is needed to reassess the child and advise on management. It is also wise to seek anaesthetic or intensive care advice as the child will need anaesthetising and intubating if this step is unsuccessful
- Give phenytoin (20 mg/kg by IV infusion over 20 minutes)
- Whilst this is being prepared, **consider** giving a dose of rectal paraldehyde (0.4 ml/kg) mixed with an equal volume of olive oil (i.e. a total of 0.8ml/kg of the paraldehyde+oil mixture)
- If the convulsion stops before phenytoin is started, the infusion should not be commenced without specialist advice
- If the convulsion stops after phenytoin has been started, the complete dose should still be given, as this will have an anticonvulsant effect for up to 24 hours
- In the case of children already receiving phenytoin as maintenance treatment for their epilepsy, phenobarbitone (20 mg/kg IV over 20 minutes) could be used in place of phenytoin. Alternatives that senior staff may recommend include IV levetiracetam or sodium valproate

STEP 4
- *If 20 minutes after step 3* has started the child remains in CSE, an anaesthetist must be present
- Check airway, breathing and circulation
- Take blood for glucose, arterial blood gas, urea, electrolytes and calcium
- Treat any vital function problem and correct metabolic abnormalities slowly
- Treat pyrexia with paracetamol or diclofenac rectally
- Consider mannitol (250–500 mg/kg IV over 30–60 minutes) or (2.7) 3% saline (3 ml/kg) if signs of increased intracranial pressure are present
- Rapid sequence induction of anaesthesia is performed with thiopentone and a short-acting paralysing agent and the child should be transferred to the paediatric intensive care unit. Midazolam (0.1 mg/kg/h up to doses of 1 mg/kg/h) is a valuable alternative and relatively easy to use. When midazolam fails to achieve seizure control, thiopentone can be used
- Further advice on management should be sought from a paediatric neurologist
- In children under 3 years with a history of chronic, active epilepsy, a trial of pyridoxine should be considered

Drugs

Lorazepam

Lorazepam is equally or more effective than diazepam and possibly produces less respiratory depression. It has a longer duration of action (12–24 hours) than diazepam (less than 1 hour). It appears to be poorly absorbed from the rectal route. Lorazepam is not available in every country. If this is the case, diazepam can be substituted at a dose of 0.25 mg/kg IV/IO or midazolam at a dose of 0.1 mg/kg IV/IO.

Midazolam

This is an effective, quick-acting anticonvulsant, that takes effect within minutes but has a shorter lasting effect than lorazepam. It can be given by IV/IO/IM routes or via buccal or nasal mucosa. Buccal/nasal midazolam may be twice as effective as rectal diazepam, but both drugs produce the same level and degree of respiratory depression. Most children do not convulse again once the seizure has been terminated. It has a depressant effect on respiration, but this occurs only in about 5% of patients, is short lived and is usually easily managed with bag–valve–mask ventilatory support.

If using the buccal route, use the licensed preparation (Buccolam®) available in pre-filled syringes of 2.5, 5, 7.5 and 10 mg midazolam. The tip of the syringe is inserted into the buccal area between the lower bottom lip and the gum margin at the side of the mouth. If the licensed preparation is not available draw up the higher dose (0.5 mg) of the IV preparation using a needle (to avoid any fragments of glass from the ampoule), after removing the needle, inject the drug in the same way. For nasal application, commercially available nasal spray can be used or the dose can be given using a MAD (mucosal atomisation device) on a standard syringe.

Continuous midazolam IV/IO is often used as a first line treatment in step 4 because of its relative ease of use, its high response rate and low complication rate. The starting dose is 0.1 mg/kg/h, increased in steps of 0.1 mg/kg/h up to a maximum of 1 mg/kg/h.

Diazepam

This is also an effective, quick-acting anticonvulsant with similar characteristics to midazolam. It is widely used but may now be superseded by the more effective midazolam where the latter is available. The rectal dose is well absorbed.

Paraldehyde

The dose is 0.8 ml/kg per rectum of the pre-mixed 50:50 solution in olive oil or normal saline. Arachis oil should be avoided because children with peanut allergy may react to it. Paraldehyde can cause rectal irritation, but intramuscular paraldehyde causes severe pain and may lead to sterile abscess formation. Paraldehyde causes little respiratory depression. It should not be used in liver disease.

Paraldehyde takes 10–15 minutes to act and its action is sustained for 2–4 hours. Do not leave paraldehyde standing in a plastic syringe for longer than a few minutes. If paraldehyde is given, this should be at the same time as the phenytoin is being drawn up or infused. It is also important that the infusion of phenytoin must not be delayed because the paraldehyde has been given.

Phenytoin

The dose is 20 mg/kg IV/IO with a rate of infusion no greater than 1 mg/kg/min. The infusion should be made up in normal saline to a maximum concentration of 10 mg in 1 ml. Phenytoin can cause dysrhythmias and hypotension, therefore monitor the ECG and blood pressure (BP). It has little depressant effect on respiration.

Thiopental (thiopentone) sodium

The induction dose is 4–8 mg/kg IV/IO. It is an alkaline solution, which will cause irritation if the solution leaks into subcutaneous tissues. It has no analgesic effect and is a general anaesthetic agent. Repeated doses have a cumulative effect. It is a potent drug with marked cardiorespiratory effects and must be used only by experienced staff who can intubate a child. It is not an effective long-term anticonvulsant and its principal use in status epilepticus is to facilitate ventilation and the subsequent management of cerebral oedema due to the prolonged seizure activity. Other antiepileptic medication must be continued.

The child should not remain paralysed as continued seizure activity cannot universally be adequately monitored by cerebral function analysis monitoring. When the child is stable he or she will need transfer to a paediatric intensive care unit (PICU). A paediatric neurologist should continue to give clinical advice and support. There are several regimes for continued drug control of the convulsions but they are outside the scope of this text.

General measures

- Maintain a normoglycaemic state:
  - Use 5% glucose solutions (10% in young infants), increasing as needed.
  - Be cautious of administering insulin to hyperglycaemic patients, as this may be stress induced.
- Give normal fluid maintenance unless there is evidence of raised intracranial pressure or increased antidiuretic hormone secretion.
- Assess and maintain electrolyte balance:
  - Keep serum sodium in the normal range of 135–145 mmol/l.
  - Avoid hyponatraemia by using normal saline or adding extra sodium in the maintenance fluids.

- Insert a gastric tube to aspirate the stomach contents. Regulate temperature, ensuring temperatures above 37.5°C are avoided.
- Undertake appropriate medical management of raised intracranial pressure, if noted:
  - Support ventilation (maintain a PCO_2 of 4.5–5.5 kPa (34-41 mmHg).
  - Maintain a 20° head-up position with the head in-line.
  - Give hypertonic (3%) saline 3 ml/kg followed by a continuous infusion of 0.1–1.0 ml/kg/h of the same solution. Serum osmolality should be maintained at less than 360 mOsm/L. Mannitol can be used as an alternative (250–500 mg/kg; i.e. 1.25–2.5 ml of 20% solution IV over 15 minutes), given 2-hourly as required, provided serum osmolality is not greater than 325 mOsm/l.
  - Consider dexamethasone (only for oedema surrounding a space-occupying lesion) 0.5 mg/kg 6-hourly.
  - Catheterise the bladder (bladder distension may aggravate raised intracranial pressure).

The role of cerebral function analysis monitoring is still unclear. Currently, clinical features and standard electroencephalography (EEG) are the preferred methods of assessing seizure activity.

Frequent reassessment of ABC is mandatory as therapy may cause depression of ventilation or hypotension. This particularly applies when treatment with benzodiazepines or barbiturates has been used to control the fit. Although it is appropriate to continue face mask oxygen treatment, its use may mask hypoventilation if breathing efficacy is being monitored by SpO_2. Either assess carbon dioxide levels or ensure that SpO_2 is assessed regularly while breathing room air. Support ventilation if hypoventilation is present.

After the fit has been controlled the clinician must consider the underlying cause of the convulsion. In many cases there will be an infectious cause: either a benign, self-limiting infection causing 'febrile status' or possibly meningitis (see Chapter 8). Additional treatments will depend on the clinical situation.

9.6 Approach to the child with systemic hypertensive crisis

Hypertension is uncommon in children. Renal disorders such as dysplastic kidneys, reflux nephropathy or glomerulonephritis account for the majority of children presenting with severe hypertension. Coarctation of the aorta is another important cause. Blood pressure is rarely measured routinely in otherwise healthy children and therefore hypertension usually presents with symptoms that may be diverse in nature. Neurological symptoms are more common in children than in adults. There may be a history of severe headaches, with or without vomiting, suggestive of raised intracranial pressure. Children may also present acutely with convulsions or in coma. Some children will present with a facial palsy or hemiplegia, and small babies may even present with apnoea or cardiac failure.

Blood pressure measurement

This may be difficult in small children and misleading if not done correctly. The following guidelines should be observed:

- Always use the biggest cuff that will fit comfortably on the upper arm. A small cuff will give erroneously high readings.
- The systolic BP may give a more reliable reading than the diastolic because the fourth Korotkoff sound is frequently either not heard or is audible down to zero.
- When using an electronic device, if the result is unexpected recheck it manually before acting on it.
- Raised BP in a child who is fitting, in pain or screaming must be rechecked when the child is calm.

Blood pressure increases with age – the reading should be checked against normal ranges for the child's age (see Table 1.1). Any BP over the 95th centile should be repeated and if persistently raised will need treatment. Blood pressures leading to symptomatology will be grossly elevated for the child's age and the diagnosis should not be difficult.

9.7 Hypertension emergency treatment

Reassess ABC

Initial treatment will be that of the presentation. Airway, breathing and circulation should be assessed and managed in the usual way and neurological status assessed and monitored. Convulsions usually respond to lorazepam, midazolam or diazepam and patients with clinical signs of raised intracranial pressure should be managed with intubation, maintenance of normal PCO_2, a 20° head-up position for nursing and hypertonic saline or mannitol (see Chapter 8).

Once the patient has been resuscitated, management of the hypertension is urgent, but should only be commenced after discussion with a paediatric nephrologist, cardiologist or intensivist. The aim of treatment is to achieve a safe reduction in BP to alleviate the urgent presenting symptoms whilst avoiding the optic nerve or neurological damage that may occur with too rapid a reduction. Typically, the aim is to bring the BP down to the 95th centile for age (or height) over 24–48 hours, with perhaps one-third of the reduction in the first 8 hours. This must be undertaken in conjunction with close BP monitoring and a titratable infusion of the antihypertensive drug. PICU admission is mandatory.

Monitoring of visual acuity and pupils is crucial during this time as lowering the BP may lead to infarction of the optic nerve heads. Any deterioration must be treated by urgently raising the BP by lowering the antihypertensive treatment and/or using IV crystalloids or colloids. Some children may be anuric – renal function (serum creatinine, urea and electrolytes) should be analysed promptly.

Some drugs commonly used to achieve BP reduction in children are shown in Table 9.1.

Table 9.1 Drug therapy of severe hypertension

Drug	Dose	Comments
Labetalol	Loading dose: 0.25–1 mg/kg in 5 min (max. 20 mg) Maintenance: 0.25–3 mg/kg/h	α- and β-blocker Titratable infusion Do not use in patients with fluid overload or acute heart failure
Sodium nitroprusside	0.2–1 micrograms/kg/min	Vasodilator. Very easy to adjust dose. Titratable infusion. Protect from light. Monitor cyanide levels
Nifedipine	0.25-0.50 mg/kg	Fluid can be drawn up from capsules and squirted into mouth sublingually. Better to bite the capsule and swallow. May be difficult to control BP drop because it is given as a bolus

Some specialists may recommend the use of sublingual nifedipine as a temporary measure before transfer; if any drug is used, the child should have their BP monitored as above and an IV infusion in place.

These children should be cared for in a unit experienced in managing paediatric hypertension. This will usually be the regional paediatric nephrology (or paediatric cardiology) centre. It is essential that adequate consultation takes place before transfer.

9.8 Summary

You should use the structured approach in the assessment and management of the convulsing child:

- Primary assessment
- Resuscitation
- Secondary assessment and looking for key features
- Emergency treatment
- Stabilisation and transfer to definitive care

PART 3
The seriously injured child

CHAPTER 10
Introduction to the seriously injured child

Learning outcomes

After reading this chapter, you will be able to:
- Identify the importance of injury prevention
- Recognise the advocacy role of clinicians in preventing injury
- Describe the role of trauma systems and some aspects of trauma teams

---

10.1 Introduction

In 2012, World Health Organisation (WHO) data showed that injury caused the death of 740 062 children worldwide, and that 670 863 of these were due to unintentional injuries. Millions more children are injured in accidents that, although not causing death, cause pain, distress and permanent disability. The majority of these events are predictable and preventable. This introduction to the seriously injured child will consider the important role of injury prevention, trauma systems and some specifics about trauma teams.

10.2 Injury prevention

Over the last few decades, injury prevention programmes in some countries have succeeded in halving childhood death rates from injury by introducing key legislation such as child restraints, speed restrictions and laws on the use of motorcycle helmets. This is a remarkable achievement. Injury prevention is a multifaceted, multidisciplinary process that provides many opportunities for clinicians, who are primarily involved in the management of acutely injured children, to play a major role.

10.3 Epidemiology

Circumstances and type of incident

A multitude of injury scenarios are possible, each of which involve the child interacting with their environment. The commonest injuries that cause death are those resulting from motor vehicle accidents, drownings, burns, falls from a height and poisonings. Children in urban environments are at particular risk of motor vehicle accidents and playground falls whilst children in a rural environment are at risk of farm equipment injuries, unintentional chemical exposure and, in some countries, snakebites. Exposure to different circumstances also varies with age. Children under 5 years of age experience injuries at home. School-age children experience injuries at school, sport and play, and are especially at risk of death as pedestrians and cyclists. Adolescents may deliberately place themselves at risk of injury, especially where alcohol and drugs may impair their judgement.

Advanced Paediatric Life Support: A Practical Approach to Emergencies, Sixth Edition. Edited by Martin Samuels and Sue Wieteska.
© 2016 John Wiley & Sons, Ltd. Published 2016 by John Wiley & Sons, Ltd.

Sex

Boys are more frequently injured than girls. The difference emerges at 1–2 years of age. How much of this difference is innate and how much cultural is a subject for speculation. Girls may mature more rapidly in terms of perception and coordination.

Age

The type of injury sustained is closely related to the child's stage of development. Take falls as an example. A newborn baby can only fall if dropped, or if a parent falls holding the baby. An older baby can wriggle and roll off a changing table or a bed. A crawling baby can climb upstairs and fall back. A small child can climb and fall out of a window. An older child can climb a tree or fall in a playground.

Social class

As with so many other health problems, injuries are linked to inequalities in environments. Children in social class V, derived from the occupation of the head of the household, are twice as likely to die from an injury as children in social class I and, for some injury types, such as burns, the chances are six times higher. This does not mean that working class parents care less about their children than middle class parents, or that they do not know about risk. It may mean that there are other pressures such as overcrowding, lack of money or poor housing, and there is less ability for financial reasons to make safety-related changes.

Psychological factors

Injuries are more common in families where there is stress from mental illness, substance abuse, marital discord, moving home or a variety of similar factors.

10.4 Levels of injury prevention

There are three levels of injury prevention. Primary injury prevention is any measure designed to reduce the incidence of injury. Examples of this are the use of speed limits, cycle lanes, pool fences, fireguards and child-resistant medication closures and road safety campaigns. Secondary injury prevention is any measure designed to minimise injury even though an incident has occurred. Examples of this are the proper use of seat belts, bicycle helmets and other personal protective clothing. Tertiary injury prevention is any measure designed to limit the extent or consequences of an injury that has already occurred. Examples include the application of cold water to burns and scalds, or direct pressure on a laceration.

Whilst injury prevention can be addressed on an individual level it is most effective for the community as a whole when viewed as a public health issue. The most successful injury prevention campaigns have a number of common attributes. Firstly, they are carefully planned, with attention given to data collection and the identification of specific issues in the target population. Secondly, they attempt to permanently change behaviour by the use of education and enforcement. Finally, they include methods to monitor effectiveness, provide feedback and modify the campaign as necessary.

Clinicians involved in the acute management of injured children are in a unique position to be able to assist in injury prevention. Their daily work gives them first-hand knowledge of injured children and credibility with parents and government. Some of the ways that clinicians may be involved include the following.

Data collection and analysis

The provision of accurate and reliable data regarding incidence and circumstances of child injury occurring in a particular city or country underpins any injury prevention strategy. It identifies areas of high priority and enables the monitoring of effectiveness. In addition, it assists in the recognition of local and national factors that contribute to injury that may need to be specifically addressed. The power of the information and the ability to identify trends will be increased if the data are pooled into a national database that is accessible by many sources.

Education

Parents, community groups and politicians need information regarding childhood injuries and the methods likely to prevent them. Information can be delivered directly face to face in talks and interviews or by posters, books, pamphlets and the internet. The information must be relevant, accurate and presented at a level appropriate to the target group. Information based on local data presented by a credible person is most likely to be well received.

Publicising cases in the media can be an effective strategy to convey messages to parents, especially if the topic is newsworthy. Such publicity tends to be immediate and short lived but may be particularly useful in certain circumstances such as at the start of summer (e.g. snakebites, drowning).

The Injury Minimisation Programme for Schools (IMPS) provides an education pack with accident lessons drawn from the national curriculum in the UK and includes a hospital visit. Health professionals are actively encouraged to contact this group as its reach through schools in the UK has expanded and requires further support from interested health professionals.

Advocacy for legislation and design

Child injury prevention is all about changing behaviour. Whist education is the preferred way of encouraging people to do this, the introduction of legislation, regulations and enforceable standards have been an extremely effective adjunct. For example, legislation regarding pool fencing and regulations concerning the packaging of medications are two important legal measures specifically directed at child safety.

Whilst clinicians do not generally draft and enact legislation and regulations they can play an important role in convincing politicians that such measures are necessary and in ensuring that they are enforced. People must not only have the knowledge of what is safe, they must have the ability to select safe products and be protected against things that are inherently unsafe. Safe design of products designed for use by and around children is essential. Clinicians have a responsibility to notify authorities when they become aware of a dangerous toy that has injured a child.

Involvement with child safety organisations

Many countries have organisations dedicated to preventing childhood injuries. These organisations are often involved in all facets of injury prevention and provide ideal vehicles for individuals to work within. Be prepared to participate in working groups and campaigns. Healthcare professionals have special expertise and influence to offer. Local initiatives involving health professionals have had an impact, for example work in bicycle helmet use and playground safety has led to a better understanding of the effects of altering the environment and on implementing advances in design.

The collection of data about accidents can lead to a decrease in childhood injury; for example, by identifying accident black spots and collaborating with police and local council authorities, effective safety changes can be implemented. Similarly, types of frequently occurring domestic injuries can lead to targeted campaigns.

Children's accidents and injuries are the major public health problem for children in developed and developing countries today. All healthcare workers can learn more about them, and can be active in reducing their toll. Healthcare professionals can form powerful alliances with heads of schools, playgroup leaders, local media, police and local councils to launch injury-prevention schemes. Support for such initiatives can be given by charitable agencies such as the Child Accident Prevention Trust, the Gloucestershire Home Safety Check and the Royal Society for the Prevention of Accidents in the UK and Kidsafe in Australia.

Prevention measures (*Continued overleaf*)

Primary prevention measures

- Parental knowledge regarding behaviour and supervision of young children
- Fencing around domestic swimming pools
- Child-resistant closures on medication containers
- Fireguards surrounding open fireplaces
- Motor vehicle speed limits around schools
- Automatic water temperature regulation in bathrooms
- Use of stair guards, window guards and toughened glass
- Installation of electrical safety switches
- Removal of unsafe toys from retail outlets

Secondary prevention measures

- Properly fitted child restraints in motor vehicles
- Wearing of bicycle helmets at all times
- Personal protective equipment such as mouth guards and wrist guards
- Installation of domestic smoke alarms, fire extinguishers and fire blankets

Tertiary prevention measures

- Cardiopulmonary resuscitation training
- Compressive bandage in snake bites
- Rapidly responding, well-trained ambulance service
- Excellent trauma care from retrieval to rehabilitation

10.5 Trauma systems

A trauma system is described as an organised, coordinated effort in a defined geographic area that delivers the full range of care to all injured patients and is integrated with the local healthcare system. Trauma systems are hubs and make efficient use of health care resources. After pre-hospital assessment ambulance crews may bypass hospitals to reach those trauma centres with specialised care, investigations and interventions 24/7.

If a trauma system is in place, then the response to a seriously injured child will be adapted to take into account the pathway for major trauma patients in a certain area. This includes the recognition that secondary transfer of children may become more prevalent. This may also increase the number of time-critical transfers as children are transferred to the place where definitive care for the life-threatening condition can be delivered. Pre-hospital practitioners may consider going directly to a hub trauma centre or moving on at the earliest possibility. The 'moving on' should potentially be seen as an extension of the pre-hospital phase and clinicians should start discharge planning as soon as the child arrives and make contact early with the place where definitive care for the life-threatening condition can be delivered. The phrase 'Stop/Sort/Go' emphasises this point.

As you read the chapters in this section, it is important that you place them in the context of your local trauma system.

Irrespective of the presence of a trauma system, it is essential that hospitals that receive paediatric traumas should have:

- Specific paediatric guidelines and protocols (see box)
- Standard operating procedures and pathways (see box)
- Paediatric equipment and monitoring
- Immediate access to staff with paediatric expertise

Paediatric guidelines, protocols, procedures and pathways

- Trauma team activation
- Head injury management
- Pelvic fracture management
- Open fracture management
- Penetrating cardiac injury management
- Drowning pathway
- Burns referral pathway
- Massive transfusion protocol:
  - recombined factor VIIa
  - tranexamic acid
  - Quickclot®
- Analgesia
- Imaging:
  - CT guidance
  - X-ray guidance
  - head and neck
  - abdominal injury
- Urethrogram and cystogram
- Tetanus prevention
- Safeguarding

10.6 Trauma teams

Teams will receive a paediatric major trauma patient infrequently and, therefore, it is important that they are familiar with all of the elements listed above and that they receive regular training and practice. The roles required in a trauma team are detailed in the box below. Considerations of non-technical skills are to be found in Chapter 3. The specifics of the trauma alert, team briefing and preparation are found in Chapter 11.

Trauma team roles

Team leader	Radiologist
Operating department practitioner	Lead nurse
Anaesthetist	Specialists:
Nurse 1	◦ Trauma and orthopaedics
Nurse 2	◦ Surgery
Doctor 1	◦ Paediatric intensive care
Doctor 2	Radiographer
Scribe	Emergency department assistant

10.7 Summary

- Injury prevention is important in reducing the number of children dying of injuries
- Clinicians have an important advocacy role in preventing injury
- Trauma systems, where implemented, will impact on pathways of care and management of the seriously injured child
- Trauma teams need regular training and practice

CHAPTER 11
Structured approach to the seriously injured child

Learning outcomes

After reading this chapter, you will be able to:
- Describe the structured approach to the seriously injured child

11.1 Introduction

In 2012, injury was the cause of death for 740 062 children worldwide. In all age groups this is 9.25% of deaths; in 5–14-year-olds it is the leading cause at 25.41%.

Children with major injuries are affected differently – physically, physiologically and psychologically. Initial presentation can be deceptive because the relative elasticity of their tissues allows more energy to be transmitted to other body parts, with less being dissipated at the impact site. This will influence your assessment and management.

Understanding the mechanism of injury will help you assess how likely it is that a child has major injuries. For example, a fall from above the child's head height is much more significant than a fall from ground level.

Trauma alert, team briefing and preparation

Preparation is the key to effective and efficient trauma management. Capturing the information given when you receive the trauma alert using a structured approach, for example ATMISTER, enables appropriate briefing and planning prior to the arrival of the child. It also allows the team leader to decide on the appropriate response, either a full paediatric trauma team or a targeted specialty response.

After the call has been received from ambulance control, the team leader should complete the following actions.

Team leader actions: Assimilate information – ATMISTER

A Age/sex
T Time of incident
M Mechanism of injury
I Injury suspected
S Signs including vital signs, Glasgow Coma Scale
T Treatment so far
E Estimated time of arrival to emergency department
R Requirements, i.e. bloods, specialist services, tiered response, ambulance call sign

Advanced Paediatric Life Support: A Practical Approach to Emergencies, Sixth Edition. Edited by Martin Samuels and Sue Wieteska.

> **Team leader actions: Plan and review**
>
> Remember early management of catastrophic haemorrhage requires urgent blood products
>
> Make plan and back-up plan according to age and mechanism
>
> Child arrives: 5-second review and adapt plan accordingly

In role allocation consideration must be given to specific roles, including primary survey, airway, breathing and circulation, plus scribe, family support and drug management.

On arrival, unless the child has a catastrophic haemorrhage, traumatic cardiac arrest or obstructed airway, a controlled 'hands-off' handover occurs. At this point, the team leader completes a 5-second review and adapts the plan accordingly. The form of the structured approach is shown in the box.

> **Structured approach**
>
> **Immediate**
>
> - Primary survey (immediate life threats)
> - Resuscitation
>
> **Focused**
>
> - Secondary survey (key features)
> - Emergency treatment
>
> **Detailed review**
>
> - Reassessment (system control)
> - Continuing stabilisation and definitive care

11.2 Primary survey and resuscitation

> During the primary survey life-threatening problems should be treated as they are identified.

> **<C>ABCDE**
>
> <Catastrophic external haemorrhage>
> Airway (with cervical spine control)
> Breathing with ventilatory support
> Circulation with haemorrhage control
> Disability with prevention of secondary insult
> Exposure with temperature control

<Catastrophic external haemorrhage>

In major trauma <C>ABC has become the established approach. Obvious external exsanguinating haemorrhage becomes the immediate priority.

> Simple direct pressure, specialised haemostatic dressings or a tourniquet must be applied instantly in these circumstances.
>
> Tranexamic acid should be given 15 mg/kg as soon as possible.

The assessment can then continue with the ABC sequence.

Airway and cervical spine

Look for anything compromising the airway.

- Material in the lumen (blood, vomit, teeth or a foreign body)
- Damage to or loss of control of the structures in the wall (the mouth, tongue, pharynx, larynx or trachea)
- External compression or distortion from outside the wall (e.g. compression from a pre-vertebral haematoma in the neck or distortion from a displaced maxillary fracture)

> Problems can develop after the primary survey e.g. bleeding or progressive swelling in facial trauma or burns.
>
> A child with a GCS score of 8 or less is unlikely to be adequately protecting their airway.
>
> The commonest cause is from occlusion by the tongue in an unconscious, head-injured child.

Whatever the cause, airway management should follow the structured sequence (see Chapter 19), bearing in mind the need to protect the cervical spine. This is summarised in the box.

> **Airway management sequence**
> - Jaw thrust
> - Suction/removal of foreign body under direct vision
> - Oro-/nasopharyngeal airways
> - Tracheal intubation
> - Surgical airway

Head tilt/chin lift is not recommended following trauma, because this manoeuvre can move the cervical spine and may exacerbate an injury. For any mechanism of injury capable of causing spinal injury (or in cases with an uncertain history), the cervical spine is presumed to be at risk, until it can be cleared. Children (and adults) can suffer spinal cord injury despite normal plain radiographs. If ignored, ligamentous instability in the absence of radiological evidence of a fracture can have devastating consequences.

If protection is considered necessary, start with manual in-line stabilisation (MILS) by a competent assistant or, if this is not possible, consider using a head block and appropriate strapping (Figure 11.1). Rigid immobilisation of the head risks increasing leverage on the neck as the child struggles. Minimise anxiety by avoiding unnecessary interventions and encouraging the parents to remain at the bedside.

Vomiting poses an obvious threat to the unprotected airway, especially if there is also a risk of spinal injury. Before providing airway suction, tilt the patient trolley head down, ensuring they are secure.

The child should be taken off the scoop stretcher as soon as possible, using the 20° tilt method (see Chapter 23), and placed directly onto a trauma board or an emergency department trolley. If the spine has not been cleared, manual in-line immobilisation will be needed for intubation if indicated. If the child is paralysed, sedated and ventilated the cervical spine cannot be cleared, and spinal immobilisation needs to be maintained until definitive imaging (see Chapter 24) and neurological examinations can take place.

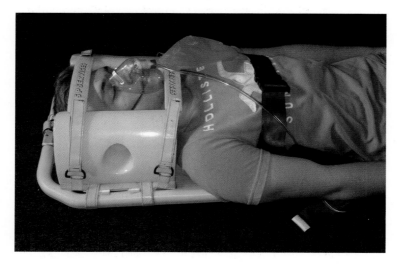

Figure 11.1 Child on a scoop stretcher

Breathing

Adequacy of breathing is checked in three domains (see Chapter 5):

- Effort
- Efficacy
- Effects on other organ systems

When examining the chest, look, listen and feel:

Look and listen – remembering asymmetry and asymmetrical movement (flail chest)
Feel – remember to check for crepitus (surgical emphysema), tracheal deviation, and percuss to distinguish a tension pneumothorax from a massive haemothorax

Conditions identified

By the end of the primary survey, the following conditions may have been recognised and treatment should be initiated as soon as they are found:

- **A**irway obstruction
- **T**ension pneumothorax
- **O**pen pneumothorax
- **M**assive haemothorax
- **F**lail chest
- **C**ardiac tamponade

If breathing is inadequate, commence ventilation with a bag–mask and prepare for intubation, which is likely to be required. The indications for intubation and mechanical ventilation are summarised in the box.

Indications for intubation and ventilation

- Persistent airway obstruction
- Predicted airway obstruction, e.g. inhalational burn
- Loss of airway reflexes
- Inadequate ventilatory effort or increasing fatigue

- Disrupted ventilatory mechanism, e.g. severe flail chest
- Persistent hypoxia despite supplemental oxygen
- Controlled ventilation required to prevent secondary brain injury (see Chapter 14)

If breath sounds are unequal consider and institute correct management (see Chapter 12):

- Pneumothorax
- Haemopneumothorax
- Misplaced tracheal tube
- Blocked main bronchus or pulmonary collapse
- Diaphragmatic rupture
- Pulmonary contusion
- Aspiration of vomit or blood

The normal resting respiratory rate changes with age. These changes are summarised in Table 1.1.

Circulation

Circulatory assessment in the primary survey involves the rapid assessment of heart rate and rhythm, pulse volume and peripheral perfusion including colour, temperature and capillary return and blood pressure (Table 11.1). Circulatory assessment must take into account the fact that resting heart rate, blood pressure and respiratory rate vary with age (see Table 1.1).

Table 11.1 Recognition of clinical signs indicating blood loss requiring urgent treatment

Sign	Indicator
Heart rate	Marked or increasing tachycardia or relative bradycardia
Systolic blood pressure	Falling
Capillary refill time (normal <2 sec)	Increasing
Respiratory rate	Tachypnoea unrelated to thoracic problem
Mental state	Altered conscious level unrelated to isolated head injury

Additionally in trauma:

- Check peripheral pulses in limb injury
- Look for internal haemorrhage (chest, abdomen, pelvis and femurs), including consideration of bleeding from multiple sites and progressive deterioration
- Apply pressure to significant external haemorrhage (if appropriate)
- Remember that exposure to cold prolongs the capillary refill time in healthy people
- Check lactate and haemoglobin as early indicators of circulatory compromise

All seriously injured children require vascular access to be established urgently using two relatively large intravenous cannulae. Peripheral veins are preferred; other options are:

- Intraosseous cannulation of the tibia, femur or humerus
- If there is no suspicion of a cervical spine injury – direct cannulation of the external jugular vein
- Indirect or direct cannulation of the femoral vein using the Seldinger technique ('wire through needle' followed by 'catheter over wire')
- Cut-down onto the cephalic vein at the elbow or the long saphenous vein at the ankle

Vascular access techniques are discussed in detail in Chapter 22. When vascular access is achieved, bloods should be taken, prioritising an urgent cross-match as well as a blood gas for haemoglobin and lactate. If there are signs of circulatory compromise, uncontrolled bleeding must be considered and appropriate teams summoned, if they are not already part of the trauma team. If the child is stable with no signs of shock, an immediate fluid bolus is not required. The principles behind this are '**the first clot is the best clot**'.

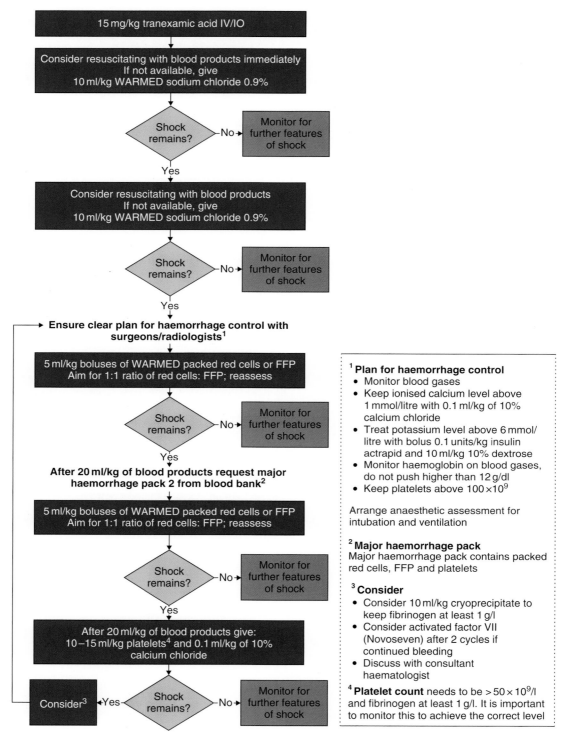

Figure 11.2 Blood and fluid therapy in severe uncontrolled haemorrhage after trauma. [FFP, fresh frozen plasma]

Major haemorrhage following injury is not common in children. Its management requires an understanding of concepts that have become standard in adult trauma care (Figure 11.2):

- Use of tranexamic acid (dose 15 mg/kg)
- Effective use of adjuncts (e.g. tourniquets, pelvic splints)

- Implementation of massive haemorrhage protocols (MHP)
- Avoidance of hypothermia using airflow heating devices
- Maintenance of an adequate haematocrit used to aid clotting by promoting platelet aggregation in small blood vessels, by use of optimal ratios of red cells to other blood products
- Prompt restoration of perfusion after controlling haemorrhage (monitored by the lactate level returning to normal within a few hours)
- Damage control interventions, involving surgery and interventional radiology

If abdominal haemorrhage is suspected, CT with contrast should be performed. In children, FAST (focused abdominal with sonography for trauma) has very limited application and there is limited evidence of its worth in detecting abdominal haemorrhage.

> The child's condition should be constantly reassessed and surgical intervention considered.

Disability

The assessment of disability during the primary survey consists of a brief neurological examination to determine the conscious level and to assess pupil size and reactivity.

The conscious level is described by the child's response to voice and (where necessary) to pain. The AVPU method describes the child as **a**lert, responding to **v**oice, responding to **p**ain or **u**nresponsive and is a rapid, and simple, assessment.

A	**A**lert
V	Responds to **V**oice
P	Responds only to **P**ain
U	**U**nresponsive to all stimuli

A children's GCS score should be performed as soon as possible (see Table 8.1).

> Agitation in a child may suggest cerebral hypoxia.

If the primary survey reveals that the child has a decompensating head injury, neurological resuscitation is required. If the GCS score is less than 8 and/or AVPU equivalent of 'P' or 'U', immediate intervention is necessary. Remember that the GCS is modified in the smaller child (see Table 8.1).

Interventions to be considered whilst organising urgent transfer (if required) include:

- Oxygenation with 15 l/min
- Head tilt 30°
- Control of carbon dioxide levels (by controlling ventilation)
- Maintenance of normal blood pressure to support cerebral perfusion including use of inotropes
- Hypertonic saline or mannitol osmotic diuretics to help reduce (if indicated) the intracranial pressure
- Anaesthesia/paralysis/sedation/analgesia to reduce cerebral metabolism
- Prompt treatment of any seizures and raised temperature

See further details in Chapter 14.

> As soon as a serious head injury is suspected, a CT scan of the brain should be ordered and the neurosurgical team (which may be off-site) alerted.

If the child is deteriorating neurologically, the child might need urgent transfer to a neurological centre prior to CT.

Exposure

In order to assess a seriously injured child fully, it is necessary to take their clothes off. Children become cold very quickly, and may be acutely embarrassed when undressed in front of strangers. Although exposure is necessary the duration should be minimised, and a blanket provided at all other times.

Ensure that the child's temperature is maintained and hypothermia is prevented.

This is achieved by having a warm resuscitation area and tasking one or more of the nursing team members to keep the child covered with a blanket or hot air warming device at all times and to warm all fluids given.

Other procedures carried out during the resuscitation phase

Imaging

See Chapter 24.

Investigations

When venous access is achieved and blood is taken for cross-matching, samples for other investigations should be taken at the same time, including full blood count, clotting screen, amylase/trypsinogen, urea and electrolytes and clotting (where available thrombelastograph (TEG®) and thromboelastometry (ROTEM®) analysis may be used). Remember to measure the glucose, especially in adolescents (who are prone to both injury and hypoglycaemia after drinking alcohol) and in very small children. Blood gas, lactate and β-human chorionic gonadotrophin should also be taken in adolescent females.

Nasogastric tube placement

Acute gastric dilatation is common in children and the stomach should be decompressed. If there is evidence or suspicion of base of skull fracture, the tube should not be passed by the nasal route. In the intubated patient, the oral route is a simple alternative. Gastric stasis is a frequent consequence of major trauma.

Analgesia

Analgesia can usually be administered just after completing the primary survey and resuscitation. See Chapter 2.

11.3 Secondary survey and looking for key features

Having finished the primary survey and set in place appropriate resuscitative measures, focused care is the next phase of management. The central diagnostic process during this phase is the secondary survey, a systematic clinical examination to identify injuries. It is supplemented by observations, imaging and other investigations. Further information is gathered at this time, especially the history of the events leading up to the injury and the presence of any co-morbid factors.

History

History should be sought from the child, ambulance personnel, relatives and witnesses of the accident. An AMPLE history can be used to obtain relevant information pertaining to:

AMPLE history
A Allergies
M Medication
P Previous medical history (pre-existing medical conditions and immunisations)
L Last meal
E Environment and events

In addition, consider the mechanism of injury. The following should cause concern and increase the likelihood of significant injury:

- Death or serious injury of an occupant of the vehicle
- Ejection from vehicle
- Prolonged extrication
- >40 mph head-on collision

Secondary survey

The secondary survey is a thorough head to toe, front to back examination searching for key anatomical features of injury. It is helpful to think in terms of:

- Surface (head to toe, front and back)
- Orifice (mouth, nose, ears, orbits; rectum, genitals)
- Cavity (chest, abdomen, pelvic cavity, retro-peritoneum)
- Extremity (upper limbs including shoulders; lower limbs including pelvic girdle)

Occasionally, a full secondary survey may be delayed if immediate life-saving interventions are required. Ensure that this decision is clearly documented and a secondary survey carried out at a later stage.

Throughout this stage of management, the vital signs and neurological status should be continually reassessed, and any deterioration should lead to an immediate return to the primary survey.

Special considerations in injury

- Perform otoscopy (for haemotympanum) and ophthalmoscopy (for retinal haemorrhage)
- Inspect the mouth inside and out – intraoral bruising may represent fractures
- Palpate the teeth for looseness
- Assess for nasal septal haematoma
- Assess for midface stability
- Look for signs of base of skull injury (panda eyes, mastoid bruising)
- Perform a full neurological examination
- Inspect neck veins and pulses if there is a neck injury
- Observe for movement
- Inspect for any external evidence of injury – tyre marks, bruising, lacerations and swelling
- Note unusual injury and bruising patterns suggesting non-accidental injury
- Inspect the perineum
- Inspect the external urethral meatus for blood

Investigations

See Chapter 24 for details on requesting and interpreting trauma imaging. An ECG should be performed in children with chest trauma or unexplained collapse/seizure.

11.4 Emergency treatment

Emergency treatment represents the early response to key findings in the secondary survey and its adjunct investigations. While the interventions are less urgent than those in the resuscitation phase, they will still need to be carried out promptly to minimise the risk of deterioration or unnecessary morbidity. The emergency treatment plan will include treatments for any potentially life-threatening or limb-threatening injuries discovered during the secondary survey. If it does not put the child at undue risk, this plan may be extended to include definitive care of other (more minor) injuries discovered at the same time.

Emergency treatments are discussed in more detail in subsequent chapters.

> In the face of a serious deterioration, return to the primary survey.

11.5 Continuing stabilisation

Continuing stabilisation and definitive care constitute the final part of the structured approach to trauma care. Good note taking and appropriate, timely referral are essential. If definitive care is to be undertaken in a specialist centre then transfer may be necessary at this stage.

The initial emphasis was on crude physiological assessment (<C>ABCDE) in the primary survey, followed by focusing on the anatomical evaluation of injuries in the secondary survey. From the time of the initial resuscitation, pulse rate, blood pressure, respiratory rate, oxygen saturation and temperature (avoid hypo- and hyperthermia) should be measured and charted frequently (every 5 minutes initially). Beyond these continuing observations, there is now a need to return to overall physiological control by considering the following systems in more detail, especially in a critically injured child:

- Respiration
- Circulation
- Nervous system
- Metabolism
- Host defence

Respiration (A and B)

The airway should be rechecked. If intubated, is the endotracheal tube of an expected length at the teeth (for the size of the child)? Are the breath sounds symmetrical? Could the tube have migrated into a main-stem bronchus?

Arterial blood gas analysis provides essential information in the child with serious head, chest or multiple injuries (arterial oxygen and CO_2 tensions) or in any child who has been intubated. Inserting an arterial line facilitates repeated measurements; in an un-intubated child, a venous blood gas should suffice.

Pulse oximetry readings should be displayed continuously. End-tidal CO_2 monitoring is mandatory in the ventilated child. It shows that the breathing circuit is still connected and that the endotracheal tube has not become dislodged. The end-tidal CO_2 should not be regarded as a reliable indicator of arterial CO_2 tension, especially in a shocked child. Ventilation–perfusion mismatch causes it to under-represent the arterial level. It can be regarded as a crude indicator of pulmonary perfusion.

Circulation (C)

This system comprises the three 'haems': haemodynamics, haemoglobin and haemostasis. In a child with serious injuries, the pulse rate and rhythm should be monitored electrocardiographically. Non-invasive blood pressure readings are generally reliable, although in serious head injuries and multiple injuries, it is better to monitor on a beat-to-beat basis using direct arterial measurements via an arterial line usually at the radius. This also allows estimation of the haemoglobin (or haematocrit) at hourly intervals to help detect ongoing bleeding and to determine the requirement for further transfusion. Base-deficit (or lactate) measurements indicate the adequacy of tissue perfusion, although it is still important to reassess the child clinically. Other invasive techniques, such as central venous pressure monitoring, may be considered at this stage, but should only be undertaken by appropriately trained personnel.

Urinary catheterisation

In a child, a urinary catheter should only be inserted if the child cannot pass urine spontaneously or if continuous accurate output measurement is required to achieve stabilisation after a serious physiological insult. The route (urethral or suprapubic) will depend on factors related to signs of urethral, bladder, intra-abdominal or pelvic injury (such as blood at the external meatus, or bruising in the scrotum or perineum; see Chapter 13). If a boy requires urethral catheterisation, urethral damage must be excluded first. The smallest possible silastic catheter should be used in order to reduce the risk of subsequent urethral stricture formation. If any doubt exists then the decision to catheterise the child can be left to the responsible surgeon. Urine should be stick-tested and sent for microscopy.

In seriously injured children, the urinary output serves as an indicator of systemic perfusion and should be recorded hourly. It should be maintained at 1–2 ml/kg/h, or higher if there has been a major crush injury or electrical burn with a high risk of myoglobinuria. If it is low, hypovolaemia is the likely cause, although other causes should be considered. If it is high, it may reflect excessive fluid therapy, but remember that diabetes insipidus can occur within a few hours of a serious head injury. After major blood loss, fresh frozen plasma and platelets may be needed to correct coagulopathy following the measurement of clotting times and platelet count. Remember that hypothermia affects clotting. Also consider TEG®/ROTEM®.

Nervous system (D)

Pupil size and reactivity and the GCS score should be checked and recorded every 15 minutes initially. Any deterioration should prompt the need to discuss the case with a neurosurgeon or consider a CT scan (or repeat one). Intracranial pressure (ICP) monitoring is an important means of identifying life-threatening rises in pressure. In conjunction with invasive blood pressure measurements, it provides a means of tracking cerebral perfusion pressure. ICP monitoring can be established in the operating theatre or the intensive care unit. Its use should be confined to hospitals with appropriately skilled personnel, but the importance of cerebral perfusion pressure should be understood by all those who deal with critical head injuries in children. See further details in Chapter 14.

Metabolism (electrolytes, fluid balance, gut and hormones)

This system refers to biochemical processes and includes renal, hepatic, gastrointestinal and endocrine problems. Glucose control ('don't ever forget glucose', especially in very young children and in adolescents who may have have taken alcohol or an overdose of unknown drugs) and urine output are key issues (see Circulation section just above).

Host defence (injury, infection, immunity, intoxication)

Host defence represents the interaction between the body as a whole and external influences. As such, it encompasses injury (including injury from poor positioning and thermal injury), infection (including wound care), immunity (including need for tetanus prophylaxis) and intoxication (including alcohol and drugs that may be present in the circulation).

Thermal injury is an important concern: hypothermia hinders blood clotting and predisposes to infection, while fever must be avoided in the severely head-injured child. Wound care, antibiotic prophylaxis for open fractures, and checking that tetanus immunisations are up to date (has the child been immunised at all?) are all considered at this stage, as is careful positioning to avoid problems such as pressure injury from a badly fitting collar. Consider tetanus toxoid and tetanus immunisation in a heavily contaminated wound (soil or faeces) as per national guidelines.

The 'tertiary survey'

In addition to physiological system control, it is essential for transport escorts, intensive care staff or receiving unit medical staff, who may take over care at this stage, to re-examine the child and review the investigations (especially the imaging) from an anatomical viewpoint to seek out any missed injuries.

Returning to the primary survey

Any sudden deterioration in the child's condition should trigger an immediate reassessment of the airway, breathing, circulation and disability so resuscitation can once more be undertaken.

Note taking

The structured approach discussed in this chapter can provide a framework for the writing of notes. It is recommended that these should be set out as shown in Table 11.2.

Referral

Many teams may be involved in the definitive care of a seriously injured child. It is essential that referrals are made appropriately, clearly and early. Guidance about which children to refer to which team is given in subsequent chapters.

Transfer

Injured children may require transfer either within the hospital or to another centre to deliver life-saving and definitive care. In either case, thorough preparation of equipment, patient and documentation is essential. A careful balance must be achieved between delaying such care and setting off with an inadequately stabilised child. Transport of children is discussed in more detail in Chapter 25.

Table 11.2 Template for note taking
History
Mechanism of injury and pre-hospital/pre-major trauma centre interventions
Past history
Primary survey and resuscitative interventions
<C>
A
B
C
D and E
Secondary survey and emergency treatment of injuries
Head
Face
Neck
Chest
Abdomen
Pelvis
Spine/back
Extremities
Continuing stabilisation
Respiration
Circulation
Nervous system
Metabolism
Host defence

11.6 Summary

The structured approach to initial assessment and management allows the clinician to care for the seriously injured child in a logical, effective way.

Assessment of vital functions (airway, breathing, circulation and disability) is carried out first and resuscitation for any problems found is instituted immediately:

- Primary survey
- Resuscitation

A complete head-to-toe examination is then carried out, adjunct investigations are performed and emergency treatment is instituted:

- Secondary survey and the search for key features
- Emergency treatment

Finally, a detailed review is undertaken and definitive care is provided:

- Reassessment and physiological system control
- Continuing stabilisation and definitive care

CHAPTER 12
The child with chest injury

Learning outcomes

After reading this chapter, you will be able to:
- Identify the chest injuries that pose an immediate threat to life and those that are discovered later
- Describe how to manage these injuries

12.1 Introduction

Isolated chest injuries are uncommon in children; they are usually associated with multisystem injury. Problems may result directly from chest injury or be secondary to other injuries. Consequences of severe trauma, such as gastric dilatation or pulmonary aspiration after vomiting or regurgitation, may further compromise respiratory function.

Children have relatively elastic tissues. Substantial amounts of kinetic energy may be transferred through a child's chest wall to deep structures with little or no external sign of injury and without rib fractures. A lack of evident rib fractures on the chest radiograph does not exclude major thoracic visceral disruption; conversely, the presence of rib fractures indicates high-energy transfer.

Children have relatively little respiratory reserve. Their high metabolic rate and small functional residual capacity allow them to desaturate more rapidly – when their oxygen supply is curtailed. Their horizontal ribs and underdeveloped musculature make them tolerate chest wall disruption badly. Flail chest, for example, is poorly tolerated.

The risk of iatrogenic chest problems must be appreciated. The child's relatively short trachea allows the endotracheal tube to become easily displaced into a main-stem bronchus or into the oesophagus. Mask ventilation can cause inadvertent gastric distension and overinflation of the lungs can result in a pneumothorax (especially after intubation, if the endotracheal tube has migrated beyond the carina). If a traumatic pneumothorax already exists, ventilation will cause it to increase in size and turn it into a tension pneumothorax.

Thoracic injuries must be considered in all children who suffer major trauma. Some may be life threatening and require immediate resuscitative therapy during the primary survey and resuscitation. Others may be discovered during the secondary survey (and its associated investigations) and be dealt with by emergency treatment. Some situations will need prompt, specialist surgical intervention, but most chest injuries can be managed in the first hour using general advanced life support skills. Practical procedures are described in detail in Chapter 23. During subsequent detailed review, attention will be redirected to the chest to maintain respiratory control and to search for missed injuries.

12.2 Injuries posing an immediate threat to life

The following conditions are life threatening. They should be identified during the primary survey and treated immediately. They do not need to be confirmed by adjunct investigations.

Advanced Paediatric Life Support: A Practical Approach to Emergencies, Sixth Edition. Edited by Martin Samuels and Sue Wieteska.
© 2016 John Wiley & Sons, Ltd. Published 2016 by John Wiley & Sons, Ltd.

A – Airway obstruction
T – Tension pneumothorax
O – Open pneumothorax
M – Massive haemothorax
F – Flail chest
C – Cardiac tamponade

Airway obstruction

The management of airway obstruction is discussed in Chapter 19.

Tension pneumothorax

This is a life-threatening emergency that can be rapidly fatal if not treated promptly. Air accumulates under pressure in the pleural space. This pushes the mediastinum across the chest and kinks the great vessels, compromising venous return to the heart and reducing cardiac output. The diagnosis is a clinical one.

Signs

- The child will be hypoxic and may be shocked
- Unless the child is deeply unconscious, there will be signs of respiratory distress
- There will be decreased air entry and possible asymmetrical air movement on inspection, with hyper-resonance to percussion on the side of the pneumothorax
- Distended neck veins may be apparent in some children
- The trachea deviates away from the side of the pneumothorax, although this is not always easy to identify clinically

Resuscitation

- High-flow oxygen should be given through a reservoir mask
- Immediate needle thoracocentesis or thoracostomy (a small incision to allow continuous drainage) should be performed to relieve the tension (Figure 12.1)
- A chest drain should be inserted urgently to prevent recurrence or progression to a tension pneumothorax

---

Air may be forced into the pneumothorax by positive pressure ventilation. If the child is ventilated, a simple pneumothorax is very likely to progress rapidly into a tension pneumothorax.

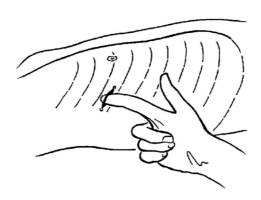

Figure 12.1 Thoracostomy

Open pneumothorax

In this situation there is a penetrating wound in the chest wall with associated pneumothorax. The wound may be obvious, but if it is on the child's back it will not be seen unless actively looked for. If the diameter of the defect is greater than about one-third of the diameter of the trachea, air will preferentially enter the pleural space via the defect rather than be drawn into the lungs via the trachea when the child takes a breath. It is then referred to as a sucking chest wound.

Signs

- Air may be heard sucking and blowing through the wound
- The other signs of pneumothorax will be present
- There may be an associated haemothorax (i.e. a haemopneumothorax)

Resuscitation

- High-flow oxygen should be given through a reservoir mask.
- The immediate treatment for a sucking wound is to occlude the wound site completely with an occlusive dressing. Another solution is to use a ported chest seal, provided that the defect is not larger than the base of this device (Figure 12.2).
- Whichever immediate treatment option is undertaken, a chest drain will be required as part of emergency treatment. It should not be inserted through the defect itself as this may spread contamination and restart bleeding.

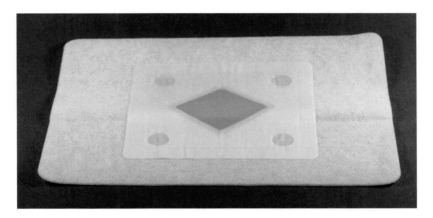

Figure 12.2 Ported chest seal

Massive haemothorax

A massive haemothorax will be identified during the B (breathing) stage of the primary survey, although it is even more of a circulatory problem than a respiratory one.

Blood accumulates in the pleural space. This may result from damage to blood vessels (arteries or veins from the pulmonary or systemic vessels) within the lung, the mediastinum or the chest wall (or from a combination). The hemithorax can contain a substantial proportion of a child's blood volume, causing haemorrhagic shock as well as local pressure effects.

Signs

- The child will show signs of shock and may be hypoxic despite added oxygen
- There will be decreased chest movement, decreased air entry and dullness to percussion on the side of the haemothorax

Resuscitation

- High-flow oxygen should be given through a reservoir mask
- Intravenous access ×2 should be established and volume replacement commenced
- A relatively large chest drain should be inserted urgently

Flail chest (or chest wall instability or deformity)

If a number of adjacent ribs are fractured in two or more places, a segment of the chest wall may be free-floating, moving inwards with inspiration and outwards with expiration (paradoxical movement). Such a flail segment is rare in children because of the elasticity of the child's chest wall. When it does occur, we expect major force to have been involved and serious underlying lung (and mediastinal) injury should be anticipated. If the reported mechanism does not involve significant force, suspect an erroneous history (remember non-accidental injury) or, more rarely, osteogenesis imperfecta.

Flail segments may not be noticed on initial examination for three separate reasons: firstly, severe pain on breathing will cause the child to splint the chest wall (this may be unmasked by analgesia); secondly, a child who has already been intubated will be receiving positive pressure ventilation, which moves the floating segment in unison with the rest of the chest wall; or thirdly, the flail segment may be posterior and unnoticed if the back of the chest is not examined carefully. Rib fractures do not always show up well on the chest radiograph, so imaging should not be relied upon in making the diagnosis.

Signs

- The child may be hypoxic despite added oxygen and in considerable pain
- Paradoxical chest movement is characteristic, but may not be obvious as indicated above. A high index of suspicion should be retained
- Other evidence of rib fractures (e.g. crepitus on palpation) may be seen

Resuscitation

- High-flow oxygen should be given through a reservoir mask.
- Tracheal intubation and ventilation should be considered immediately if the child is compromised. If ventilation is necessary, it may need to be continued for up to 2 weeks before the flail segment becomes 'sticky' and stabilises. On the other hand, minor cases may do well simply with good pain relief and with oxygen by face mask. Nasal or facial continuous positive airway pressure (CPAP), combined with pain relief, may be effective in intermediate cases.
- Pain relief should be given using titrated intravenous opioids in the first instance. Local or regional neural blockade avoids the respiratory depressant effects of opioids and should be considered. However, intercostal blocks and epidural catheters are hazardous in the uncooperative patient and sedation may be needed to achieve safety – the risks and benefits of the decision must be carefully considered. Epidural analgesia in children should be carried out by an expert and only after injury to the spine has been ruled out formally.

Cardiac tamponade

Cardiac tamponade can occur after both penetrating and blunt injury, though it is much more common after penetrating trauma. The blood that accumulates in the fibrous pericardial sac reduces the volume available for cardiac filling during diastole. As more blood accumulates, the cardiac output is progressively reduced.

Signs

- The child will be in shock
- The heart sounds may be muffled
- The neck veins may be distended, although this will not be apparent if the child is also hypovolaemic

Resuscitation

- High-flow oxygen should be given through a reservoir mask.
- Intravenous access should be established and volume replacement commenced. This may temporarily increase cardiac filling.
- An emergency thoracotomy will generally be required. A cardiothoracic surgeon (or a paediatric or general surgeon, in centres without cardiothoracic surgery) should be involved as soon as the diagnosis is suspected.

If personnel are not available to carry out an emergency thoracostomy, an emergency needle pericardiocentesis should be considered. Removing even a small volume of fluid from within the pericardial sac can dramatically increase cardiac output.

12.3 Serious injuries discovered later

These conditions will generally be discovered during the secondary survey and its associated investigations, but delayed presentation and masking by other injuries can occur, demanding continual vigilance into the detailed review phase and beyond.

Pulmonary contusion

Children have a high incidence of pulmonary contusion. Energy is readily transmitted to the lungs as the ribs are elastic and do not easily dissipate energy by fracturing. If the ribs do fracture, the degree of force is such that pulmonary contusion is likely too. Pulmonary contusion usually results from blunt trauma, although the shock wave from a high-speed bullet can also cause it. At the microscopic level, pulmonary contusion manifests itself as oedema and interstitial and intra-alveolar haemorrhage.

Clinical features include hypoxia, dyspnoea and haemoptysis, but are not specific. Initially, there may be little to show on the chest radiograph, although an area of non-segmental opacification may be clearly visible from the outset. It is important to realise that the clinical features and radiological findings may progress over the next few hours. The appearance on the plain chest film is not specific and may be confused with aspiration, other causes of consolidation/collapse and even with haemothorax (on a supine film). A CT scan, when indicated for other reasons, helps to distinguish pulmonary contusion from other diagnoses, but it is not warranted for this purpose alone. There are simpler means of demonstrating a haemothorax, for example clinical examination and bedside ultrasound.

Treatment consists of the administration of high-flow oxygen and artificial ventilation if necessary. Uncomplicated contusions will largely resolve within the next 36 hours. Physiotherapy plays an important role in reducing the risk of pulmonary collapse and secondary infection.

Tracheal and bronchial rupture

Tracheobronchial disruption has a high mortality and requires prompt referral to a specialist cardiothoracic surgeon. It presents as a pneumothorax or haemopneumothorax, typically with a persistent (and often vigorous) air leak after the insertion of a chest drain. Subcutaneous emphysema is frequently present.

Emergency care may involve the insertion of more than one chest drain (with suction applied). When intubation is required, the passage of the endotracheal tube may further disrupt a tracheal tear. When mechanical ventilation is needed, it is important to limit the pressure applied to the airway. This requires specialist ventilation techniques. Unless the leak is small enough to seal spontaneously, definitive surgical repair will be needed.

Disruption of great vessels

This is usually due to a high-speed motor vehicle crash and is generally fatal at the scene. A child with aortic rupture who survives to get to hospital has a tear that has tamponaded itself within an intact adventitial (outermost) layer and will require urgent specialist intervention.

The patient may be shocked and peripheral pulses may be poorly palpable. On the other hand, if the leak has (temporarily) sealed itself with little blood loss, relative hypertension can occur. Symptoms are generally non-specific. The diagnosis should be suspected if the mediastinum is widened or has an abnormal profile on chest radiograph. Remember that a supine anteroposterior film will increase the apparent width of the mediastinum and that the thymus is shown as a prominent mediastinal mass in small children. Sternal and spinal fractures can also cause apparent mediastinal widening.

Arch angiography remains the cornerstone of definitive diagnosis, although multislice CT promises to serve as an alternative. It is important to avoid surges in blood pressure that could precipitate rebleeding. Definitive repair requires cardiothoracic surgery.

Ruptured diaphragm

Diaphragmatic rupture is a rare blunt injury in children. It is generally thought to be more common on the left side, although some recent studies have questioned this. Penetrating trauma may also involve the diaphragm, usually in the form of knife stab wounds entering the chest or abdomen. Unless other structures are damaged at the same time, such knife wounds may be asymptomatic, only to present many years later as diaphragmatic hernias.

The child with a ruptured diaphragm may be hypoxic due to diaphragmatic dysfunction and to pulmonary compression from a herniated viscus. Shock may result from mediastinal distortion that affects venous return or result from haemorrhage from adjacent structures. The plain chest radiograph may show an apparently raised hemidiaphragm or evidence of abdominal contents within the chest, e.g. bowel shadowing or a nasogastric tube. Surgical referral should be made. Most ruptures can be repaired from the abdomen, without the need for thoracotomy.

12.4 Other injuries

Simple pneumothorax

Air is present in the pleural space with some degree of lung collapse, but it is not yet under pressure (tension). Signs of hypoxia with decreased chest wall movement, diminished breath sounds and normal or increased resonance to percussion on the side of the pneumothorax may be found, but the signs may be subtle or barely perceptible compared with tension pneumothorax. The diagnosis is usually made on the plain chest radiograph as a lung edge with no lung markings beyond it. However, an anterior pneumothorax is often difficult to recognise. The increasing use of thoracic CT scanning in severe blunt trauma is picking up injuries that may have been missed on plain films.

As traumatic pneumothoraces may not resolve spontaneously, a chest drain should be considered, even if the child is relatively asymptomatic. If the patient needs to be ventilated, a chest drain must be inserted as a matter of urgency to avoid a simple pneumothorax developing into a tension pneumothorax.

12.5 Practical procedures

Needle thoracocentesis, chest drain insertion and pericardiocentesis are described in Chapter 23. Clamshell thoracotomy should only be performed by those with expertise and therefore it is not described in detail within the practical procedures. It is not a procedure that is recommended for the non-expert.

12.6 Referral

A competent clinician, trained in advanced life support skills, can provide immediate management for most of the life-threatening injuries discovered during the primary survey. Emergency cardiothoracic surgical involvement will be needed if cardiac tamponade is diagnosed. Other serious injuries discovered during the secondary survey will need cardiothoracic referral (see indications in box).

Indications for cardiothoracic surgical referral

- Continuing massive air leak after chest drain insertion
- Continuing haemorrhage after chest drain insertion
- Cardiac tamponade
- Disruption of the great vessels

Patients who require ventilation as part of the treatment of their chest injury (such as those with significant pulmonary contusion) will need transfer to a paediatric intensive care unit. Critical care management will be needed for transfer and as part of continuing stabilisation in general. Appropriate medical and nursing referrals should be made.

12.7 Continuing stabilisation

In serious chest injuries, the oxygen saturation and pulse rate must be continuously monitored through to the detailed review stage and beyond. The respiratory rate and blood pressure need to be checked frequently. Chest drains must be well secured. Arterial blood gas monitoring is invaluable in severe cases for confirming adequate oxygenation and adjusting carbon dioxide tensions (particularly if there is a concomitant head injury). Remember that many conditions worsen with time, especially pulmonary contusion. An arterial line will also allow haemoglobin, base deficit and lactate to be tracked.

Continual clinical review is required. Changes in the respiratory pattern and in the apparent degree of illness, in conjunction with trends in the monitoring data, will alert the vigilant clinician to new problems and missed injuries.

12.8 Summary

- A clear airway must be established before attending to chest injuries
- All children should receive high-concentration oxygen through a reservoir mask (if breathing spontaneously), through a mask and self-inflating bag with an oxygen reservoir (if receiving assisted ventilation) or via a ventilator (if intubated)
- Chest injuries are life threatening, but most can be managed successfully by any clinician capable of performing the following techniques:
  - needle thoracocentesis
  - chest drain insertion
  - intubation and ventilation
  - fluid replacement
  - pericardiocentesis
- Clamshell thoracotomy can be life-saving, but it is not a procedure recommended for the non-expert
- Cardiothoracic surgical referral may be necessary once the immediate management of life-threatening conditions has been carried out
- Intensive care involvement will be needed for the continuing stabilisation of severe cases

CHAPTER 13
The child with abdominal injury

Learning outcomes

After reading this chapter, you will be able to:
- Describe how to assess the injured abdomen
- Identify the options for definitive care

13.1 Introduction

Blunt trauma causes the majority of abdominal injuries in children. Most occur because of accidents on the roads, although a significant number happen during recreational activities. It is important to consider non-accidental injury. A high index of suspicion is necessary if some injuries are not to be missed.

The abdominal contents are susceptible to injury in children for a number of reasons:

- The abdominal wall is thin and offers relatively little protection
- The diaphragm is more horizontal than in adults, causing the liver and spleen to lie lower and more anteriorly
- The ribs, being very elastic, offer less protection to these organs
- The bladder is intra-abdominal, rather than pelvic, and is therefore more exposed when full

> The management of children with abdominal injury may be complicated by respiratory compromise because of diaphragmatic irritation or splinting.

13.2 History

A precise history of the mechanism of injury may help in diagnosis. Rapid deceleration, such as experienced during road accidents, causes abdominal compression or sheering of fixed organs. The solid organs and duodenum especially are at risk from such forces. Direct blows, such as those caused by punching (consider non-accidental injury if history is not compatible) or impact with bicycle handlebars, readily injure the underlying solid organs. Injury to the pancreas or duodenum is a particular feature of handlebar injury due to their fixed position anterior to the spine. Finally, straddling injuries associated with a significant perineal haematoma or urethral bleeding suggests urethral injury.

13.3 Assessment of the injured abdomen

Initial assessment and management must be structured and directed to the care of the airway, breathing and circulation as discussed in Chapter 11.

Advanced Paediatric Life Support: A Practical Approach to Emergencies, Sixth Edition. Edited by Martin Samuels and Sue Wieteska.
© 2016 John Wiley & Sons, Ltd. Published 2016 by John Wiley & Sons, Ltd.

Examination

If shock is not amenable to fluid replacement during the primary survey and resuscitation, and no obvious site of haemorrhage exists, then intra-abdominal injury may be the cause of blood loss. The abdomen should be assessed urgently to establish whether early surgical or interventional radiological management is necessary. In other circumstances, the abdominal examination is carried out during the secondary survey.

The abdomen should be inspected for bruising, lacerations and penetrating wounds. Although major intra-abdominal injury can occur without obvious external signs, visible bruising increases the likelihood of significant injury. A high index of suspicion and frequent, repeated clinical assessment is appropriate in such cases. The external urethral meatus should be examined for blood.

Gentle palpation should be carried out. This will reveal areas of tenderness and rigidity. Care should be taken not to hurt the child because his or her continued cooperation is important during the repeated examinations that form an important part of management.

Aids to assessment

Rectal and vaginal examinations are rarely required in the injured child. Internal digital examination therefore should be limited to the surgeon who has overall responsibility for the child. Adequate analgesia and both gastric and urinary bladder drainage may help the assessment by decompressing the abdomen.

Gastric drainage

Air swallowing during crying with consequent acute gastric dilatation is common in children. Early passage of a nasogastric/orogastric tube of an appropriate size is essential. If there is a possibility of a basal skull fracture this should be by the oral rather than nasal route. The tube should be aspirated regularly and left on free drainage at other times. A massively distended stomach can mimic intra-abdominal pathology needing laparotomy, and cause serious diaphragm splintage with consequent respiratory compromise.

Urinary catheterisation

Catheterisation of a child should only be performed if the child cannot pass urine spontaneously or if continuous accurate output measurement is required. The route (urethral or suprapubic) will depend on factors related to signs of urethral, bladder, intra-abdominal or pelvic injury (such as blood at the external meatus, or bruising in the scrotum or perineum). If a boy requires urethral catheterisation, urethral damage must be excluded first. The catheter should be silastic and as small as possible in order to reduce the risk of subsequent urethral stricture formation.

Investigations

Blood tests

Intravenous access will have already been secured during the primary survey and resuscitation, and at that time blood will have been drawn for baseline blood counts, urea and electrolytes and cross-matching. An amylase/tryptase estimation should be requested and can usually be performed on the sample sent for urea and electrolytes. Repeated monitoring of blood parameters may be appropriate in some patients.

Imaging

See Chapter 24 for the guidelines on requesting and interpreting trauma imaging.

13.4 Definitive care

Many children can be managed without surgical intervention. For this to be undertaken the following are essential:

- Adequate observation and frequent monitoring
- Precise fluid management
- The immediate availability of a paediatric surgeon (a good interventional radiology service may limit the requirement for surgery)

As well as avoiding the morbidity associated with laparotomy, this approach also reduces the number of children at risk of overwhelming, potentially fatal sepsis following splenectomy.

Indications for surgical intervention

In the face of uncontrolled or significant haemorrhage despite appropriate resuscitation, damage control surgery should be undertaken by a paediatric trained surgeon. The purpose of this is to reduce the progression of acidosis, hypothermia and coagulopathy, the main causes of death in trauma. Children with penetrating injuries or evidence of intestinal perforation should also be considered for urgent surgery. The majority of solid organ injuries should be managed conservatively in an appropriately staffed, paediatric high-dependency area. This has a lower morbidity, mortality and blood use than an operative approach.

13.5 Summary

- The assessment and management of airway, breathing and circulation must be carried out first. Abdominal assessment is only carried out at this stage if there is a high index of clinical suspicion of injury or shock is refractory
- Abdominal assessment consists of careful observation and gentle, repeated palpation. Gastric and urinary drainage aid this assessment
- Abdominal CT scan with contrast is the investigation of choice
- The majority of children with solid organ injury may be managed non-operatively. Urgent intervention is required when children with solid organ injury have persisting haemodynamic instability despite adequate blood replacement, or for penetrating abdominal injury, or signs of a perforated viscus

CHAPTER 14

The child with traumatic brain injury

Learning outcomes

After reading this chapter, you will be able to:
- Describe the structured approach to the child with traumatic brain injury

---

14.1 Introduction

Epidemiology

Head injury is the most common single cause of trauma death in children aged 1–15 years. It accounts for 27% of deaths from injury and many (but largely unstudied) cases of permanent brain injury, probably up to 2000 or even 3000 children per year in the UK alone. Head injury deaths in children most commonly result from road traffic accidents – pedestrians are the most vulnerable, followed by cyclists and then passengers in vehicles. Falls are the second most common cause of fatal head injuries. In infancy, the most common cause is child abuse.

Pathophysiology

Primary traumatic brain injury is the damage incurred as a direct consequence of the impact. Neurones, axonal sheaths and blood vessels may be physically disrupted at the moment of impact, often with irreversible cell damage. **Secondary** brain injury represents further damage to central nervous system tissue by secondary insults, and adverse physiological events that can occur minutes, hours or days after the initial injury. Such insults include hypotension, hypoxia, raised intracranial pressure and seizures. A key aim of head injury management is to prevent or minimise secondary brain injury.

Primary damage

- Injury to neural tissue:
  - focal cerebral contusions and lacerations (direct impact and contrecoup)
  - diffuse axonal injury (shearing injury)
- Injury to intracranial blood vessels:
  - extradural haematoma (especially middle meningeal artery)
  - subdural haematoma (especially dural bridging veins)
  - intracerebral haematoma
  - subarachnoid haemorrhage

Injury to the cranium and to the dural sac may be associated with the above neural and vascular injuries. Open skull fractures, where there is a breach in the skull (vault or base) and in the dural membrane, allow brain tissue to come into contact with the external environment (directly or via the sinuses), with consequent risk of infection.

Advanced Paediatric Life Support: A Practical Approach to Emergencies, Sixth Edition. Edited by Martin Samuels and Sue Wieteska.
© 2016 John Wiley & Sons, Ltd. Published 2016 by John Wiley & Sons, Ltd.

Secondary damage

This may result from either the direct secondary effects of cerebral injury or from the cerebral consequences of associated injuries and stress.

- Ischaemia from poor cerebral perfusion secondary to raised intracranial pressure:
  - expanding intracranial haematoma (exacerbated by coagulopathy)
  - cerebral swelling/oedema
- Ischaemia secondary to hypotension and anaemia:
  - haemorrhage with hypovolaemia or dilutional anaemia
  - other causes of hypotension (spinal cord injury, drug-induced vasodilatation or later sepsis)
- Hypoxia:
  - airway obstruction
  - inadequate respiration (loss of respiratory drive or mechanical disruption of chest wall or diaphragm)
  - shunt from pulmonary contusion or later respiratory failure
- Hypoglycaemia and hyperglycaemia
- Fever
- Convulsions
- Later infection

Raised intracranial pressure

Once sutures have closed at 12–18 months of age, the child's cranial cavity behaves like an adult's with a fixed volume. If cerebral oedema worsens or if intracranial haematomas increase in size, the pressure within the cranium increases. Initial compensatory mechanisms include diminution in the volume of cerebrospinal fluid and venous blood within the cranial cavity. When these mechanisms fail, ICP rises, compromising cerebral perfusion:

$$\text{Cerebral perfusion pressure} = \text{Mean arterial pressure} - \text{Mean intracranial pressure}$$

Normal cerebral blood flow is 50 ml of blood per 100 g brain tissue per minute. A fall in cerebral perfusion pressure decreases cerebral blood flow. A flow below 20 ml/100 g brain tissue/min will produce ischaemia. This in turn increases cerebral oedema, causing a further rise in ICP. A cerebral blood flow of below 10 ml/100 g brain tissue/min leads to electrical dysfunction of the neurones and loss of intracellular homeostasis.

A generalised increase of ICP in the supratentorial compartment initially causes transtentorial (uncal) herniation, leading to transforaminal (central) herniation and death. In uncal herniation, the third nerve is nipped against the free border of the tentorium, causing ipsilateral pupillary dilatation secondary to loss of parasympathetic constrictor tone to the ciliary muscles. In central herniation, also known as *coning*, the cerebellar tonsils are forced through the foramen magnum.

In childhood, the most common cause of raised ICP following head injury is cerebral oedema. Children are especially prone to this problem. They may, of course, also have expanding extradural, subdural or intracerebral haematomas that require prompt surgical treatment. Depending on the aetiology of the raised ICP, treatment is either aimed at preventing it rising further or removing its cause (by surgical evacuation of haematomas).

There are special considerations in infants with head injuries. Unfused sutures allow the cranial volume to increase initially. Large extradural or subdural bleeds may occur before neurological signs or symptoms develop. Such infants may show a significant fall in haemoglobin concentration. In addition, the infant's vascular scalp may bleed profusely, causing shock. In children aged over 1 year with shock associated with head injury, serious extracranial injury should be sought as the cause of the shock.

14.2 Triage

Head injuries vary from the trivial to the fatal. Triage is necessary in order to give more seriously injured patients a higher priority. Factors indicating a potentially serious injury are shown in the box.

Factors indicating a potentially serious injury

- History of substantial trauma such as involvement in a road traffic accident or a fall from a height
- A history of loss of consciousness
- Children who are not fully conscious and responsive
- Any child with obvious neurological signs/symptoms such as headache, convulsions or limb weakness

---

14.3 Primary survey and resuscitation

The first priority is to assess and stabilise the airway, breathing and circulation as discussed in Chapter 11. Head injury may be associated with cervical spine injury, and stabilisation must be achieved as previously described.

Pupil size and reactivity should be examined and a rapid assessment of conscious level should be made. In the first place, the AVPU classification may be used.

A	**A**lert
V	Responds to **V**oice
P	Responds only to **P**ain
U	**U**nresponsive to all stimuli

In a time-limited situation, it is not essential to work out the numerical Glasgow Coma Scale (GCS) score immediately, although the EMV (eye, motor, verbal) responses will have been noted. But it is important to note the response to voice or pain (if not responding to voice) in more detail using the GCS before proceeding with neurological resuscitation. The assessment serves as a baseline for continuing care and as a key indicator of the need to intervene immediately.

Resuscitation of a child with a traumatic brain injury requires good coordination and you should have a low threshold for calling the trauma team. Immediate control of the airway, breathing and circulation should be carried out in response to the primary survey findings, according to the general approach in Chapter 11. This support will help to prevent secondary cerebral damage caused by hypoxia and shock arising from both the head injury and other coexistent injuries. Throughout the resuscitation process, the team leader must be aware of the need for urgent neurosurgical intervention or the timely transfer to a neurosurgical centre (within the first hour of a child's attendance).

During the primary survey assessment of disability, evidence of decompensating head injury will have been recognised. In the severely injured child, extra information from blood gas sampling will be obtained during the resuscitation phase or ongoing monitoring. On the basis of simple clinical evaluation, supported when necessary by blood gas data, a set of indications for immediate intubation and ventilation in severe head injury have been recommended (in the UK, the National Institute for Health and Care Excellence (NICE) has produced evidence-based guidelines for treatment, imaging and referral).

Indications for immediate intubation and ventilation

- Coma – not obeying commands, not speaking, not eye opening (equivalent to a GCS score of <8)
- Loss of protective laryngeal gag reflexes
- Ventilatory insufficiency as judged by blood gases: hypoxaemia (PaO_2 <9 kPa (68 mmHg) on air or <13 kPa (98 mmHg) with added oxygen) or hypercarbia ($PaCO_2$ >6 kPa (45 mmHg))
- Spontaneous hyperventilation (causing $PaCO_2$ <3.5 kPa (26 mmHg))
- Respiratory irregularity

Other indications
- Significantly deteriorating conscious level
- Unstable facial fractures
- Copious bleeding into the mouth
- Seizure

14.4 Secondary survey and looking for key features

History

The history of the injury itself and the child's course since the injury should be established from bystanders and pre-hospital personnel. Other history should be obtained from parents or carers.

Examination

The head should be carefully observed and palpated for bruises and lacerations to the scalp and for evidence of a depressed skull fracture. Look for evidence of a basal skull fracture, such as blood or CSF from the nose or ear, haemotympanum, panda eyes or Battle's sign (bruising behind the ear over the mastoid process).

The conscious level should be reassessed using the modified GCS if the child is less than 4 years old, or using the standard scale in older children. These scales are shown in Table 14.1. It should be noted that the coma scales reflect the degree of brain dysfunction at the time of the examination. Assessment should be repeated frequently – every few minutes if the level is changing. Communication with the child's care-givers is required to establish the child's best usual verbal response. A 'grimace' alternative to verbal responses should be used in pre-verbal or intubated patients (Table 14.2).

The pupils should be re-examined for size and reactivity. A dilated, non-reactive pupil indicates third nerve dysfunction due to an ipsilateral intracranial haematoma until proven otherwise.

The fundi should be examined using an ophthalmoscope. Papilloedema will not be seen in acute raised ICP, but the presence of retinal haemorrhage may indicate non-accidental injury in a young infant.

Motor function should be assessed. This includes examination of extraocular muscle function and facial and limb movements. Limb tone, movement and reflexes should be assessed and any focal or lateralising signs noted.

Table 14.1 Glasgow Coma Scale and Children's Glasgow Coma Scale

Glasgow Coma Scale (4–15 years)		Children's Glasgow Coma Scale (<4 years)	
Response	Score	Response	Score
Eye opening		Eye opening	
Spontaneously	4	Spontaneously	4
To verbal stimuli	3	To verbal stimuli	3
To pain	2	To pain	2
No response to pain	1	No response to pain	1
Best motor response		Best motor response	
Obeys verbal command	6	Spontaneous or obeys verbal command	6
Localises to pain	5	Localises to pain or withdraws to touch	5
Withdraws from pain	4	Withdraws from pain	4
Abnormal flexion to pain (decorticate)	3	Abnormal flexion to pain (decorticate)	3
Abnormal extension to pain (decerebrate)	2	Abnormal extension to pain (decerebrate)	2
No response to pain	1	No response to pain	1
Best verbal response		Best verbal response	
Orientated and converses	5	Alert; babbles, coos words to usual ability	5
Disorientated and converses	4	Less than usual words, spontaneous irritable cry	4
Inappropriate words	3	Cries only to pain	3
Incomprehensible sounds	2	Moans to pain	2
No response to pain	1	No response to pain	1

Table 14.2 The best grimace response

Grimace response	Score
Spontaneous normal facial/oromotor activity	5
Less than usual spontaneous ability or only response to touch stimuli	4
Vigorous grimace to pain	3
Mild grimace to pain	2
No response to pain	1

Investigations

Blood tests

Blood for full blood count, clotting, glucose, urea and electrolytes should already have been taken during the immediate care phase. Blood for cross-matching should have been sent off at the same time. Blood gases should be taken in head-injured patients to allow careful control of $PaCO_2$ and PaO_2, as well as to check pH and base deficit or lactate. End-tidal CO_2 should also be monitored.

Imaging

Refer to Chapter 24.

Indications for performing an emergency head CT scan within 1 hour

For children who have sustained a head injury and have any of the following risk factors, perform a CT head scan within 1 hour of the risk factor being identified:
- Suspicion of non-accidental injury
- Post-traumatic seizure but no history of epilepsy
- On initial emergency department assessment GCS score <14, or for children under 1 year GCS (paediatric) score<15
- At 2 hours after the injury, GCS score <15
- Suspected open or depressed skull fracture or tense fontanelle
- Any sign of basal skull fracture (haemotympanum, panda eyes, cerebrospinal fluid leakage from the ear or nose, Battle's sign)
- Focal neurological deficit
- For children under 1 year, presence of bruise, swelling or laceration of more than 5 cm on the head

For children who have sustained a head injury and have more than one of the following risk factors, perform a CT head scan within 1 hour of the risk factors being identified;
- Loss of consciousness lasting more than 5 minutes
- Abnormal drowsiness
- Three or more discrete vomiting episodes
- Dangerous mechanism of injury
- Amnesia retrograde or antegrade lasting more than 5 minutes

---

14.5 Emergency treatment

The initial aim of management for a child with a traumatic brain injury is prevention of secondary brain damage. The key aims are to maintain oxygenation, ventilation and circulation, and institute neuro-protective measures, to avoid rises in intracranial pressure.

These can best be achieved by paying attention to the <C>ABCs. If the airway is at risk, it should be secured. Children with a GCS score of 8 or less or who appear agitated/combative should be intubated and ventilated without delay. There is good evidence to suggest that ketamine and rocuronium should be the induction agents of choice as they offer a degree of neuro-protection and avoid the risk of sudden hypotension (see Chapter 21). Capnography must be used immediately after intubation to confirm endotracheal tube placement, to serve as a disconnection monitor, and to help maintain normocapnia or mild hypocapnia if there is evidence of a raised ICP. Remember that the end-tidal CO_2 level may differ significantly from the arterial level, especially in the shocked child – **it is essential to check the PCO_2 level with a blood gas sample. The PaO_2 should be maintained at a level greater than 13 kPa (98 mmHg) with an oxygen saturation >98%.** While routine hyperventilation has not been shown to improve outcome, arterial PCO_2 levels of 4–4.5 kPa (30–34 mmHg) are considered to be appropriate in the presence of an acutely rising ICP. Lower levels may adversely affect cerebral perfusion in the areas of brain still responsive to changes in PCO_2. Hypotension should be treated vigorously to avoid hypoperfusion of the brain, initially with normal saline; consider early inotropic support and the use of blood products. A systolic blood pressure above the 95th centile for age should be maintained to ensure adequate cerebral pressure. Tranexamic acid (15 mg/kg) may be useful in preventing progressive intracranial haemorrhage in traumatic brain injuries; however further trials are ongoing to evaluate its use.

Systolic blood pressure targets (age specific)

<1 year	>80 mmHg
1–5 years	>90 mmHg
5–14 years	>100 mmHg
>14 years	>110 mmHg

To avoid an increase in raised ICP, further neuro-protective measures must be undertaken. The child's bed must be tilted to 30° elevation, maintaining the head and neck in a midline position. Hypertonic saline 3% (3 ml/kg) should be administered, maintaining the serum sodium greater than 135 mmol/l. The use of mannitol 0.25–0.5 g/kg may be indicated to reduce the level of intracranial oedema. Immediate transfer to a neurosurgical unit must be organised and the child transferred without any unnecessary delay. A loading dose of phenytoin may be useful to avoid any risk of convulsion or seizure activity. It is important to keep the child normothermic throughout avoiding any dramatic changes in core temperature.

Analgesia

Following initial assessment, sufficient analgesia should be administered by careful titration. There have been concerns that opioid analgesic agents will lower the conscious level, cause respiratory depression and conceal pain in the abdomen and elsewhere. However, withholding analgesia may contribute to deterioration of the child's condition by leading to a rise in ICP. Failing to control pain will leave the child agitated and uncooperative, making any assessment of the pain more difficult, rather than easier.

It is important to appreciate that head-injured children are often more sensitive to opioids. If the child's conscious level is normal, despite other evidence of head injury, IV morphine in an initial standard dose of 100–200 micrograms/kg (<1 year: 80 micrograms/kg) (administered in increments) is appropriate. In obtunded children, particularly if the GCS score is 8 or less, intubation and ventilation will have a higher priority than analgesia alone. In intermediate cases, a useful rule of thumb is to expect that half the standard dose may be sufficient in the first instance.

Remember that opioids can be rapidly reversed with naloxone if necessary, although it is clearly better to avoid overadministration by cautious titration. Alternative opioids such as fentanyl that act more quickly when given intravenously or that can be given by an alternative route (e.g. mucosal) may be considered, as described in Chapter 2. Local anaesthetic techniques such as femoral nerve block may also be used to good effect, avoiding opioid side effects.

Management of specific problems

Deteriorating conscious level

If airway, breathing and circulation are satisfactory and hypoglycaemia has been excluded, then a deteriorating conscious level is assumed to be due to increased ICP, resulting from an intracranial haematoma or cerebral oedema. A CT scan and urgent neurosurgical referral are indicated and the temporising manoeuvres shown in the box may be instituted.

Measures to increase cerebral perfusion temporarily

- Nurse in the 30° head-up position and head in midline to help venous drainage
- Ventilation to achieve a $PaCO_2$ of 4.0–4.5 kPa (30–34 mmHg)*
- Infusion of intravenous mannitol 0.25–0.5 g/kg or 3% hypertonic saline (3 ml/kg)
- Combat hypotension if present with crystalloid/blood infusion and inotropes if necessary

*Note this level is lower than normal because it is a temporary, short-term, urgent intervention.

Signs of uncal or central herniation

These signs (see Chapter 8) should lead to immediate institution of the measures in the box above and emergency neurosurgical referral.

Convulsions

A focal seizure should be regarded as a focal neurological sign of considerable concern. A generalised convulsion, while also worrying, has less prognostic significance in children. Seizure activity raises ICP in both non-paralysed and paralysed patients, as well as causing an acidosis and increased cerebral metabolic demand. The lack of limb or facial movement makes it more difficult to recognise a seizure if the child has been paralysed, but fitting should still be suspected if there is a sharp increase in heart rate and blood pressure, with dilatation of the pupils.

Seizures due to head injury should be controlled promptly. Hypoglycaemia should be excluded, especially in small children and in adolescents who have been drinking alcohol. Phenytoin should be used to control the seizure. The dose is 20 mg/kg intravenously over 20 minutes, with appropriate monitoring for rhythm irregularities and hypotension.

Neurosurgical referral

Agreed indications for neurosurgical referral are shown in the box below (NICE guidelines).

Indications for referral to a neurosurgeon

- Persisting coma (GCS score <8) after initial resuscitation
- Unexplained confusion lasting for more than 4 hours
- Deteriorating conscious level (especially motor response changes)
- Focal neurological signs
- Seizure without full recovery
- Definite or suspected penetrating injury
- A cerebrospinal fluid leak

Other cases may be discussed to consider referral and to ensure optimal management, such as when there is evidence of a depressed or basal skull fracture or if the initial GCS score is between 8 and 12. In general, the care of all children with new, surgically significant abnormalities on imaging should be discussed with a neurosurgeon.

14.6 Detailed review and continuing stabilisation

Review anatomical injuries and physiological system control. It is easy to miss injuries in the face of an altered conscious level. A high index of suspicion is essential. Reconsider the mechanism of injury, review the physical and radiological findings, and make sure that the appropriate specialists have been involved.

In the severely head-injured child, physiological system control is of critical importance in preventing secondary insults. The airway and ventilation have been dealt with as part of emergency treatment. The position of the endotracheal tube should now be checked on a chest radiograph and the tube fixation adjusted and re-secured, if necessary. Attention to detail in adjusting the ventilator settings, according to repeated arterial blood gas sampling, is vital. A systolic blood pressure above the 95th centile fo age should be maintained to ensure adequate cerebral pressure. Sedation and paralysis play an important role in tolerating the endotracheal tube and in suppressing rises in ICP, but must not be allowed to cause hypotension. A morphine and midazolam infusion should be initiated immediately after intubation. Bleeding from other injuries should already have been stopped and the blood volume restored. Normoglycaemia and a normal or slightly reduced temperature help to guarantee an optimal outcome.

Vigilance is needed to recognise any significant deterioration in the child's condition. If any of the following examples of neurological deterioration are present, this should prompt urgent reappraisal by the supervising medical team (NICE guidelines).

Examples of neurological deterioration prompting urgent reappraisal

- Development of agitated or abnormal behaviour
- A sustained (>30 minutes) drop of 1 point in the GCS (especially in the motor score)
- Any drop of 2 points in the GCS
- Severe/increasing headache/vomiting
- New neurological signs

14.7 Transfer to definitive care

Children with a traumatic brain injury often require time-critical transfers for timely surgical intervention. In such circumstances, the delay in waiting for a retrieval team to arrive may be unacceptable, so that the responsibility for transfer may revert to the primary hospital. Where this timely surgical intervention is not required there may be time to wait for a team from the receiving hospital. For further details information on transfer see Chapter 25.

14.8 Summary

- The aim of initial management is to prevent secondary damage
- This is achieved by attention to airway, breathing and circulation, and by prompt neurosurgical referral and transfer for operative decompression or neurocritical care, when indicated

---

Treatment of children with severe head injury includes management of the following:

- Early consideration for intubation and ventilation
- Avoid desaturation: PaO_2 >13 kPa (98 mmHg) and $PaCO_2$ 4.5–5.0 kPa (34–38 mmHg)
- Avoid hypotension and maintain cerebral perfusion
- Avoid raised intracranial pressure: 30° head-up tilt, 3% NaCl (if required)
- Avoid and manage seizure(s): phenytoin 20 mg/kg
- Maintain normothermia
- Ensure normoglycaemia
- Analgesia, sedation and neuromuscular blockade

CHAPTER 15

The child with injuries to the extremities or the spine

Learning outcomes

After reading this chapter, you will be able to:
- Identify the extremity injuries that pose an immediate threat to life and limb
- Describe how to manage these extremity injuries
- Recognise the incidence of spinal cord injury
- Identify the steps necessary to prevent exacerbation of an underlying cord injury
- Describe the structured approach to the stabilisation of the cervical spine

15.1 Extremity trauma: introduction

Skeletal injury accounts for 10–15% of all childhood injuries – of these, 15% involve physeal disruptions. It is uncommon for extremity trauma to be life threatening in the multiply injured child. It is crucial to recognise and treat associated life-threatening injuries before assessing and managing the skeletal trauma. Although rarely life threatening, fractures and associated extremity trauma must be managed well or they can have devastating implications for subsequent rehabilitation. This chapter deals with problems from the perspective of multiple injury; the principles apply equally to individual injuries. It should be remembered that children's bones can absorb more force than adults and this may result in an underestimation of the degree of trauma to associated soft tissues.

15.2 Assessment of extremity trauma

Unless extremity injury is life threatening, evaluation is carried out during the secondary survey and treatment commenced during the definitive care phase. Single, closed extremity injuries may produce enough blood loss to cause hypovolaemic shock, but this is not usually life threatening. Pelvic fractures are relatively uncommon in children – the energy that would have fractured a pelvis in an adult may have been transmitted to vessels within the pelvis of a child, leading to disruption and haemorrhage. Closed fractures of the femur may cause loss of approximately 20% of the intravascular volume into the thigh, and blood loss from open fractures can be even more significant. This blood loss begins at the time of the injury, and it can be difficult to estimate the degree of pre-hospital loss.

15.3 Primary survey and resuscitation of extremity trauma

All multiply injured children should be approached in the structured way discussed in Chapter 11. Relevant history should be sought from relatives and pre-hospital staff. Extremity deformity and perfusion prior to arrival at hospital are especially important, and information concerning the method of injury is helpful.

Advanced Paediatric Life Support: A Practical Approach to Emergencies, Sixth Edition. Edited by Martin Samuels and Sue Wieteska.
© 2016 John Wiley & Sons, Ltd. Published 2016 by John Wiley & Sons, Ltd.

Life-threatening injuries

These include the following:

- Massive haemorrhage
- Crush injuries of the abdomen and pelvis
- Traumatic amputation of an extremity

They should be dealt with immediately and take precedence over any other extremity injury.

Crush injuries to the abdomen and pelvis

The pelvic bones of a child are much more cartilaginous and thus more flexible than those of an adult; therefore if fractures occur it will only be after significant impact. A child's pelvis tends to be narrower than that of an adult and thus does not offer the same protection to the internal structure and organs. The significance of a fracture in itself is not important but the subsequent damage caused to the associated organs and structures can be life threatening and must be treated accordingly. Pelvic disruption can lead to life-threatening blood loss. The child will present with hypovolaemic shock; this may remain resistant to treatment until either the pelvic disruption is stabilised or the injured vessels are occluded.

Initial treatment during the primary survey and resuscitation phase consists of splinting of the pelvis with a pelvic splint (or improvised device), tranexamic acid administration (15 mg/kg) and initiation of the massive haemorrhage algorithm (see Figure 11.2). The diagnosis may be obvious if disruption is severe or if fractures are open. More often this cause of resistant hypovolaemia is discovered when the pelvic radiograph is taken. If a pelvic fracture or injury is suspected, manual handling should be kept to the minimum (using the 20° tilt if necessary) and CT should be considered for first line imaging rather than X-ray. Emergency orthopaedic opinion should be sought, and interventional radiology considered if no laparotomy is indicated for abdominal injuries.

Traumatic amputation

Traumatic amputation of an extremity may be partial or complete. Paradoxically, it is usually the former that presents the greatest initial threat to life. This is because completely transected vessels go into spasm, whereas partially transected vessels may not. Blood loss can be large and the pre-hospital care of these injuries is critical; an exact history of this should be sought.

Once in hospital, exsanguinating haemorrhage must be controlled. Two wide-bore cannulae should be inserted and pneumatic tourniquets applied to the injured limb. If the child is in shock, but the bleeding points are well controlled, vigorous fluid therapy may be instituted. If the bleeding is still uncontrolled, fluid boluses should be commenced in 5–10 ml/kg aliquots, and the massive haemorrhage algorithm should be initiated as soon as possible (see Chapter 11).

On the basis of experience from land-mine injuries, an elasticated compression bandage and dressing, if applied carefully, may help stem the haemorrhage and better preserve tissue viability. Emergency orthopaedic and plastic surgical opinions should be sought. If no active bleeding is taking place, the stump should be dressed with a sterile dressing soaked in normal saline and the limb splinted and elevated. The child should receive intravenous antibiotic prophylaxis within an hour of their arrival to hospital and their tetanus status should be checked.

Reimplantation techniques are available in specialist centres. The success rate is improving, particularly in children. Urgent referral and transfer are necessary – the amputated part will only remain viable for 8 hours at room temperature, or for 18 hours if cooled. The amputated part should be cleaned, wrapped in a moist, sterile towel, placed in a sterile, sealed plastic bag and transported in an insulated box filled with crushed ice and water in the same vehicle as the child. Care should be taken to avoid direct contact between the ice and tissue. If, after discussion with the specialist centre, it is decided that reimplantation is not appropriate, the amputated part should still be saved because it may be used for grafting of other injuries.

Massive, open, long-bone fractures

The blood loss from any long-bone fractures may be significant; open fractures bleed more than closed ones because there is no tamponade effect from surrounding tissues. As a general rule, an open fracture causes twice the blood loss of a corresponding closed fracture. Thus a single, open, femoral shaft fracture may result in 20–30% loss of circulating blood volume. This in itself is life threatening.

On arrival at hospital during the initial resuscitation phase, two relatively large-bore cannulae should be inserted and fluid boluses should be commenced according to the child's overall circulatory state (see Chapter 11). Exsanguinating haemorrhage should be controlled both by the application of pressure at the fracture site, and by correct splinting of the limb; in certain cases the use of tourniquets may be indicated. The child should receive prophylactic antibiotics within the hour and their tetanus status checked.

Emergency orthopaedic opinion should be sought. Angiography may be necessary to examine whether any major vessel rupture has occurred, and if such an injury is considered likely then a vascular surgical opinion should be obtained immediately.

15.4 Secondary survey and looking for key features of extremity trauma

Limb-threatening injury

The viability of a limb may be threatened by vascular injury, compartment syndrome or open fractures. These situations are discussed below.

Vascular injury

Assessment of the vascular status of the extremity is a vital step in evaluating an injury. Vascular damage may be caused by traction (resulting in intimal damage or complete disruption), or by penetrating injuries caused by either a missile or the end of a fractured bone. Brisk bleeding from an open wound or a rapidly expanding mass is indicative of active bleeding. Complete tears are less likely to bleed for a prolonged period due to contraction of the vessel. It should be remembered that nerves usually pass in close proximity to vessels and are likely to have been damaged along with the vessel.

The presence of a pulse, either clinically or on Doppler examination, does not rule out a vascular injury. A diminished pulse should not be attributed to spasm.

The signs of vascular injury are shown in the box below.

Signs of vascular injury

- Abnormal pulses
- Impaired capillary return
- Decreased sensation
- Rapidly expanding haematoma
- Bruit

If these signs are present, urgent investigation and emergency treatment should be commenced. The fracture should be aligned and splints checked to ensure that they are not restrictive. If no improvement occurs a vascular surgeon should be consulted and angiography considered. Vascular damage may not always be immediately apparent so constant reassessment is essential.

Compartment syndrome

If the interstitial pressure within a fascial compartment rises above capillary pressure, then local muscle ischaemia occurs. If this is unrecognised, it eventually results in Volkmann's ischaemic contracture. Compartment syndrome usually develops over a period of hours and is most often associated with crush injuries. It may, however, occur following simple fractures and also as a result of misplaced intraosseous infusions. The classic signs are shown in the box.

Classic signs of compartment syndrome

- Pain, accentuated by passively stretching the involved muscles
- Decreased sensation
- Swelling
- Pallor of limb
- Paralysis
- Pulselessness

Distal pulses only disappear when the intracompartmental pressure rises above arterial pressure; by this time irreversible changes have usually occurred in the muscle bed. Initial treatment consists of releasing any constricting bandages and splints. If this is ineffective, then urgent surgical fasciotomy should be performed.

Open fractures

Any wound within the vicinity of a fracture should be assumed to communicate with the fracture. Open wounds are classified according to the degree of soft tissue damage, the amount of contamination and the presence or absence of associated neurovascular damage. Initial treatment includes removal of gross contamination and covering the wound with a sterile, saline-soaked dressing. A photograph of the wound should be taken to reduce the number of times the dressing is removed. No attempt should be made to ligate bleeding points because associated nerves may be damaged as this is done. Bleeding should be controlled by direct pressure. Broad-spectrum antibiotics should be given, and tetanus immunisation status checked (consult the British Orthopaedic Association Standards for Trauma (BOAST4) guidelines for the most up-to-date antibiotic advice). Further management is surgical debridement which should be carried out within 6 hours by orthopaedic and plastic surgeons under operating theatre conditions.

Non-accidental injury must always be considered if the history is not consistent with the injury pattern. It is discussed in detail in Appendix C.

15.5 Emergency treatment of extremity trauma

Life-threatening problems identified during the primary survey in the multiply injured patient are managed first. Only then should attention be turned to the extremity injury. The specific management of complications such as vascular injury, compartment syndrome, traumatic amputation and open wounds have been discussed earlier in this chapter.

15.6 Extremity trauma: summary

- Extremity trauma is rarely life threatening per se, unless exsanguinating haemorrhage ensues. Multiple fractures can cause significant blood loss.
- The first priority is assessment of the airway, breathing and circulation.
- Full assessment of the extremities takes place during the secondary survey. Limb-threatening injuries should be identified at this stage and further investigation and management begun. Other injuries should be treated by splintage.

15.7 Spinal trauma: introduction

Spinal injuries are rare in children (31 children in 2013 in the UK according to UK TARN data, only nine with cervical spinal cord injury). For any mechanism of injury capable of causing cervical spine damage (or in cases with uncertain history), the cervical spine is presumed to be at risk. A high index of suspicion, correct management and prompt referral are necessary in order to prevent exacerbation of underlying cord injury (Figure 15.1).

Immobilisation

If the child is unconscious, uncooperative or has had a significant mechanism of injury that makes it possible to have a spinal injury, the head and neck should be stabilised initially by manual immobilisation. Head block and tape should be considered to assist with stabilisation of the neck and to provide staff and carers with a visual indicator that the neck has not been cleared.

Some situations are particularly difficult. An injured child may be uncooperative for many reasons including fear, pain or hypoxia. Manual immobilisation should be maintained and the contributing factors addressed. Too rigid immobilisation of the head in such cases may increase leverage on the neck as the child struggles.

Once a child has been immobilised, a member of staff must remain with the child at all times for reassurance, and to ensure there is minimal movement and that the airway remains patent. Immobilisation of the cervical spine can be very frightening and disorientating to a child and thus must be carried out supportively and sensitively with careful explanation appropriate to the child's age and cognitive level throughout the procedure.

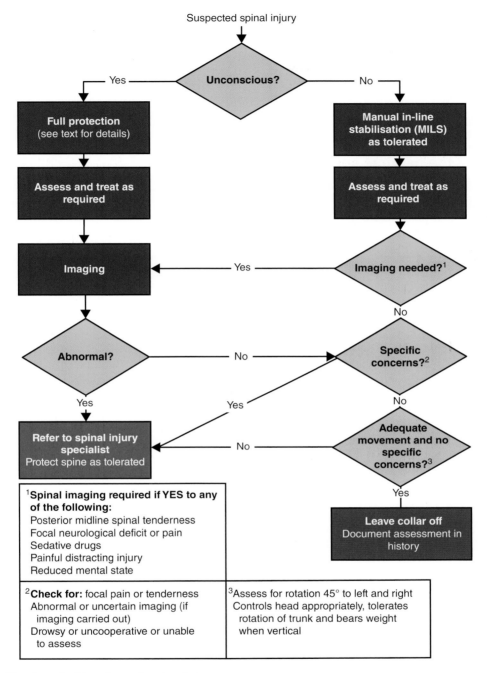

Figure 15.1 Algorithm for spinal imaging, referral and clearance

Children being transported between institutions may require additional immobilisation. This may involve head blocks, sand bags or a vacuum mattress, where possible axial loading must be avoided. Spinal boards should only be used in the short term for extrication: scoop stretchers should be used to assist with transportation and transfer.

If guidelines for clinically clearing the cervical spine are met (see box), indicating a low risk of cervical spine injury, the patient should be asked to rotate their neck 45° to the left and right. If any of these manoeuvres cause midline posterior pain the neck should be immobilised again and the spine imaged. If there is no pain on movement, immobilisation is no longer required.

Guidelines for clinically clearing a cervical spine

- No midline cervical tenderness on direct palpation
- No focal neurological deficit
- Normal alertness
- No intoxication
- No painful distracting injuries

15.8 Injuries of the cervical spine

Injuries to the cervical spine are rare in children; however they are associated with substantial levels of impact. The upper three vertebrae are usually involved – injury is more common in the lower segments of an adult. The low incidence (0–2% of all children's fractures and dislocations) of bony injury is explained by the mobility of the cervical spine in children, which dissipates applied forces over a greater number of segments.

Cervical spine imaging

Imaging must be taken in all children who cannot have their spine cleared clinically. Children with a GCS score of 15 who need imaging and have no features suggestive of cord or nerve root injury can generally be imaged with plain spinal radiographs initially. These children should have a full cervical spine series including lateral, anteroposterior and odontoid peg views (the latter only if they can open their mouth). Injury must be presumed until excluded radiologically and clinically. Spinal injury may be present even with a normal radiograph. The development of the cervical vertebrae is complex. There are numerous physeal lines (which can be confused with fractures), and a range of normal sites for ossification centres. Pseudosubluxation of C2 on C3 and of C3 on C4 occurs in approximately 9% of children; particularly those aged 1–7 years. Interpretation of cervical radiographs can therefore be difficult even for the most experienced (50% sensitivity) and there is growing support for just ordering MRI scans in preference to plain films or CT.

Indirect evidence of trauma can be detected by assessing retropharyngeal swelling. At the inferior part of the body of C3, the pre-vertebral distance should be one-third the width of the body of C2. This distance varies during breathing and is increased in a crying child. Cervical spine X-rays are discussed in more detail in Chapter 24. Some children will require further imaging and specialist consultation depending on their clinical and radiological features.

Proceed to an MRI scan if the plain views are abnormal or inadequate. Children with a GCS score of <13 require a CT scan of the entire cervical spine, as well as a head CT scan. It is a matter of clinical judgement whether children with a GCS score of 13–14 should have a CT scan of the upper or entire cervical spine, balancing the risk of missing an injury against unnecessary radiation to the thyroid and other tissues. Whether the rest of the spine needs CT scanning or plain views requires clinical judgement and depends on the overall clinical assessment.

After a high-energy mechanism of injury, if there is evidence of a serious trunk injury or cardiorespiratory instability, a CT scan from the occiput to the pelvis should be considered, irrespective of the conscious level. This will encompass the entire spine. Plain spinal films are not then required.

If there are features suggestive of cord or nerve root injury an MRI scan is indicated. The timing is a matter of clinical judgement by a spinal injury specialist.

Injury types

Atlantoaxial rotary subluxation is the most common injury to the cervical spine. The child presents with torticollis following trauma. Radiological demonstration of the injury is difficult, and CT or MRI may be necessary. Other injuries of C1 and C2 include odontoid epiphyseal separations and traumatic ligament disruption. It should be noted that significant cervical cord injuries have been reported without any radiological evidence of trauma.

Immediate treatment

Despite the rarity of fractures, a severely injured child's spine should be protected until spinal injury has been excluded. If in any doubt, the child should continue to be protected and senior help sought.

15.9 Injuries of the thoracic and lumbar spine

Injuries to the thoracic and lumbar spine are rare in children; they are most common in the multiply injured child. In the second decade, 44% of reported injuries result from sporting and other recreational activity. Some spinal injuries may result from non-accidental injury. When an injury does occur, it is not uncommon to find multiple levels of involvement because the force is dissipated over many segments in the child's mobile spine. This increased mobility may also lead to neurological involvement without significant skeletal injury.

The most common mechanism of injury is hyperflexion, and the most common radiographic finding is a wedge- or beak-shaped vertebra resulting from compression.

The most important clinical sign is a sensory level – a Spinal Cord Injury Assessment Chart (ASIA) can be used to determine at what level sensory loss occurs. Neurological assessment is difficult in children, and such a level may only become apparent after repeated examinations. Because of the difficulties of assessment, a child with multiple injuries should be assumed to have spinal injury, and therefore their spines should remain protected. If injury is confirmed, further treatment is similar to that in adults. Unstable injuries may require open reduction and stabilisation with fusion.

15.10 Spinal cord injury without radiographic abnormality

Spinal cord injury without radiographic abnormality (SCIWORA) is said to have occurred when the spinal cord has been injured without an obvious accompanying injury to the vertebral column. The cervical spine is affected more frequently than the thoracic spine. Because the upper segments of the cervical spine have the greatest mobility, the upper cervical cord is most susceptible to this injury.

Children who are seriously injured should have immobilisation of the spine maintained until such time as a full neurological assessment can be carried out since normal X-rays do not exclude a cord injury. If there is any doubt, MRI scans should be obtained.

15.11 Spinal trauma: summary

- Spinal injuries are rare in children but must be considered when associated with a significant mechanism of injury
- Assessment can be difficult and significant cord damage can occur without fractures
- Spinal immobilisation must be applied until the assessment is complete and then can only be removed if the spine has been cleared

CHAPTER 16
The burned or scalded child

Learning outcomes

After reading this chapter, you will be able to:
- Describe how to use the structured approach to assess and manage a child with a burn

16.1 Introduction

Epidemiology

In 2012, 104 232 children died worldwide as a result of injuries from fire, heat and hot substances (WHO data). This is an average of 285 children each day. Sixty per cent of these were under the age of 5 years. Most children who suffer fatal burns are never admitted to hospital and house fires with smoke inhalation are the usual cause of death. The number of deaths from burns has decreased because of a combination of factors; the move away from open fires, safer fireguards, increased use of smoke alarms and more stringent low-flammability requirements for night clothes all playing a part. Non-fatal burns often involve clothing and are associated with flammable liquids.

Scalds are usually caused by hot drinks or contact burns, but bath water and cooking oil scalds are not uncommon. The improvement in survival following scalding (which followed improvements in treatment) has reached a plateau. There is a strong link between burns to children and low socioeconomic status. Family stress, poor housing conditions and overcrowding are implicated in this.

Non-accidental injury should be considered if there are inconsistencies in the history given as to how/when a burn occurred, a delay in seeking medical help, the history being incompatible with the pattern of burn, certain patterns of burn, and the pattern of burn being consistent with forced immersion. Local safeguarding procedures must be followed.

Pathophysiology

Two main factors determine the severity of burns and scalds – these are the temperature and the duration of contact. The time taken for cellular destruction to occur decreases exponentially with temperature: at 44°C contact would have to be maintained for 6 hours, at 54°C for 30 seconds, and at 70°C epidermal injury happens within a second. This relationship underlies the different patterns of injury seen with different types of burn. Scalds generally involve water at below boiling point and contact for less than 4 seconds. Scalds that occur with liquids at a higher temperature (such as hot fat or steam), or in children incapable of minimising the contact time (such as young infants and the handicapped), tend to result in more serious injuries. Flame burns involve high temperatures and consequently produce the most serious injuries of all.

It must be emphasised that the most common cause of death within the first hour following burn injuries is due to smoke inhalation. Smoke-filled rooms not only contain soot particles, hot gases and noxious substances but are also depleted of oxygen; inhalation of all or any of these can lead to cardiac arrest. Thus, as with other types of injury, attention to the airway and breathing is of prime importance.

Advanced Paediatric Life Support: A Practical Approach to Emergencies, Sixth Edition. Edited by Martin Samuels and Sue Wieteska.
© 2016 John Wiley & Sons, Ltd. Published 2016 by John Wiley & Sons, Ltd.

16.2 Primary survey and resuscitation

When faced with a seriously burned child it is easy to focus on the immediate problems of the burn, and forget the possibility of other injuries. The approach to the burned child should be the structured one advocated in Chapter 11.

Airway and cervical spine

The airway may be compromised either because of inhalational injury and oral scalds or because of severe burns to the face. The latter is usually obvious, whereas the former two may not be and a high index of suspicion is required. The presence of inhalation injury is directly related to mortality – an observational study carried out in the USA found that there was a 15% higher mortality rate where inhalation injury was present. The indicators of inhalational injury are shown in the box.

Indications of inhalational injury

- History of exposure to smoke in a confined space
- Deposits around the mouth and nose
- Carbonaceous sputum

Because oedema occurs following thermal injury, the airway can deteriorate rapidly. Thus even suspicion of airway compromise, or the discovery of injuries that might be expected to cause problems with the airway at a later stage, should lead to immediate consideration of tracheal intubation. This procedure increases in difficulty as oedema progresses; it is therefore important to perform it as soon as possible. All but the most experienced should seek expert help urgently, unless apnoea requires immediate intervention.

If there is any suspicion of cervical spine injury, or if the history is unobtainable, appropriate precautions to immobilise the neck should be taken until such injury is excluded (see Chapters 11 and 15).

Breathing

Once the airway has been secured, the adequacy of breathing should be assessed. Signs that should arouse suspicion of inadequacy include abnormal rate, abnormal chest movements and cyanosis (a late sign). Circumferential burns to the chest or abdomen (the latter in infants) may cause breathing difficulty by mechanically restricting chest movement.

All children who have suffered significant burns should be given high-flow oxygen. If there is evidence of increased work of breathing then senior anaesthetic help should be sought and intubation and ventilation should be considered.

Circulation

In the first few hours following injury signs of hypovolaemic shock are rarely attributable to burns. Therefore, any such signs should raise the suspicion of bleeding from elsewhere, and the source should be actively sought. Intravenous access should be established with two cannulae during resuscitation, and fluids started. If possible, drips should be put up in unburnt areas, but burned skin (eschar) can be perforated if necessary. Remember that the intraosseous route can be used to administer fluid and drugs. Blood should be taken for blood glucose, carboxyhaemoglobin level, haemoglobin, electrolytes and urea and cross-matching at this stage.

Disability

Reduced conscious level following burns may be due to hypoxia (remember smoke-filled rooms may contain little oxygen), head injury or hypovolaemia. It is essential that a quick assessment is made during the primary survey as described in Chapter 11, because this provides a baseline for later observations.

Exposure

Exposure should be complete remembering that burned children lose heat particularly rapidly, and should be kept in a warm environment and covered with blankets when not being examined. Remove all jewellery including piercings as soon as possible prior to digit and/or limb swelling.

16.3 Secondary survey and looking for key features

As well as being burned, children may suffer the effects of blast, be injured by falling objects or may fall while trying to escape from the fire. Thus other injuries are not uncommon and a thorough head-to-toe secondary survey must be carried out. This is described in Chapter 11. Any injuries discovered, including the burn, should be treated in order of priority.

Assessing the burn

The severity of a burn depends on its relative surface area and depth. Burns to particular areas require special attention.

Surface area

The surface area is usually estimated using burns charts. It is particularly important to use a paediatric chart when assessing burn size in children, because the relative surface areas of the head and limbs change with age. This variation is illustrated in Figure 16.1 and the table accompanying it.

Another useful method of estimating relative surface area relies on the fact that the patient's palm and adducted fingers cover an area of approximately 1% of the body surface. This method can be used when charts are not immediately available, and is obviously already related to the child's size. Note that the 'rule of 9s' cannot be applied to a child who is less than 14 years old. There are a number of apps available to help assess burned surface area and these include the Mersey Burns app.

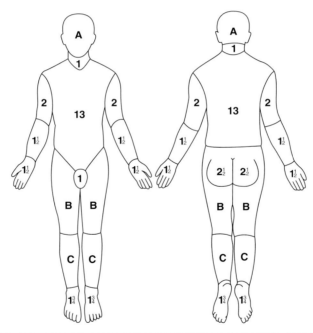

Area indicated	Surface area at				
	0	1 year	5 years	10 years	15 years
A	9.5	8.5	6.5	5.5	4.5
B	2.75	3.25	4.0	4.5	4.5
C	2.5	2.5	2.75	3.0	3.25

Figure 16.1 Differences in body surface area (per cent) in children. (Source: Artz, 1969. Reproduced with permission of Elsevier)

Depth

Burns are classified as being superficial epidermal, superficial dermal, mid-dermal, deep dermal, partial thickness and full thickness. Superficial dermal burns present with pale pink skin with blisters; mid-dermal burns have sluggish capillary refill, are dark pink in colour and sensation to touch may be decreased; deep dermal burns have blotchy, red skin and may or may not have blisters and the hallmark of these burns is the loss of capillary blush phenomenon. Partial-thickness burns cause some damage to the dermis, blistering is usually seen and the skin is pink or mottled. Deeper, full-thickness burns damage both the epidermis and dermis, and may cause injury to deeper structures as well. The skin looks white or charred, and is painless and leathery to the touch.

Special areas

Burns to the face and mouth have already been dealt with above. Burns involving the hands or feet can cause severe functional loss if scarring occurs. Perineal burns are prone to infection and present particularly difficult management problems. Circumferential, full- or partial-thickness burns of the limbs or neck may require urgent incision to relieve distal ischaemia. Similarly, circumferential burns to the torso may restrict ventilation and also require urgent incision. This procedure is called escharotomy and usually needs to be done before transfer to a burns centre.

16.4 Emergency treatment

Analgesia

Most children with a burn will be in severe pain, and this should be dealt with urgently. Older children may manage to use Entonox®, but most will not. Any child with more than a minor burn should be given intranasal diamorphine initially and then further pain can be controlled with intravenous morphine at a dose of 100 micrograms/kg (<1 year: 80 micrograms/kg), if needed, as soon as possible. Further doses are often required but must be titrated against pain and sedation.

> There is no place for the administration of intramuscular analgesia in burns because it is painful and absorption is unreliable.

Fluid therapy

Two cannulae should already have been sited during the primary survey and resuscitation and therapy for shock (10 + 10 ml/kg) commenced if indicated. Children with burns of 10% body surface area or more will require intravenous fluids as part of their burns care. This fluid is in addition to their normal maintenance fluid requirement. The additional fluid (in ml) required per day to treat the burn can be estimated using the following modified Parkland formula:

$$\text{Percentage burn} \times \text{Weight}(\text{kg}) \times 3 = \text{Total fluid replacement for burn in 24 hours}$$

Half of this should be given in the first 8 hours following the time of their burn. The fluid given is usually crystalloid. Remember that this is only an initial guide; subsequent therapy will be guided by urine output, which should be kept at 1 ml/kg/h or more; in children who have sustained greater than 15% burns it should be 2 ml/kg/h or more. Urethral catheterisation should be considered early to help with fluid management.

Wound care

Infection is a significant cause of mortality and morbidity in burns victims, and wound care should start as early as possible to reduce this risk. Furthermore, appropriate wound care will reduce the pain associated with air passing over burned areas. The burned area should be cooled immediately for 20 minutes. Although cold compresses and irrigation with cold water may reduce pain and can be useful for several hours after the injury, it should be remembered that burned children lose heat rapidly. Children should never be transferred with cold soaks in place.

Burns should then be covered with non-adhesive sterile towels or cling film. Cling film is often used as a sterile dressing, and can be applied loosely onto the burned area. No additional ointments or creams should be applied. Unnecessary re-examination should be avoided and blisters should be left intact. Photographs taken prior to applying the dressing can aid this process and allow others to assess the burn without disturbing the child. Provide tetanus prophylaxis if required.

Management of carbon monoxide poisoning

During a fire, burning of organic compounds in a low-oxygen environment produces carbon monoxide. Inhalation by the victim induces the production of carboxyhaemoglobin, which has a 200-fold greater affinity for oxygen molecules than haemoglobin. A high level will therefore cause cellular hypoxia as oxygen will not be given up to cells. Children who have been in house fires should have their blood carboxyhaemoglobin measured. (Note: most pulse oximeters show the oxygen saturation, regardless of haemoglobin concentration, i.e. normal SpO_2 does not exclude carbon monoxide poisoning.)

Levels of 5–20% are treated with oxygen (which speeds up the removal of CO). Levels over 20% should prompt consideration of hyperbaric oxygen chamber treatment – discuss with the paediatric burns service. In some environments the burning of plastics, wool and silk can produce cyanide. Assessment and treatments are complex. Be aware of the possibility of cyanide poisoning and consider it in a child from a house fire who is in a coma or presents with a severe metabolic acidosis without apparent cause. In general, antidotes are used when blood levels of cyanide are greater than 3 mg/l. Discuss treatment immediately with a poisons centre if cyanide poisoning is suspected as other factors such as the concomitant presence of carboxyhaemoglobin are contraindications for some antidotes.

16.5 Continuing stabilisation and transfer to definitive care

Definitive care requires transfer to a paediatric burns service. Criteria for transfer are shown in the box.

Initial indication for referral to a specialised burns service

1. A child with a partial-thickness burn greater than 2% total body surface area (TBSA)
2. In addition, any child with a burn injury regardless of age and %TBSA who presents with any of the following should be discussed with the local burns service and consideration given for the need for referral:
   - Inhalation injury (defined as either visual evidence of suspected upper airway smoke inhalation, laryngoscopic ± bronchoscopic evidence of tracheal/bronchial contamination/injury or suspicion of inhalation of products of incomplete combustion)
   - Full-thickness burn greater than 1% TBSA
   - Burns to special areas (hands, face, neck, feet, perineum)
   - Burns to an area involving a joint that may adversely affect mobility and function
   - Electrical burns
   - Chemical burns
   - Any burn with suspicion of non-accidental injury should be referred to a specialised burns service for an expert assessment within 24 hours
   - Burns associated with major trauma
   - Burns associated with significant co-morbidities
   - Circumferential burns to the trunk or limbs

If in doubt, discuss the child with the specialist paediatric burns service team who will advise the level of care required (at a centre, unit or facility).

As with any injury in childhood, consider the possibility of non-accidental injury. Note the timeliness of presentation, and assess whether the history given to account for the burn or scald fits in with the clinical appearance of the injury in size, shape, age and location. Consider whether the injury is consistent with the child's development. If concerned or in doubt, consult with a safeguarding specialist.

16.6 Toxic shock syndrome

Toxic shock syndrome (TSS) is a toxin-mediated disease that can occur in children, usually following relatively small burns. It causes significant mortality, and therefore any child presenting unwell within a few days post burn who has a fever and a rash or diarrhoea and vomiting should be urgently investigated and treated if TSS is suspected. Urgent senior help should be sought for children suspected of having TSS. Any child discharged home with a small burn should be given written information about TSS.

16.7 Summary

- Initial assessment and management of the burned child should be directed towards care of the airway, breathing and circulation. Intubation and ventilation should be performed early if indicated
- Assessment of the area and depth of the burn should be undertaken during the secondary survey
- Fluid replacement should be used initially to treat shock. Additional maintenance fluids will be needed for burns. Urine output should be used as an indicator of the efficacy of treatment. Beware over-resuscitation, which is more common than under-resuscitation
- Specialist burns centres should be contacted, and transfer arranged if indicated

CHAPTER 17
The child with an electrical injury or drowning

Learning outcomes

After reading this chapter, you will be able to:
- Demonstrate the assessment and management of the child with an electrical injury or drowning using the structured approach

17.1 Electrical injuries: introduction

Epidemiology

Many minor electrical injuries do not require medical treatment and the incidence of this sort of injury is unknown. Only a small percentage of electrical injuries requiring hospital attention occur in children. Electrical injuries usually occur in the home and involve relatively low currents and voltage. The mortality from electrical injuries from high-power external sources such as electrified railways is high.

Other injuries may occur during the event: for example, the child may fall or be thrown from the source. As with all injuries, a systematic approach is required.

Pathophysiology

Alternating current (AC) produces cardiac arrest at lower voltages than does direct current (DC). Regardless of whether the electrocution is caused by AC or DC, the risk of cardiac arrest is related to the size of the current and the duration of exposure. The current is highest when the resistance is low and the voltage is high.

Current

A lightning strike is a massive direct current of very short duration which can depolarise the myocardium and cause an immediate asystole.

The typical effects of an increase in current are given in the following list:

- Above 10 mA: tetanic contractions of muscles may make it impossible for the child to let go of the electrical source
- 50 mA: tetanic contraction of the diaphragm and intercostal muscles leads to respiratory arrest, which continues until the current is disconnected. If hypoxia is prolonged, secondary cardiac arrest will occur
- Over 100 mA to 50 A: primary cardiac arrest may be induced (defibrillators used in resuscitation deliver around 10 A)
- 50 A to several 100 A: massive shocks cause prolonged respiratory and cardiac arrest and more severe burns

Advanced Paediatric Life Support: A Practical Approach to Emergencies, Sixth Edition. Edited by Martin Samuels and Sue Wieteska.
© 2016 John Wiley & Sons, Ltd. Published 2016 by John Wiley & Sons, Ltd.

Resistance

The resistance of the tissues determines the path that the current will follow. Generally, the current will follow the path of least resistance from the point of contact to the earth. The relative resistance of the body tissues is in increasing order: tissue fluid, blood, muscle, nerve, fat, skin and bone. Electrocution generates heat, which causes a variable degree of tissue damage. Nerves, blood vessels, the skin and muscles are damaged the most. Swelling of damaged tissues, particularly muscle, can lead to a crush or compartment syndrome requiring fasciotomy. Water decreases the resistance of the skin and will increase the amount of current that flows through the body. Some of the effects may be hidden and you should, therefore, look for them.

Voltage

High-voltage sources such as lightning or high-tension cables cause extremely high currents and severe tissue damage. However, very high voltages can cause severe superficial burns without damage to deeper structures (flash burns and arcing).

17.2 Initial treatment of electrical injuries

The first priority is to disconnect the current. Be aware that high-voltage sources can discharge through several centimetres of air.

17.3 Primary survey of electrical injuries and resuscitation

The upper airway should be opened and secured, especially if this is compromised by facial or other injuries. The cervical spine should be immobilised, especially in an unconscious child (see Chapter 11). Other injuries should be treated in an appropriate and structured manner. The entry and exit point of the current should be sought in order to determine the sort of possible internal injuries that could have occurred.

17.4 Secondary survey and looking for key features of electrical injuries

Associated injuries are common in electrocution. Almost all possible injuries can occur as a result of falls or being thrown from the source. Burns are particularly common and are caused either by the current itself or by burning clothing. Tetanic contraction of muscles can cause fractures, luxations or muscle tearing.

Associated problems

Burns cause oedema and fluid loss. Myoglobinuria occurs after significant muscle damage. In this case it is important to maintain a urine production of more than 2 ml/kg/h with the judicious use of diuretics such as mannitol and appropriate fluid loading. Alkalisation of the urine with sodium bicarbonate increases the excretion of myoglobin. Children with significant internal injuries have a greater fluid requirement than one would suspect on the basis of the area of the burn.

17.5 Stabilisation of electrical injuries and transfer to definitive care

A significant electrical burn is an indication for transfer to a burns centre.

17.6 Electrical injuries: summary

- The first priority in electrical injuries is to switch off the current
- The management of electrocution should be structured according to the ABCDE principle, including the appropriate treatment of a possible cervical spine injury
- Electrocution can be associated with injuries to any system
- The entry and exit wounds should be sought in order to form a picture of the possible internal injuries
- Myoglobinuria should be treated aggressively

17.7 Drowning: introduction

The International Liaison Committee on Resuscitation (ILCOR) defines drowning as 'a process resulting in primary respiratory impairment from submersion/immersion in a liquid medium'. The term 'near drowning' and 'wet' or 'dry' drowning are no longer official terms, mainly because they have been used differently worldwide, which has caused confusion.

Epidemiology

According to the annual WHO report, 140 220 children under the age of 15 years died in 2012 as a result of drowning worldwide, which makes it the leading cause of accidental death in this age group. Male victims are more likely to die from drowning than female victims (63% from WHO 2012 data). Infants die most commonly in bathtubs, older children die in private swimming pools, garden ponds and other inland waterways. It is estimated that up to 80% of drowning incidents are preventable. Prevention strategies like fencing of private pools and reinforcing the importance of adult supervision may reduce this number.

Pathophysiology

Bradycardia and apnoea occur shortly after submersion as a result of the diving reflex. As apnoea continues, hypoxia and acidosis causes tachycardia and a rise in blood pressure. Between 20 seconds and 5 minutes later a breakpoint is reached, and breathing occurs. Fluid is inhaled and on touching the glottis causes immediate laryngeal spasm. After a variable but short period of time, the laryngospasm subsides and fluid is aspirated into the lungs, resulting in alveolitis and pulmonary oedema. Hypoxia is by this time severe and the patient will have lost consciousness. Bradycardia and other dysrhythmias can also occur and may be fatal (ventricular fibrillation is rare). Hypoxia is thus the key pathological process that ultimately leads to death and needs to be corrected as quickly as possible.

Children who survive because of interruption of this chain of events not only require therapy for drowning, but also assessment and treatment of concomitant hypothermia, hypovolaemia and injury (particularly spinal). Major electrolyte abnormalities due to the amount of water swallowed seldom occur.

The type of water – freshwater or saltwater – does not predict the clinical course of drowning and should not influence treatment. However, immersion in severely contaminated water is associated with infections with unusual organisms, and aspiration of water contaminated with petroleum products can lead to severe acute respiratory distress syndrome (ARDS).

Submersion injuries are generally associated with hypothermia. The large body surface area to weight ratio in infants and children put them at particular risk. Hypothermia may have a protective effect against the neurological sequelae following hypoxia and ischaemia but is also associated with life-threatening dysrhythmias, coagulation disorders and susceptibility to infections.

The initial approach to drowning patients focuses on the correction of hypoxia, hypothermia and the treatment of associated injuries, which are common in older children and are often overlooked. Cervical spine injury should always be suspected in drowning victims for whom the mechanism of injury is unclear, although these are rare (0.5% overall, and much rarer in children under 5 years).

17.8 Primary survey of drowning and resuscitation

The first priority is to move the victim from the water as quickly as possible without risk to the rescuer in order to allow cardiopulmonary resuscitation and ABC stabilisation without delay. Immobilisation of the neck should be instigated as soon as practicable until injury is excluded, although cervical spine injury is uncommon except after diving or traffic accidents. Rescue of the victim in a vertical position may lead to cardiovascular collapse due to venous pooling. However, horizontal rescue or cervical spine immobilisation in the water must not be allowed to delay the rescue. The initiation of early and effective basic life support (BLS) reduces the mortality drastically and is the most important factor for survival. Rescue breaths must be commenced as early as possible even in shallow water if this can be done without risk to the rescuer. Mouth-to-nose ventilation may be easier in this situation. BLS then proceeds according to the standard paediatric algorithm even in hypothermia. The presence of cardiac arrest can be difficult to diagnose as pulses are difficult to feel. If in doubt chest compressions should be given and continued. If an automatic external defibrillator (AED) is used it is vital to first dry the chest before applying the electrodes.

Following a submersion episode, the stomach is usually full of swallowed water. The risk of aspiration is therefore increased and the airway must be secured as soon as possible, usually by endotracheal intubation using a rapid sequence induction. Following this an oro- or nasogastric tube should be inserted. Ventilate the child to achieve an SpO_2 of 94–98% using additional oxygen and positive end-expiratory pressure (PEEP) as required.

Respiratory deterioration can be delayed for 4–6 hours after submersion and even children who have initially apparently recovered should be observed for at least 8 hours. Chest X-ray changes may occur even later. Advanced life support proceeds according to the standard algorithm except for slight modifications in cases of hypothermia.

Hypothermia

A core temperature reading (rectal or oesophageal) should be obtained as soon as possible and further cooling prevented. Hypothermia is common following drowning and adversely affects resuscitation attempts unless treated. Not only are arrhythmias more common but some, such as ventricular fibrillation, may be refractory at temperatures below 30°C, when defibrillation should be limited to three shocks and inotropic or antiarrhythmic drugs should not be given. If unsuccessful the patient should be warmed to above 30°C as quickly as possible, when further defibrillation may be attempted. The dose interval for resuscitation drugs is doubled between 30°C and 35°C. Resuscitation should be continued until the core temperature is at least 32°C or cannot be raised despite active measures. If a child requires endotracheal intubation, the advantages outweigh the small risk of precipitating malignant arrhythmias.

Rewarming strategies (see box) depend on the core temperature and signs of circulation. External rewarming including a warm air system is usually sufficient if the core temperature is above 30°C. Active core rewarming should be added in patients with a core temperature of less than 30°C. Extracorporeal warming is the preferred method in circulatory arrest.

Rewarming

External rewarming
- Remove cold, wet clothing
- Supply warm blankets
- Warm air system
- Heating blanket
- Infrared radiant lamp

Core rewarming
- Warm intravenous fluids to 39°C to prevent further heat loss
- Warm ventilator gases to 42°C to prevent further heat loss
- Gastric or bladder lavage with normal (physiological) saline at 42°C
- Peritoneal lavage with potassium-free dialysate at 42°C, 20 ml/kg with a 15-minute cycle
- Pleural or pericardial lavage
- Endovascular warming
- Extracorporeal blood rewarming (i.e. extracorporeal membrane oxygenation or bypass)

The temperature is generally allowed to rise by 0.25–0.5°C per hour to reduce haemodynamic instability. Most hypothermic patients are hypovolaemic. During rewarming, vasodilatation occurs, resulting in hypotension that requires large quantities of warmed intravenous fluids while avoiding overfilling and pulmonary oedema. Continuous haemodynamic monitoring is essential. Therapeutic hypothermia (32–34°C) for at least 24 hours has been shown to improve neurological outcome in some patients and may be of benefit in children who remain comatose.

17.9 Secondary survey and looking for key features in drowning

During the secondary survey, the child should be carefully examined from head to toe. Any injury may have occurred during the incident that preceded immersion, including spinal injuries. Older children may have ingested alcohol and/or drugs.

Investigations
- Blood glucose
- Blood gas analysis and blood lactate
- Urea and electrolytes
- Coagulation status
- Blood and aspirate cultures

- Chest X-ray
- Electrocardiogram
- Cervical spine imaging, if indicated (see Chapter 24)

17.10 Emergency treatment and stabilisation in drowning

The brain is the most vulnerable organ for asphyxia, and cerebral impairment occurs before cardiac problems in submersion. Except for early BLS and possibly therapeutic hypothermia, there are few effective measures for reducing brain damage in drowning.

It is essential to monitor the vital functions closely, especially during the first couple of hours. Early suggestions of respiratory insufficiency, haemodynamic instability or hypothermia are indications for admission to the intensive care unit.

Prophylactic antibiotics have not been shown to be helpful but are often given after immersion in severely contaminated water. Fever is common during the first 24 hours but is not necessarily a sign of infection, which usually becomes manifest later. Gram-negative organisms, especially *Pseudomonas aeruginosa*, are common and *Aspergillus* species have been reported. When an infection is suspected broad-spectrum intravenous antibiotic therapy (such as cefotaxime) should be started after repeating blood and sputum cultures.

Signs of raised intracranial pressure may develop as a result of a post-hypoxic injury, and this should be treated, although aggressive treatment to lower a raised ICP has not been shown to improve the prognosis. Other therapeutic measures, such as barbiturates, calcium channel blockers, surfactants, steroids and free-radical scavengers, have not been shown to be of benefit. However, keeping the patient normoglycaemic is important for the neurological outcome. Unless obvious, a careful search should be made for a precipitating cause of the drowning such as a channelopathy, particularly long QT-syndrome.

17.11 Prognostic indicators in drowning

The clinical course of drowning is determined by the duration of hypoxic–ischaemic injury and the adequacy of initial resuscitation. It is assumed that hypoxic brain damage is reduced when the brain cools before the heart stops. No single factor can predict good or poor outcome in drowning reliably; however, the factors listed in Table 17.1 may give an indication of outcome.

Table 17.1 Prognostic indicators in drowning

Immersion time	Most children who have been submerged for more than 10 minutes have a very small chance of intact neurological recovery or survival. Details of the incident are therefore vital *Time to basic life support*: starting basic life support at the scene greatly reduces mortality, whereas a delay of more than 10 minutes is associated with a poor prognosis
Time to first respiratory effort	If this occurs within 3 minutes after the start of basic cardiopulmonary support, the prognosis is good. If there has been no respiratory effort after 40 minutes of full cardiopulmonary resuscitation, there is little or no chance of survival unless the child's respiration has been depressed (e.g. by hypothermia, medication or alcohol)
Core temperature	Pre-existing hypothermia and rapid cooling after submersion also seems to protect vital organs and can improve the prognosis. A core temperature of less than 33°C on arrival and a water temperature of less than 10°C have been associated with increased survival. This effect is more pronounced in small children because of their large surface area to weight ratio
Persisting coma	A persistent Glasgow Coma Scale (GCS) score of less than 5 indicates a bad prognosis
Arterial blood pH	If this remains below 7.1 despite treatment, the prognosis is poor
Arterial blood PO_2	If this remains below 8.0 kPa (60 mmHg) despite treatment, the prognosis is poor
Type of water	Whether the water was salt or fresh has no bearing on the prognosis

The duration of resuscitation efforts may not be a helpful prognostic factor. The decision to discontinue resuscitation attempts is particularly difficult in cases of drowning, and should be taken only after all the prognostic factors discussed above have been considered carefully. Resuscitation should only be discontinued out of hospital if there is clear evidence of futility such as massive trauma or rigor mortis.

17.12 Outcome of drowning

Seventy per cent of children survive drowning when BLS is provided at the scene, whereas only 40% survive without early BLS, even with maximum therapy. Of those who do survive, having required full cardiopulmonary resuscitation in hospital, around 70% will make a complete recovery and 25% will have a mild neurological deficit. The remainder will be severely disabled or remain in a persisting vegetative state.

17.13 Drowning: summary

- Starting BLS as soon as possible is crucial to the outcome after drowning
- Many associated injuries and underlying illnesses may be associated with submersion
- If cervical injury cannot be excluded, stabilisation should be initiated as soon as practical but should not delay rescue and the start of BLS
- Hypothermia should be actively sought and treated
- Prolonged resuscitation may be necessary and the decision to stop resuscitation should be taken after all prognostic indicators have been considered

PART 4
Life support

CHAPTER 18
Basic life support

Learning outcomes

After reading this chapter, you will be able to:
- Demonstrate how to assess the collapsed patient and perform basic life support

---

18.1 Introduction

Paediatric basic life support (BLS) is not simply a scaled-down version of that provided for adults, although, where possible, guidelines are the same for all ages to aid teaching and retention. Some of the techniques employed need to be varied according to the size of the child. A somewhat artificial line is drawn between infants (less than 1 year old) and children (between 1 year and puberty), and this chapter follows that approach. The preponderance of hypoxic causes of paediatric cardiorespiratory arrest means that oxygen delivery rather than defibrillation is the critical step in children and even in adolescence. This underlines the major differences with the adult algorithm.

By applying the basic techniques described, a single rescuer can support the vital respiratory and circulatory functions of a collapsed child with no equipment. However, health professionals who treat children should use bag–mask ventilation to deliver rescue breaths, if provided (see Section 21.1). Basic life support is the foundation on which advanced life support is built. Therefore it is essential that all advanced life support providers are proficient at basic techniques, and that they are capable of ensuring that basic support is provided continuously and well during resuscitation.

18.2 Primary assessment and resuscitation

Once the child has been approached safely and been tested for unresponsiveness, assessment and treatment follow the familiar ABC pattern. The overall sequence of BLS in paediatric cardiopulmonary arrest is summarised in Figure 18.1. Note: this guidance is for one or more health professionals. BLS guidance for lay people can be found later in this section.

The initial approach: safety, stimulate, shout (SSS)

In the external environment, it is essential that the rescuer does not become a second victim, and that the child is removed from continuing danger as quickly as possible. These considerations should precede the initial airway assessment. Within a healthcare setting the likelihood of risk is decreased and help should be summoned as soon as the victim is found to be unresponsive. The steps are summarised in Figure 18.2.

When more than one rescuer is present one starts BLS while another activates the emergency medical services (EMS) system and then returns to assist in the BLS effort. If there is only one rescuer and no help has arrived after 1 minute of cardiopulmonary resuscitation (CPR), then the rescuer must activate the EMS system him- or herself before returning to CPR. In the case of a baby or small child the rescuer will probably be able to take the victim with him or her to a telephone whilst attempting to continue CPR on the way.

Advanced Paediatric Life Support: A Practical Approach to Emergencies, Sixth Edition. Edited by Martin Samuels and Sue Wieteska.
© 2016 John Wiley & Sons, Ltd. Published 2016 by John Wiley & Sons, Ltd.

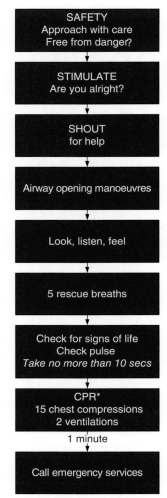

*CPR = Cardiopulmonary resuscitation

Figure 18.1 Basic life support algorithm

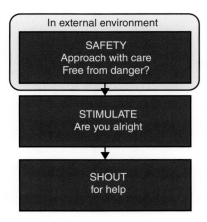

Figure 18.2 The initial SSS approach

Phone first

In a few instances the sequence in the above paragraph is reversed. As previously described, in children, respiratory and circulatory causes of cardiac arrest predominate, and immediate respiratory and circulatory support as provided by the breaths and chest compressions of BLS can be life saving. However, there are circumstances in which early defibrillation may be life saving, i.e. cardiac arrests caused by arrhythmia. On these occasions, where there is more than one rescuer, one may start BLS and another summons the emergency medical services. But if there is a lone rescuer then he or she should activate the EMS system first on witnessing the collapse and then start BLS afterwards.

The clinical indication for EMS activation before BLS by a lone rescuer include:

- Witnessed sudden collapse with no apparent preceding morbidity
- Witnessed sudden collapse in a child with a known cardiac condition and in the absence of a known or suspected respiratory or circulatory cause of arrest

The increasingly wide availability of public access defibrillation programmes with automatic external defibrillators (AEDs) may result in a better outcome for this small group (see the section on AEDs in children in this chapter).

Are you alright?

The initial simple assessment of responsiveness consists of asking the child loudly 'Are you alright?' and gently applying a stimulus such as holding the head and shaking the arm. This will avoid exacerbating a possible neck injury whilst still waking a sleeping child. Infants and very small children who cannot talk yet, and older children who are very scared, are unlikely to reply meaningfully, but may make some sound or open their eyes to the rescuer's voice or touch.

Airway (A)

An obstructed airway may be the primary problem, and correction of the obstruction can result in recovery without further intervention. If a child is not breathing it may be because the airway has been blocked by the tongue falling back and obstructing the pharynx. An attempt to open the airway should be made using the head tilt/chin lift manoeuvre. The rescuer places the hand nearest to the child's head on the forehead and applies pressure to tilt the head back gently. The different anatomy of the infant and child makes the desirable degrees of tilt neutral in the infant and 'sniffing' in the child. These are shown in Figures 18.3 and 18.4.

If a child is having difficulty breathing, but is conscious, then transport to hospital should be arranged as quickly as possible. A child will often find the best position to maintain his or her own airway, and should not be forced to adopt a position that may be less comfortable. Attempts to improve a partially maintained airway in a conscious child in an environment where immediate advanced support is not available can be dangerous, because total obstruction may occur.

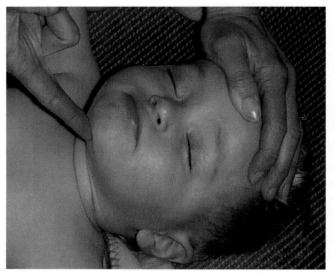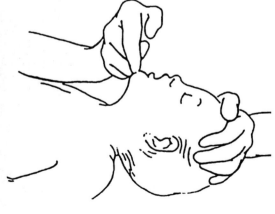

Figure 18.3 Head tilt and chin lift in infants: neutral position in an infant

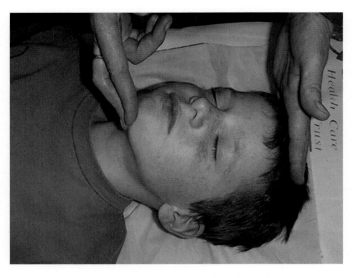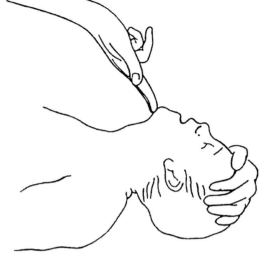

Figure 18.4 Head tilt and chin lift: sniffing position in a child

Place the hand nearest to the child's head on the forehead and apply pressure to tilt the head back gently. The fingers of your other hand should then be placed under the chin and the chin should be lifted upwards. Care should be taken not to injure the soft tissue by gripping too hard. As this action can close the child's mouth, it may be necessary to use the thumb of the same hand to part the lips slightly. In the infant, the head is placed in the neutral position; in the child, the head should be in the 'sniffing' position.

The patency of the airway should then be assessed. This is done by:

LOOKing	for chest and/or abdominal movement
LISTENing	for breath sounds
FEELing	for breath

This is best achieved by the rescuer placing his or her face above the child's, with the ear over the nose, the cheek over the mouth and the eyes looking along the line of the chest for up to 10 seconds (Figure 18.5).

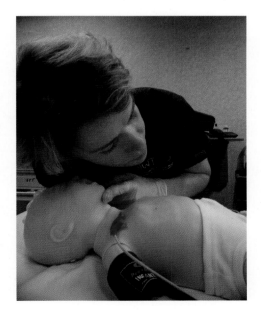

Figure 18.5 Looking, listening, feeling

If the head tilt/chin lift manoeuvre is not possible or is contraindicated because of suspected neck injury, then the jaw thrust manoeuvre can be performed. This is achieved by placing two or three fingers under the angle of the mandible bilaterally and lifting the jaw upwards. This technique may be easier if the rescuer's elbows are resting on the same surface as the child is lying on. A small degree of head tilt may also be applied if there is no concern about neck injury. This is shown in Figure 18.6.

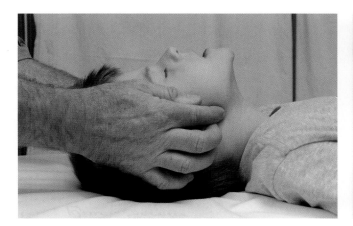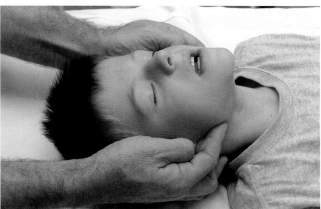

Figure 18.6 Jaw thrust

As before, the success or failure of the intervention is assessed using the technique described above:

- LOOK
- LISTEN
- FEEL

It should be noted that, if there is a history of trauma, then the head tilt/chin lift manoeuvre may exacerbate cervical spine injury. In general, the safest airway intervention in these circumstances is the jaw thrust without head tilt. However, on rare occasions, it may not be possible to control the airway with a jaw thrust alone in trauma. In these circumstances, an open airway takes priority over cervical spine risk and a gradually increased degree of head tilt may be tried. Cervical spine control should be achieved by a second rescuer maintaining in-line cervical stabilisation throughout.

The blind finger sweep technique for removal of a foreign body (see Section 18.4) should not be used in children. The child's soft palate is easily damaged, and bleeding from within the mouth can worsen the situation. Furthermore, foreign bodies may be forced further down the airway; they can become lodged below the vocal cords (vocal folds) and be even more difficult to remove. In the child with a tracheostomy, additional procedures are necessary (see Section 21.8).

Breathing (B)

If normal breathing starts after the airway is open, turn the child onto his or her side in the recovery position, maintaining the open airway. Send or go for help and continue to monitor the child for normal breathing. If the airway-opening techniques described above do not result in the resumption of adequate breathing within 10 seconds, exhaled air resuscitation should be commenced. The rescuer should distinguish between adequate breathing and ineffective, gasping or obstructed breathing. If in doubt, attempt rescue breathing.

Five initial rescue breaths should be given

While the airway is kept open as described above, the rescuer breathes in and seals his or her mouth around the victim's mouth (for a child), or mouth and nose (for an infant, as shown in Figure 18.7). If the mouth alone is used then the nose should be pinched closed using the thumb and index fingers of the hand that is maintaining the head tilt. Slow exhalation (1 second) by the rescuer should make the victim's chest visibly rise – too vigorous a breath will cause gastric inflation and increase the chance of regurgitation of stomach contents into the lungs. The rescuer should take a breath between rescue breaths to maximise oxygenation of the victim.

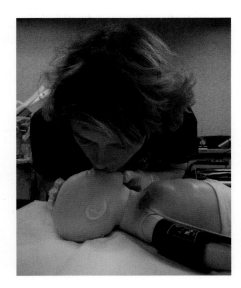

Figure 18.7 Mouth to mouth and nose in an infant

If the rescuer is unable to cover the mouth and nose in an infant, he or she may attempt to seal only the infant's nose or mouth with his or her mouth and should close the infant's lips or pinch the nose to prevent air escape.

General guidance for exhaled air resuscitation

- The chest should be seen to rise
- Inflation pressure may be higher because the airway is small
- Slow breaths at the lowest pressure reduce gastric distension
- As soon as possible change to self-inflating bag

If the chest does not rise, then the airway is not clear. The usual cause is failure to apply correctly the airway-opening techniques discussed above. Thus, the first thing to do is to readjust the head tilt/chin lift position, and try again. If this does not work, a jaw thrust should be tried. It is quite possible for a single rescuer to open the airway using this technique and perform exhaled air resuscitation; however, if two rescuers are present one should maintain the airway whilst the other breathes for the child. Five rescue breaths are given. While performing rescue breaths, note any gag or cough response to your action. These responses, or their absence, will form part of your assessment of 'signs of life' described below.

Failure of both head tilt/chin lift and jaw thrust should lead to the suspicion that a foreign body is causing the obstruction, and appropriate action should be taken (see Section 18.4).

Circulation (C)

Once the rescue breaths have been given, attention should turn to the circulation.

Assessment

Failure of the circulation is recognised by the absence of signs of circulation ('signs of life'), i.e. no normal breaths or cough in response to rescue breaths and no spontaneous movement. In addition, the absence of a central pulse for up to 10 seconds or the presence of a pulse at an insufficient rate (less than 60 with no signs of circulation) may be detected.

The absence of 'signs of life' is the primary indication to start chest compressions. Signs of life include: movement, coughing or normal breathing (not agonal gasps – these are irregular, infrequent breaths). Experienced health professionals can find it difficult to be certain that the pulse is absent within 10 seconds, therefore unless you are certain you feel a pulse, start chest compressions.

In children, the carotid artery in the neck or the femoral artery in the groin can be palpated. In infants, the neck is generally short and fat and the carotid artery may be difficult to identify. Therefore the brachial artery in the medial aspect of the antecubital fossa, or the femoral artery in the groin, can be felt.

Start chest compressions if within 10 seconds:

- There are no signs of life
- You are not certain if there is a pulse
- There is a slow pulse (less than 60 beats/min with no signs of circulation and no reaction to ventilation)

Assess the circulation (signs of life); take no more than 10 seconds to look for the following signs of life:

- Any movement
- Coughing
- Normal breathing (not abnormal gasps or infrequent, irregular breaths)

In the absence of signs of life, chest compressions must be started unless you are certain that you can feel a pulse of more than 60 beats/min within 10 seconds. 'Unnecessary' chest compressions are almost never damaging and it is important not to waste vital seconds before starting them. If the pulse is present – and has an adequate rate, with good perfusion – but apnoea persists, exhaled air resuscitation must be continued until spontaneous breathing resumes.

Chest compressions

For the best effect the child must be placed lying flat on his or her back, on a hard surface. When in a hospital bed use a backboard. Children vary in size, and the exact nature of the compressions given should reflect this. In general, infants (less than 1 year old) require a technique different from children up to puberty, in whom the method used in adults can be applied with appropriate modifications for their size. Compressions should be at least one-third of the depth of the child's (5 cm) or infant's (4 cm) chest.

Position for chest compressions

Chest compressions should compress the lower half of the sternum, but avoid placing the hand/fingers too low, thus pressing the xiphisternum in the abdomen. Of equal importance is to ensure that the chest wall fully recoils before the next compression starts – this will ensure that the coronary arteries fill.

Infants   Infant chest compression can be more effectively achieved using the hand-encircling technique: the infant is held with both the rescuer's hands encircling or partially encircling the chest. The thumbs are placed over the lower half of the sternum and compression carried out, as shown in Figure 18.8. This method is only possible when there are two rescuers, as the time needed to reposition the airway precludes its use by a single rescuer if the recommended rates of compression and ventilation are to be achieved. The single rescuer should use the two-finger method, placing two fingers on the lower half of the sternum and employing the other hand to maintain the airway position as shown in Figure 18.9.

Children   Place the heel of one hand over the lower half of the sternum. Lift the fingers to ensure that pressure is not applied over the child's ribs. Position yourself vertically above the child's chest and, with your arm straight, compress the sternum to depress it by at least one-third of the depth of the chest or by 5 cm (Figure 18.10). For larger children, or for small rescuers, this may be achieved most easily by using both hands with the fingers interlocked (Figure 18.11). The rescuer may choose one or two hands to achieve the desired compression of at least one-third of the depth of the chest.

Once the correct technique has been chosen and the area for compression identified, 15 compressions should be given to two ventilations.

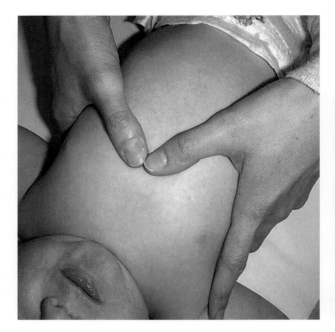

Figure 18.8 Hand-encircling technique

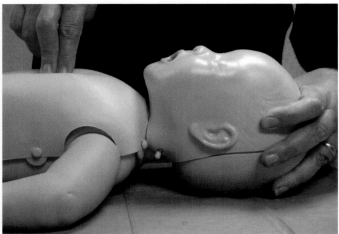

Figure 18.9 Chest compressions in an infant

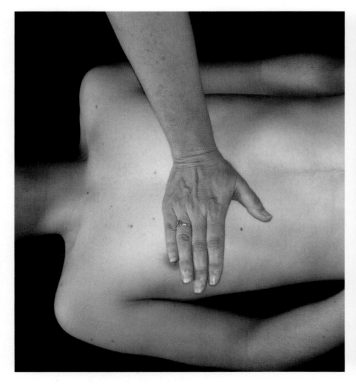

Figure 18.10 Chest compressions: one hand

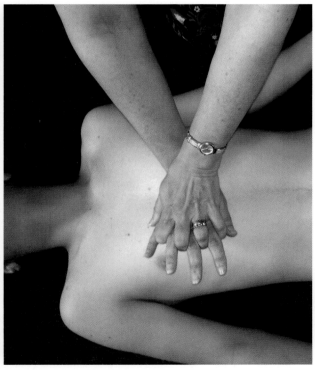

Figure 18.11 Chest compressions: two-handed

Compression:ventilation ratios

Experimental work has shown that coronary perfusion pressure in resuscitation increases if sequences of compressions are prolonged rather than curtailed. Equally, ventilations are a vital part of all resuscitation and are needed early especially in the hypoxic/ischaemic arrests characteristic of childhood. Once BLS has started, interruptions to chest compressions should only be for ventilations. Pausing compressions will decrease coronary perfusion pressure to zero and several compressions will be required before adequate coronary perfusion recurs. There is no experimental evidence to support any particular ratio in childhood but a 15:2 ratio has been validated by experimental and mathematical studies and is the recommended ratio for healthcare professionals.

Where possible once the child has been intubated during advanced life support, asynchronous compressions may be carried out with a ventilation rate of 10–12 breaths per minute.

Continuing cardiopulmonary resuscitation

The compression rate at all ages is 100–120 per minute. A ratio of 15 compressions to two ventilations is maintained whatever the number of rescuers. If possible, change rescuers every 2 minutes to maintain optimal compressions. If no help has arrived the emergency services must be contacted after 1 minute of CPR. With pauses for ventilation there will effectively be less than 100–120 compressions per minute although the **rate** is 100–120 per minute. Compressions can be recommenced at the end of inspiration and may augment exhalation. Apart from this interruption to summon help, BLS must not be interrupted unless the child moves or takes a breath.

Research on the delivery of CPR has shown that rescuers tend to compress too slowly and too gently. So the current emphasis is on CPR which is 'hard and fast', with compressions of at least one-third of the victim's anteroposterior chest diameter and a rate of between 100 and 120 compressions a minute, minimising interruptions as completely as possible. Any time spent readjusting the airway or re-establishing the correct position for compressions will seriously decrease the number of cycles given per minute. This can be a very real problem for the solo rescuer, and there is no easy solution. In the infant and small child, the free hand can maintain the head position. The correct position for compressions does not need to be re-measured after each ventilation.

In the older child biometric devices may be used which give feedback on the quality and speed of chest compressions – unless the application of such devices causes a delay in compressions.

The CPR manoeuvres recommended for infants and children are summarised in Table 18.1.

Table 18.1 Summary of basic life support techniques in infants and children

	Infant (<1 year)	Child (1 year to puberty)
Airway		
Head tilt position	Neutral	Sniffing
Breathing		
Initial slow breaths	Five	Five
Circulation		
Pulse check	Brachial or femoral	Carotid or femoral
Landmark	Lower half of sternum	Lower half of sternum
Technique	Two fingers or two thumbs	One or two hands
CPR ratio	15:2	15:2

Age definitions

As the techniques of CPR have been simplified there is now no need to distinguish between different ages of children but only between infants (under 1 year) and children (from 1 year to puberty). It is clearly inappropriate and also unnecessary to establish the physical evidence for puberty at CPR. The rescuer should use paediatric guidelines if he or she believes the victim to be a child. If the victim is, in fact, a young adult, no harm will be caused as the aetiology of cardiac arrest is, in general, similar in this age group to that in childhood, i.e. hypoxic/ischaemic rather than cardiac in origin.

Recovery position

No specific recovery position has been identified for children. An example of one recovery position is shown in Figure 18.12. The child should be placed in a stable, lateral position that ensures maintenance of an open airway with free drainage of fluid from the mouth, the ability to monitor and gain access to the patient, security of the cervical spine and attention to pressure points.

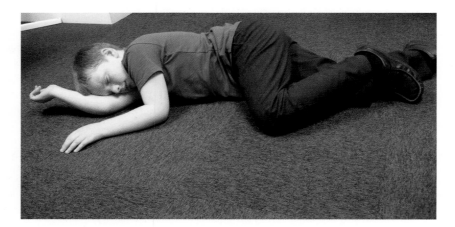

Figure 18.12 Example recovery position

The following is a description of the technique for adults and is suitable for children:

- Kneel beside the victim and make sure that both his legs are straight
- Place the arm nearest to you out at right angles to his body, elbow bent with the hand palm up
- Bring the far arm across the chest, and hold the back of the hand against the victim's cheek nearest to you
- With your other hand, grasp the far leg just above the knee and pull it up, keeping his foot on the ground
- Keeping his hand pressed against his cheek, pull on the far leg to roll the victim towards you on to his side
- Adjust the upper leg so that both the hip and knee are bent at right angles
- Tilt the head back to make sure that the airway remains open
- If necessary, adjust the hand under the cheek to keep the head tilted and facing downwards to allow liquid material to drain from the mouth
- Check breathing regularly
- If the victim has to be kept in the recovery position for more than 30 minutes turn him to the opposite side to relieve the pressure on the lower arm

Lay rescuers

Bystander CPR is associated with better neurological outcome in adults and children. However it has become clear that bystanders often do not undertake BLS because they are afraid of doing it wrongly and because of an anxiety about performing mouth-to-mouth resuscitation on strangers. For lay rescuers, therefore, the adult compression : ventilation ratio of 30 compressions to two ventilations is recommended for children as well as adults, thus simplifying the guidance. To increase the appropriateness for children, lay rescuers should be advised to precede their efforts by five rescue breaths if the victim is a child. If lay rescuers are unable or unwilling to perform mouth-to-mouth resuscitation they may perform compression-only CPR.

Single healthcare professional rescuers are encouraged to perform five rescue breaths followed by a ratio of 30 compressions to two ventilations for children if they find difficulty in the transition from compressions to ventilations.

Automatic external defibrillators in children

The use of the AED is now included in BLS teaching for adults because early defibrillation is the most effective intervention for the large majority of unpredicted cardiac arrests in adults. As has been stated, in children and young people, circulatory or respiratory causes of cardiac arrest predominate. However, in certain circumstances, children may suffer a primary cardiac cause for cardiac arrest, and the use of an AED may be life saving. Recently there has been a large increase in the number of AEDs, together with trained operators, made available in public places such as airports, places of entertainment and shops, so the opportunity for their use will correspondingly increase.

In this text, the discussion of the use of AEDs with regard to children will be found in Chapter 20.

18.3 Basic life support and infection risk

There have been a few reports of transmission of infectious diseases from casualties to rescuers during mouth-to-mouth resuscitation. The most serious concern in children is meningococcus, and rescuers involved in the resuscitation of the airway in such patients should take standard prophylactic antibiotics (rifampicin or ciprofloxacin). Tuberculosis can be transmitted during CPR and appropriate precautions should be taken when this is suspected.

There have been no reported cases of transmission of human immunodeficiency virus (HIV) through mouth-to-mouth ventilation. Blood-to-blood contact is the single most important route of the transmission of such viruses, and in non-trauma resuscitations the risks are negligible. Sputum, saliva, sweat, tears, urine and vomit are low-risk fluids. Precautions should be taken, if possible, in cases where there might be contact with blood, semen, vaginal secretions, cerebrospinal fluid, pleural and peritoneal fluids and amniotic fluid. Precautions are also recommended if any bodily secretion contains visible blood. Devices that prevent direct contact between the rescuer and the victim (such as resuscitation masks) can be used to lower risk; gauze swabs or any other porous material placed over the victim's mouth is of no benefit in this regard.

The number of children in the UK with acquired immune deficiency syndrome (AIDS) or HIV-1 infection is less than the number of adults similarly affected. If transmission of HIV-1 does occur in the UK, it is therefore much more likely to be from the adult rescuer to the child rather than the other way around.

In countries where HIV/AIDS is more prevalent, the risk to the rescuer will be greater. In South Africa, in a medical ward 25–40% of children may be HIV-positive but the prevalence is lower in trauma cases. In the Caribbean, HIV prevalence is second only to sub-Saharan Africa. The situation may change, as effective antiretroviral agents are made available to resource-poor countries.

Although practice manikins have not been shown to be a source of infection, regular cleaning is recommended and should be carried out as shown in the manufacturer's instructions. Infection rates vary from country to country and rescuers must be aware of the local risk.

18.4 The choking child

The vast majority of deaths from foreign body airway obstruction (FBAO) occur in pre-school children. Virtually anything may be inhaled, foodstuffs predominating. The diagnosis may not be clear-cut, but should be suspected if the onset of respiratory compromise is sudden and is associated with coughing, gagging and stridor.

Airway obstruction also occurs with infections such as acute epiglottitis and croup. In these cases, attempts to relieve the obstruction using the methods described below are dangerous. Children with known or suspected infectious causes of obstruction, and those who are still breathing and in whom the cause of obstruction is unclear, should be taken to hospital urgently. The treatment of these children is dealt with in Chapter 5.

If a foreign body is easily visible and accessible in the mouth then remove it, but while attempting that take great care not to push it further into the airway. Do not perform blind finger sweeps of the mouth or upper airway as these may further impact a foreign body and damage tissues without removing the object.

The physical methods of clearing the airway, described below, should therefore only be performed if:

1. The diagnosis of FBAO is clear-cut (witnessed or strongly suspected) and ineffective coughing and increasing dyspnoea, loss of consciousness or apnoea have occurred.
2. Head tilt/chin lift and jaw thrust have failed to open the airway of an apnoeic child. (The sequence of instructions is shown in Figure 18.13.)

If the child is coughing he should be encouraged. A spontaneous cough is more effective at relieving an obstruction than any externally imposed manoeuvre. An effective cough is recognised by the victim's ability to speak or cry and to take a breath between coughs. The child should be continually assessed and not left alone at this stage. No intervention should be made unless the cough becomes ineffective, that is quieter or silent, and the victim cannot cry, speak or take a breath or if he or she becomes cyanosed or starts to lose consciousness. If this happens then call for help and start the intervention.

These manoeuvres are then alternated with each other and with examination of the mouth and attempted breaths as shown in Figure 18.13.

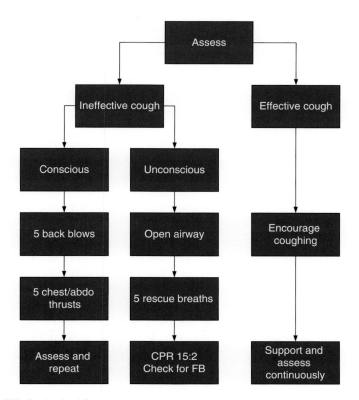

Figure 18.13 FBAO algorithm. [FB, foreign body]

Infants

Abdominal thrusts may cause intra-abdominal injury in infants. Therefore a combination of back blows and chest thrusts is recommended for the relief of foreign body obstruction in this age group.

The baby is placed along one of the rescuer's arms in a head-down position, with the rescuer's hand supporting the infant's jaw in such a way as to keep it open, in the neutral position. The rescuer then rests his or her arm along the thigh, and delivers five back blows between the shoulder blades with the heel of the free hand.

If the obstruction is not relieved the baby is turned over and laid along the rescuer's thigh, still in a head-down position. Five chest thrusts are given – using the same landmarks as for cardiac compression but at a slower rate of one per second and sharper than chest compressions. If an infant is too large to allow use of the single-arm technique described above, then the same manoeuvres can be performed by laying the baby across the rescuer's lap. These techniques are shown in Figures 18.14 and 18.15.

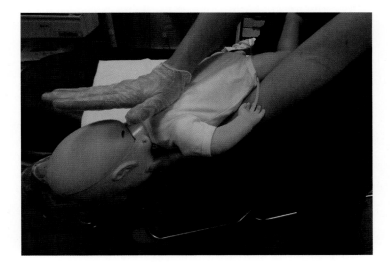

Figure 18.14 Back blows

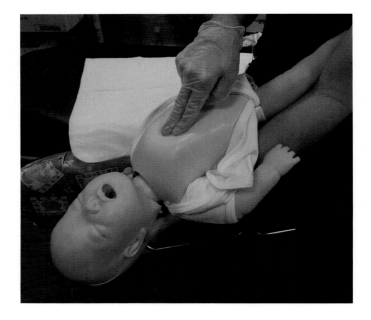

Figure 18.15 Chest thrusts

Children

Back blows can be used as in infants or, in the case of a larger child, with the child supported in a forward leaning position (Figure 18.16). In the child the abdominal thrust (Heimlich manoeuvre) can also be used. This can be performed with the victim either standing or lying, but the former is usually more appropriate.

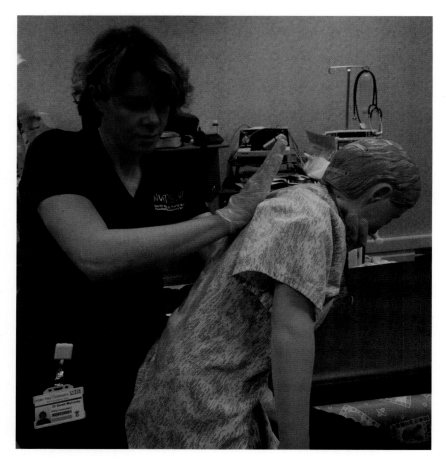

Figure 18.16 Child supported in a forward leaning position

If the Heimlich manoeuvre is to be attempted with the child standing, the rescuer moves behind the victim and passes his or her arms around the victim's body. Owing to the short height of children, it may be necessary for an adult to raise the child or kneel behind them to carry out the standing manoeuvre effectively. One hand is formed into a fist and placed against the child's abdomen above the umbilicus and below the xiphisternum. The other hand is placed over the fist, and both hands are thrust sharply upwards into the abdomen. This is repeated five times unless the object causing the obstruction is expelled before then.

To carry out the Heimlich manoeuvre in a supine child, the rescuer kneels at his or her feet. If the child is large it may be necessary to kneel astride him or her. The heel of one hand is placed against the child's abdomen above the umbilicus and below the xiphisternum. The other hand is placed on top of the first, and both hands are thrust sharply upwards into the abdomen, with care being taken to direct the thrust in the midline. This is repeated five times unless the object causing the obstruction is expelled before that. This technique is shown in Figure 18.17. When performing the abdominal thrust make sure that the pressure is not applied to the xiphisternum or the lower rib cage to avoid abdominal trauma.

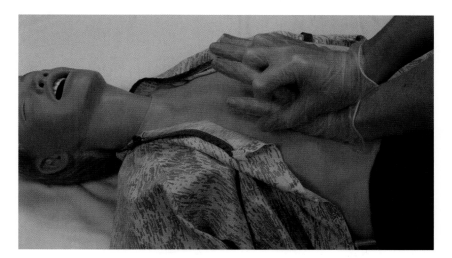

Figure 18.17 Heimlich manoeuvre in a supine child

Following successful relief of the obstructed airway, assess the child clinically. There may be still some part of the foreign material in the respiratory tract. If abdominal thrusts have been performed, the child should be assessed for possible abdominal injuries.

Each time breaths are attempted, look in the mouth for the foreign body and remove it if visible. Take care not to push the object further down and avoid damaging the tissues. If the obstruction is relieved, the victim may still require either continued ventilations if not breathing but is moving or gagging, or both ventilations and chest compressions if there are no signs of life. Advanced life support may also be needed.

If the child breathes effectively then place them in the recovery position and continue to monitor regularly.

Unconscious infant or child with foreign body airway obstruction

- Call for help
- Place the child supine on a flat surface
- Open the mouth and attempt to remove any visible object
- Open the airway and attempt five rescue breaths, repositioning the airway with each breath if the chest does not rise
- Start chest compressions even if the rescue breaths were ineffective
- Continue the sequence for single-rescuer CPR for about a minute then summon help again if none is forthcoming

Each time breaths are attempted, look in the mouth for the foreign body and remove it if visible. Take care not to push the object further down and avoid damaging the tissues.

If the obstruction is relieved the victim may still require either continued ventilations if not breathing but is moving or gagging, or both ventilations and chest compressions if there are no signs of life. Advanced life support may also be needed. If the child breathes effectively then place in the recovery position and continue to monitor regularly.

18.5 Summary

The teaching in this chapter is consistent with ILCOR's 2015 Resuscitation guidelines – the references used in this process are available on the ALSG website (see details in the prelims).

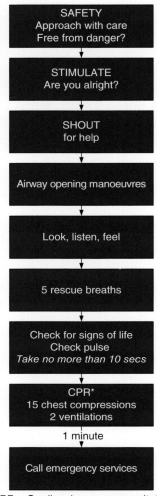

Figure 18.18 Basic life support algorithm

*CPR = Cardiopulmonary resuscitation

CHAPTER 19

Support of the airway and ventilation

Learning outcomes

After reading this chapter, you will be able to:
- Describe how to respond to airway and breathing problems with a structured approach
- Recognise equipment that may be used to assess and support airway and breathing

---

19.1 Introduction

Along with control of catastrophic haemorrhage, the management of airway and breathing has priority in the resuscitation of patients of all ages. The rate at which respiratory function can deteriorate in children is particularly high. Effective resuscitation techniques must be applied quickly and in order of priority.

The differences between adults and children must be appreciated, along with familiarity with appropriate paediatric equipment. Techniques for obtaining a patent and protected airway, and for achieving adequate ventilation and oxygenation, must be learned and practised, and competency maintained by repeated practise.

> It should be stressed that basic, simple techniques are often effective and therefore life saving. When this is the case, prolonged or repeated attempts at advanced airway techniques that interrupt ventilation or other ongoing resuscitation may be detrimental.

19.2 Airway and breathing management: principles

In order to respond urgently and yet retain thoroughness, effective emergency management demands a systematic, prioritised approach. As with other aspects of resuscitation, care can be structured into the standard ABCDE phases.

19.3 Primary assessment and resuscitation

This consists of a rapid 'physiological' examination to identify immediately life-threatening emergencies. From the respiratory viewpoint, perform the following assessments:

- Look, listen and feel for airway obstruction, respiratory arrest, depression or distress (NB: should the patient have undergone prior intubation, the correct placement and functioning of the endotracheal tube must be checked by the receiving team at this stage)
- Assess the effort of breathing
- Auscultate for breath sounds, including any stridor
- Assess skin colour

Advanced Paediatric Life Support: A Practical Approach to Emergencies, Sixth Edition. Edited by Martin Samuels and Sue Wieteska.
© 2016 John Wiley & Sons, Ltd. Published 2016 by John Wiley & Sons, Ltd.

If a significant problem is identified, management of that problem should be started immediately. After appropriate interventions have been performed, and their effect assessed, primary assessment can be resumed or repeated.

During this phase, life-saving interventions are performed. In the critically injured or sick child the resuscitation phase and primary assessment occur together, as problems are dealt with as they are found. This may include such procedures as intubation, ventilation, cannulation and fluid resuscitation. At the same time, oxygen is provided, vital signs are recorded and essential monitoring is established.

From the respiratory viewpoint, do the following:

Airway

- Perform basic airway-opening manoeuvres
- Give oxygen at high flow
- Provide suction if necessary
- Place airway adjuncts if necessary
- Proceed to advanced airway management if required

(Should a cervical collar have been placed it should be loosened if it impairs airway access.)

Breathing

- Establish adequate ventilation via a bag–valve–mask
- Intubate if necessary
- Decompress the stomach with a large-bore orogastric or nasogastric tube if necessary
- Perform chest decompression if necessary
- Consider alternative intubation techniques (or, very rarely, surgical airway)
- Monitoring: oxygen saturation monitoring should be initiated, along with capnometry, in an intubated patient

19.4 Secondary assessment

This consists of a thorough physical examination, together with appropriate investigations. Before embarking on this phase, it is important that the resuscitative measures are fully under way.

From the respiratory viewpoint, do the following:

- Perform a detailed examination of the airway, neck and chest
- Identify any swelling, bruising or wounds
- Re-examine for symmetry of chest movement and air entry
- Do not forget to inspect and listen to the back of the chest

19.5 Emergency treatment

All other urgent interventions are included in this phase. If at any time the patient deteriorates, return to the primary assessment and recycle through the system.

19.6 Team aspects of airway management

Team members will generally have agreed roles, with a team leader having a coordinating role. In many paediatric resuscitation teams an anaesthetist or paediatric intensivist will take charge of airway management. As this involves taking a position at the head of the trolley, the person in charge of the airway will also be in charge of protecting and managing the cervical spine if this is necessary. They will have a key role in the coordination of rolling manoeuvres during the secondary survey, and in any subsequent transfer of the patient, for imaging or to intensive care. Being at the patient's head, they will be in a position to see and bring to the team's attention any significant untreated scalp lacerations, which can be a cause of significant blood loss in children. The person managing the airway will need at least one skilled assistant to help with drugs and equipment if advanced airway techniques become necessary.

The decision to embark on intubation or other advanced airway techniques will be taken by the team leader, in full discussion with the member managing the airway and with other team members. Members of the airway team can prepare for intubation while other members of the team complete their part of the secondary survey. Should a person skilled in paediatric airway management not be present then every effort should be made by the team to contact an anaesthetist/Intensivist to discuss the situation and if possible wait for them to arrive before embarking on advanced airway management, except in an emergency.

Following trauma, even if the patient's airway is not compromised by the injury, many severely traumatised children may require early intubation. However, the process of intubation may cause coughing, vomiting and 'bucking', with associated harmful rises in intracranial pressure. In this situation general anaesthesia will be required to perform a smooth intubation. Induction of anaesthesia will make neurological assessment of the patient impossible, so communication between team members is essential in order for an initial neurological assessment to be performed first.

Airway and breathing management protocol (*Continued overleaf*)

Assess the airway and give oxygen

- If dealing with a trauma case:
  - control of major haemorrhage occurs simultaneously
  - consider cervical spine (see Chapters 11 and 15)
- If evidence of obstruction or altered consciousness:
  - perform airway-opening manoeuvres (**common**)
  - consider suction, foreign body removal (**common**)
- If obstruction persists:
  - consider oro- or nasopharyngeal airway or laryngeal mask airway /i-gel (**common**)
- If obstruction still persists:
  - consider intubation (**uncommon**)
- If performed, immediately check position of tracheal tube (auscultation and capnometry)
- If intubation is difficult or impossible:
  - see failed intubation algorithm (see Figure 21.7)
  - consider surgical airway (**very uncommon**)
- If stridor but relatively alert:
  - allow self-ventilation whenever possible
  - encourage oxygen but do not force to wear mask
  - do not force to lie down; sitting on parent's knee may be preferred
  - do not inspect the airway (except as a definitive procedure under controlled conditions)
  - assemble expert team and equipment

Assess the breathing

- If respiratory arrest or depression:
  - administer oxygen by bag–valve–mask
  - SpO_2 monitoring
  - consider supraglottic airway
  - consider intubation
  - check the position of tube if inserted (capnometry and auscultation)
- If sedative or paralysing drugs possible:
  - administer reversal agent
- If respiratory distress or tachypnoea:
  - administer oxygen
- If lateralised ventilatory deficit:
  - consider haemopneumothorax or inhaled foreign body
  - consider lung consolidation, collapse or effusion
- If chest injury:
  - consider tension pneumothorax and haemothorax, flail segment and open pneumothorax
- If evidence of tension pneumothorax:
  - perform immediate needle decompression
  - follow with chest drain
- If evidence of massive haemothorax:
  - insert chest drain
  - commence blood volume replacement, simultaneously if possible

- If wheeze or crackles:
  - consider asthma, bronchiolitis, pneumonia and heart failure
  - remember inhaled foreign body
- If evidence of acute severe asthma:
  - give inhaled or intravenous β-agonists
  - give steroids and consider aminophylline or magnesium
- Continue primary assessment:
  - proceed to assess the circulation and nervous system
- **If deterioration from any cause: reassess airway and breathing**

19.7 Equipment for providing oxygen and ventilation

Oxygen source

A wall oxygen supply (at a pressure of 4 bar, 400 kPa) is provided in most resuscitation rooms. A flow meter capable of delivering at least 15 l/min should be fitted. (Note that in some clinical areas 7 bar outlets may also be found – these are for powering medical equipment such as orthopaedic drills and are not for direct patient use.)

Masks for spontaneous breathing

A mask with a reservoir bag (Figure 19.1) should be used in the first instance so that a high concentration of oxygen is delivered. A simple mask or other device such as a head box may be used later if a high oxygen concentration is no longer required. Nasal prongs are often well tolerated, but they may cause drying of the airway, hence flow rates are limited. Younger children are more susceptible to the drying effect of a non-humidified oxygen supply. Devices providing high-flow, high-humidity inspired gases with air/oxygen blenders permit titration of inspired oxygen levels whilst maintaining high flow rates. These may also provide additional non-invasive respiratory support.

Face masks (for artificial ventilation)

Face masks for mouth-to-mouth or bag–valve–mask ventilation in infants are of two main designs. Some masks are shaped to conform to the anatomy of the child's face and have a low dead space. Circular, soft plastic masks give a good seal and are preferred by many. Clear masks allow the presence of vomit to be seen, and also misting during effective ventilation.

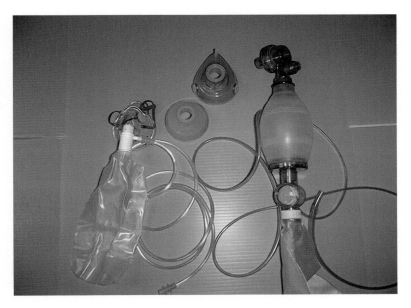

Figure 19.1 Face masks, bag–valve–mask and oxygen mask with reservoir

The pocket mask is a single-size, clear plastic mask with a cushioned rim designed for mouth-to-mask resuscitation. It is often supplied flattened in a rigid case, and needs pushing out into shape before use. It may have a port for attaching to an oxygen supply and can be used in adults and children. By using it upside down it may be used to ventilate an infant.

Self-inflating bags

Self-inflating bags come in three sizes: 250, 500 and 1500 ml. The smallest bag is ineffective except in very small babies. The two smaller sizes usually have a pressure-limiting valve set at 4.5 kPa (45 cmH$_2$O), which may occasionally need to be overridden for high-resistance/low-compliance lungs, but which protects normal lungs from inadvertent barotrauma. The patient end of the bag connects to a one-way valve of a fish-mouth or leaf-flap design. The opposite end has a connection to the oxygen supply and to a reservoir attachment. The reservoir enables high oxygen concentrations to be delivered. Without a reservoir bag, it is difficult to supply more than 50% oxygen to the patient whatever the fresh gas flow, whereas with a reservoir bag and high-flow oxygen, an inspired oxygen concentration of 98% can be achieved. Should the oxygen supply fail, ventilation continues with air.

Anaesthetic breathing systems (e.g. T-piece with open-ended bag)

This equipment may be chosen by those experienced in its use. The T-piece provides useful tactile feedback, and also allows positive end-expiratory pressure (PEEP) to be delivered either by means of an adjustable valve or by the operator varying the degree of occlusion of the bag outlet, often with the little finger. T-pieces are difficult to use by inexperienced operators, particularly if one-handed when the other hand is holding a face mask. High gas flows are necessary to prevent re-breathing, and although T-pieces could be used for patients of any size, in practice they are usually used for infants and sometimes for younger children. The open ended bag on T-piece systems is usually a small size (0.5 or 1 litre) suitable for these smaller patients. Unlike self-inflating bags, they are totally dependent on a pressurised supply of fresh gas. When in use, particularly during transportation, a back-up self-inflating bag should be available in case of gas supply failure.

Mechanical ventilators

A detailed discussion of individual mechanical ventilators is beyond the scope of this book. If a ventilator is used, frequent re-evaluation is necessary, with monitoring of expired CO$_2$ and pulse oximetry.

Chest tubes

These are included because haemothorax or pneumothorax may severely limit ventilation. They are described elsewhere (see Chapter 23).

Gastric tubes

Children are prone to air swallowing and vomiting. Air may also be forced into the stomach during bag–mask ventilation. This may cause vomiting, vagal stimulation and diaphragmatic splinting. A gastric tube will decompress the stomach and significantly improve both breathing and general well-being. Withholding the procedure 'to be kind to the child' may cause more distress than performing it.

19.8 Equipment for managing the airway

Equipment for managing the airway should be available in a variety of sizes and should be present in all resuscitation areas. Complete familiarity with airway equipment should be gained before an emergency occurs.

Airway equipment

- Face masks
- Supraglottic airways (pharyngeal airway, laryngeal mask airway/i-gel))
- Laryngoscopes with a selection of blades
- Tracheal tubes, introduces and connectors
- Suction devices

Assessment and continued monitoring is a vital part of the safe use of an airway device, and appropriate equipment for this should also be available.

Pharyngeal airways

There are two main types of pharyngeal airway:

- Oropharyngeal
- Nasopharyngeal

An oropharyngeal airway, otherwise referred to as an oral airway or Guedel airway, may be used in the unconscious or obtunded patient for short-term airway management. It is frequently used as the first intervention when a patent airway cannot be achieved by manual methods. It provides a patent airway channel between the tongue and the posterior pharyngeal wall. It may also be used to stabilise the position of an oral endotracheal tube following intubation. In a patient with an intact gag reflex it may not be tolerated; in this situation attempted forced insertion may cause vomiting. During use if the patient begins to gag as the level of consciousness improves, the airway should be removed.

A correctly sized airway when placed with its flange at the centre of the incisors, then curved around the face, will reach the angle of the mandible (Figure 19.2). This method of sizing is an estimate only, and a larger or smaller airway should be tried if no immediate improvement is seen. Too small an airway may be ineffective, too large an airway may cause laryngospasm. Either may cause oral trauma or may worsen airway obstruction.

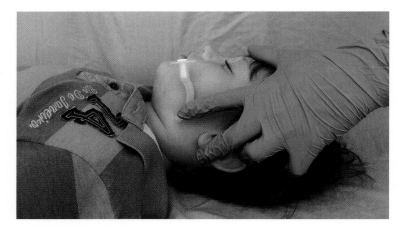

Figure 19.2 Sizing an oropharyngeal airway

A nasopharyngeal airway is often better tolerated than a Guedel airway. It is contraindicated in fractures of the anterior base of the skull. Insertion may cause haemorrhage from the vascular nasal mucosa, especially if it is not well lubricated. A suitable length can be estimated by measuring from the lateral edge of the nostril to the tragus of the ear. An appropriate diameter is one that just fits into the nostril without causing blanching. As small-sized nasopharyngeal airways may not be available, shortened endotracheal tubes may be used with a large safety pin to prevent loss into the nose.

Laryngeal mask airway and related devices

The laryngeal mask airway (LMA) was originally designed for use in elective anaesthesia, but is increasingly used for the management of the airway in emergencies. The LMA has an inflatable elliptical mask that sits around the laryngeal inlet. At the proximal end is a tube similar to a large endotracheal tube, with a pilot tube to inflate the cuff. The original LMAs were reusable, but disposable LMAs and other designs such as the intubating LMA are now available, some designs incorporating a channel for the suctioning of gastric contents.

The i-gel is based on similar design principles to the LMA, but has a soft, gel-like cuff that does not require inflation and a more rigid, flatter tube that may be less prone to rotation after insertion than the round tube of the LMA. It also incorporates a suction channel. Both the LMA and i-gel are available in paediatric sizes (Tables 19.1 and 19.2).

The LMA and i-gel have an established role in many areas, including the emergency department and in pre-hospital care, as they are relatively easy and quick to insert even for non-expert users, particularly the i-gel. Training in their use is still advisable, as in the hands of inexperienced users it is possible for them to be misplaced. Success rates are high in those experienced in their use, and reach near 100% when used electively by anaesthetists. Success rates are lower in infants.

Table 19.1 Laryngeal mask airway (LMA) sizes

Patient weight (kg)	LMA size (standard disposable LMA)	Maximum cuff volume (ml)
<5	1	5
5–10	1.5	7
10–20	2	10
20–30	2.5	15
30–50	3	20
50–70	4	30
>70	5	40

Excepting for the two smallest sizes, maximum cuff inflation volume is given by the formula:

Approx. inflation volume (ml) = (LMA size × 10) − 10

NB Recommended maximum inflation volumes vary slightly between manufacturers and different models of LMA. Check packaging.

Table 19.2 I-gel sizes

Patient weight (kg)	I-gel size
<5	1
5–12	1.5
10–25	2.0
25–35	2.5
30–60	3
50–90	4

Use of these devices may result in less gastric distension than with bag–valve–mask ventilation. This reduces, but does not eliminate, the risk of aspiration: the seal is less effective than the cuff of an endotracheal tube in protecting the trachea against contamination.

Note that the manufacturers' recommended sizes for different patient weights differ slightly between LMAs and i-gels.

Intubation

Intubation should take no longer than approximately 30 seconds, or, as a very rough guide, for how long the operator can hold their breath easily. If intubation has not been achieved within this timescale, or the child is desaturating, the child should be re-ventilated with the bag–valve–mask device before any further intubation attempt is made. Oxygen saturations should not normally fall during intubation.

Laryngoscopes

There are many designs of laryngoscope available for paediatric use, and choice is to some degree a matter of the personal preference of the user. There are two principal design categories: straight bladed and curved bladed. Most blade designs are available in varying sizes. The appropriate size of laryngoscope blade should be chosen for the age of the patient. It is possible to intubate with a blade that is too long but not one that is too short.

The straight-bladed laryngoscope (e.g. Miller, Robertshaw) may be used to directly lift the epiglottis, thereby uncovering the vocal folds. The advantage of this approach is that the epiglottis is moved sufficiently so that it does not obscure the cords.

The curved-bladed laryngoscope (e.g. Macintosh) is designed to move the epiglottis forward by lifting it from in front. The tip of the blade is inserted into the mucosal pocket, known as the vallecula (Figure 19.3), anterior to the epiglottis and the epiglottis is then moved forward by anterior pressure in the vallecula. (This has the possible advantage that less vagal stimulation ensues, as the mucosa of the vallecula is innervated by the glossopharyngeal nerve; however patients should be anaesthetised before intubation, so this should not be a major issue.)

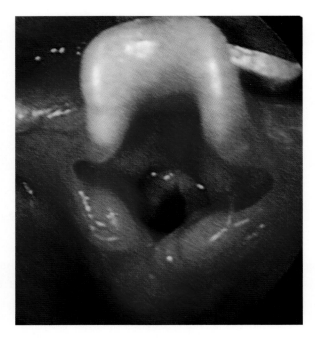

Figure 19.3 View of an infant larynx with a laryngoscope blade in the vallecula

Either technique can be equally effective at obtaining a view of the cords. In practice, either technique may be used with either type of blade according to user preference. Users should simply choose whichever combination of blade design and intubation technique gives the best view of the cords in their hands.

Modern laryngoscopes have a fibreoptic light guide carrying light to the blade from a light source in the handle. This design is replacing the former arrangement whereby small, unreliable and possibly loose light bulbs in the blade were powered by a battery in the handle. As fibreoptic laryngoscopes were introduced, blades and handles from different manufacturers were not necessarily compatible. Current standard designs have green bands in the handle and blade to show compatibility between manufacturers (Figure 19.4).

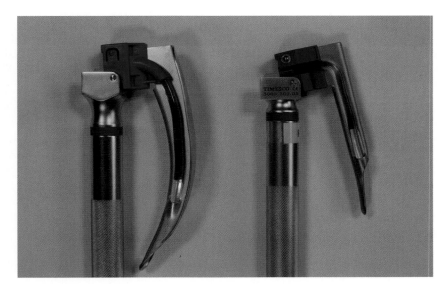

Figure 19.4 Green bands show compatibility between the fibreoptic laryngoscope blade and handle

Despite improvements in the light source, laryngoscope batteries can and do go flat, so like all emergency equipment they should be regularly checked and a spare available.

Tracheal tubes (or endotracheal tubes)

Traditionally it has been taught that uncuffed tubes should be used in paediatrics. Improvements in materials and design, and modern studies of paediatric airway anatomy, have led to a gradual change in this view, and the choice between cuffed and uncuffed tubes for infants and children is largely a matter of availability, preference and any local protocols.

An appropriately sized uncuffed tube should give a relatively gas-tight fit in the larynx but should not be so tight that no leak is audible when inflation is continued to pressures slightly over the maximum normal inflation pressure. Failure to observe this condition may lead to damage to the mucosa at the level of the cricoid ring and to subsequent oedema following extubation. An uncuffed tube that is significantly too small will have a leak of gas around it, possibly leading to difficulty achieving adequate ventilation, as well as possible problems with capnometry. In this situation the patient may need to be reintubated with a more suitably sized tube.

If a cuffed tube is used there will be no audible leak of air during ventilation after the cuff is inflated. However, overinflation of the cuff to excessive pressure may lead to mucosal damage. To prevent this, when possible, cuff pressures should be monitored.

In the circumstance of resuscitation in a young child where the lungs are very 'stiff', for example in severe bronchiolitis, a cuffed tube rather than an uncuffed tube may be preferred but the possible risk of airway damage from the cuff must be balanced against the risk of failure to inflate the lungs.

To estimate endotracheal tube size for emergency intubation use the following formula:

$$\text{Internal diameter (mm)} = (\text{Age} / 4) + 4$$

The age is in whole years, so the formula is appropriate for ages over 1 year. If a cuffed tube is chosen it may be appropriate to calculate the size using:

$$(\text{Age}/4) + 3.5$$

(Some manufacturers place an age guide on the endotracheal tube pack.)

Neonates under 3 kg usually require an uncuffed tube of size 3.0 or 3.5 mm. Pre-term neonates may require a smaller tube.

- Age 6 months – size 4
- Age 1 year – size 4.5

Note that for historical reasons endotracheal tubes are sized by the internal diameter of the tube, not the overall diameter, which will be affected by the wall thickness; this may vary slightly between manufacturer and tube type. Alternative tubes, one larger and one smaller, should always be immediately available.

To estimate endotracheal tube length, use:

$$\text{Length (cm)} = (\text{Age}/2) + 12 \text{ for an oral tube}$$

$$\text{Length (cm)} = (\text{Age}/2) + 15 \text{ for a nasal tube}$$

Knowledge of the predicted length may be of use following intubation to check that the tube has been inserted to approximately the correct length from the lips. This does not replace clinical checks of correct tube placement.

There is a risk in cutting a tube to shorten it to the predicted length. A tube that has been cut to a length that is inappropriately short for a patient may, at best, only enter the trachea for a short distance, and hence be at risk of accidentally slipping out of the trachea. At worst the tube may be too short to even reach the vocal cords, and hence be useless. For emergency use, therefore, it may be best to use a non-shortened tube.

Tracheal tube introducers

While these are not routinely necessary, intubation may be facilitated by the use of a stylet or introducer, placed through the lumen of the tracheal tube. There are two types: soft and flexible or firm and malleable. The former can be allowed to project out of the tip of the tube, as long as it is handled very gently. The latter is used to alter the shape of the tube, but can easily damage the tissues if allowed to protrude from the end of the tracheal tube. Tracheal tube introducers should not be used to force a tracheal tube into position.

It is wise to apply lubrication to the introducer before insertion into the endotracheal tube. This reduces the chance of being in the situation of having achieved tracheal placement of the endotracheal tube, but being unable to withdraw the introducer.

Tracheal tube connectors

In adults, the proximal end of the tube connectors is of standard size, based on the 15–22 mm system, ensuring that they can be connected to a standard self-inflating bag.

The same standard system exists for children, including neonates. Smaller 8.5 mm connectors may be used in some intensive care units (in infants) but should be avoided in the resuscitation setting because of the risk of incompatibility with standard resuscitation equipment.

Magill forceps

Magill forceps are angled to allow a view around the forceps when in the mouth. They may be useful to help position a tube through the cords by lifting it anteriorly, or to remove pharyngeal or supraglottic foreign bodies.

Suction devices

In the resuscitation room the usual suction device is the pipeline vacuum unit. It consists of a suction hose inserted into a wall terminal outlet, a controller (to adjust the vacuum pressure), a reservoir jar, suction tubing and a suitable sucker nozzle or catheter. In order to aspirate vomit effectively, it should be capable of producing a high negative pressure and a high flow rate, although these can be reduced in non-urgent situations, so as not to cause mucosal injury.

The Yankauer sucker is available in both adult and paediatric sizes. It may have a side hole, which can be occluded by a finger, allowing greater control over vacuum pressure. Lack of awareness of the existence of such a side hole may give the impression of suction failure. Vigorous blind sweeping with the hard Yankauer sucker may lead to intraoral damage. Partly for this reason, in small infants, a soft suction catheter and a Y-piece are often preferred, but are less capable of removing vomit.

Portable suction devices are required for resuscitation in remote locations, and for transport to and from the resuscitation room. These are usually battery powered, but foot- and hand-powered versions are also available.

Tracheal suction may be required after intubation to remove bronchial secretions or aspirated fluids. In general, the appropriate size in French gauge of the required catheter is numerically twice the internal diameter in millimetres, e.g. for a 3 mm tube the correct suction catheter is French gauge 6. Use of an excessively large tracheal suction catheter may occlude the tracheal tube, such that all the suction pressure is transmitted to the lungs, encouraging atelectasis.

Equipment for difficult intubations

Very occasionally, for example in the presence of craniofacial abnormalities, it may be difficult to visualise the vocal cords by direct line of sight. Management of the airway should be maintained by face mask with a supraglottic airway (see Chapter 21) or LMA/i-gel.

Should intubation be considered necessary, various further aids to intubation are available. Illuminated stylets or wands have a bright light at the tip. When the tip of the light-wand is in the glottis, a glow can be seen through the soft tissue of the anterior neck, and the endotracheal tube is advanced over the stylet. If the light-wand is in the oesophagus, however, no such transillumination is observed.

Also simple in concept is the intubation LMA, which is placed without direct vision of the larynx, and that then acts as a conduit to lead an endotracheal tube to the vocal cords, through which it is then pushed.

In videolaryngoscopes (e.g. the GlideScope® system) the angled laryngoscope blade has a camera situated at the angle of the blade. The operator holds and manipulates the endotracheal tube in the normal manner, but while visualising the larynx on the device's monitor screen.

The AirTraq® device is akin to a laryngoscope, with a series of prisms in the laryngoscope blade that carry the view from the blade tip to an optical eyepiece, or to a monitor screen. A channel in the handle and blade of the device guides the endotracheal tube.

In fibreoptic intubating bronchoscopes the endotracheal tube is initially placed over the flexible fibreoptic shaft. The shaft is then inserted through the mouth or nose, or alternatively inserted through an LMA that is already in place. The operator sees the view at the tip on a screen or though the bronchoscope eyepiece. Controls on the handle alter the configuration of the shaft while advancing it towards the vocal cords. Once the bronchoscope is through the vocal cords the endotracheal tube is advanced over it into the trachea.

The above devices have a significant associated learning curve. So, while these are useful aids in experienced hands, there is no place for the uninitiated to 'have a go' for the first time once a real airway emergency has developed.

19.9 Monitoring an intubated patient

Immediately following intubation, the following checks should be performed. These checks should also be performed when taking over an intubated patient, such as following an out of hospital intubation.

- Attach a pulse oximeter (if not already in place).
- Connect a capnometer if available.
- Auscultate the patient in both axillae and over the stomach.
- Pulse oximetry assesses patient oxygenation, not ventilation. In the event of a misplaced (i.e. oesophageal) endotracheal tube, the saturations may only drop slowly, not immediately. Thus pulse oximetry has limited use as a rapid check of correct intubation.
- Capnometers respond rapidly to falls in expired CO_2 and immediately indicate the absence of expired CO_2. Hence capnometry is the gold standard monitor for correct intubation: lack of expired CO_2 suggests oesophageal intubation.

When monitoring a ventilated patient, a sudden drop in expired CO_2 to zero indicates an equipment problem such as a disconnection in the breathing system, extubation or ventilator failure.

A more gradual fall in expired CO_2 suggests a patient problem such as a drop in cardiac output due to cardiac arrest, inadequate external cardiac compressions or pulmonary embolism. As the lungs are still ventilated, expired CO_2 falls more slowly as CO_2 is washed out of the lungs over several breaths.

Limits of capnometry

- There may be little or no CO_2 output in low or zero cardiac output states.
- Capnometry may not detect endobronchial intubation. Endobronchial intubation may be suspected by asymmetrical chest movement following intubation, and should be detected by auscultation.
- Ventilation of a patient with an uncuffed endotracheal tube that is significantly too small may result in a large leak with expiration around the tube rather than through it, especially if PEEP is used. As no expired gases are flowing through the breathing system, the capnometer may give a misleadingly low or even zero reading.
- Auscultation should be performed over both axillae, as in small patients breath sounds may transmit from one side of the chest to the other. Auscultation is also performed over the stomach, as the sound of air entry into the stomach may be misinterpreted as lung air entry unless the stomach is auscultated as well for comparison.

Airway and ventilator problems in an intubated patient

The DOPE mnemonic may aid assessment of potential causes (Table 19.3):

D – Displaced (endobronchial or oesophageal) endotracheal tube.
O – Obstructed endotracheal tube (blocked or kinked).
P – Pneumothorax.
E – Equipment problems (may include ventilator problems, leaks, breathing system disconnection, oxygen supply failure or disconnection).

Table 19.3 DOPE mnemonic for airway and ventilator problems in intubated patients

DOPE	Problem		Action
D Displaced endotracheal tube (ETT)	Tracheal tube is endobronchial	Asymmetrical chest movements, unilateral breath sounds, SpO_2 falling	Slightly withdraw ETT, re-auscultate
	Tracheal tube is oesophageal	Capnometry – no end tidal CO_2	Remove ETT, mask ventilate, prepare for reintubation
O Obstructed ETT	Kinked tube Plugged tube (mucus, blood)	Examine visible part of tube for kinks Have high index of suspicion of tube plugging if patient with small ETT has been ventilated with non-humidified gases. Thick mucus plugs may form near tube tip	Straighten tube, fix securely Suction full length of tube If not resolved: remove ETT, mask ventilate, prepare for reintubation
P Pneumothorax	Tension pneumothorax	See Chapters 12 and 23 High peak ventilator pressure, rapid decline in SpO_2 and cardiac output	Needle decompression
E Equipment	Equipment problems	Check breathing system for disconnection, leaks, oxygen supply, ventilator function. Check for deflated ETT cuff	If problem not immediately obvious, hand ventilate while equipment checked

19.10 Management of a blocked tracheostomy (Figure 19.5)

Many children with an established tracheostomy will improve when the blocked tube is removed, allowing them to breathe through the stoma prior to replacing the blocked tube with a new one. However, there are risks in removing the tube from a newly created tracheostomy as, until the stoma track is established, attempted replacement of a tracheostomy tube may be difficult and a blind-ending false track could be created.

Parents who routinely care for their child's tracheostomy at home may be more familiar with tube suction and tube changing for their child than hospital staff in medical areas where this is rarely performed.

Procedure
Commence basic life support.
1. Stimulate the child.
2. Shout for help.
3. Open and check airway with a head tilt/chin lift. This exposes the tracheostomy tube and opens the upper airway.
4. Apply oxygen to the face and tracheostomy.
5. Assess patency of the tracheostomy using a suction catheter.
6. If you are unable to pass the suction catheter through the tracheostomy tube, then the tube must be changed immediately with the same size tube. If this fails to relieve the obstruction, or you cannot insert it:
   - Try a half size smaller tube.
   - If it is not possible to insert this, thread a lubricated suction catheter through the size smaller tracheostomy tube. Insert the suction catheter into the stoma and then attempt to guide the new tracheostomy tube along the catheter and into the stoma.
   - If this is unsuccessful then remove the tracheostomy tube.
7. Check for breathing. Look, listen, feel: Place the side of your face over the tracheostomy tube or patient's face to listen and feel for any breaths, and at the same time look at the child's chest to observe any breathing movement. If the child is breathing satisfactorily, place them in the recovery position and continue to assess. If the child is not breathing, you will have to give rescue breaths.
8. Give five rescue breaths.
9. If you have succeeded in removing the obstructed tracheostomy and replaced it with a patent tracheostomy tube you should attach a self-inflating bag and ventilate (or, if that is not available, perform mouth-to-tracheostomy ventilation).
10. If you have failed to replace the tracheostomy tube:
   - If the child has a fully or partially patent upper airway, occlude the tracheal stoma and provide rescue breaths via the mouth by bag–valve–mask or mouth to mouth.
   - If the child does not have a patent upper airway these resuscitation breaths are applied directly to the stoma.

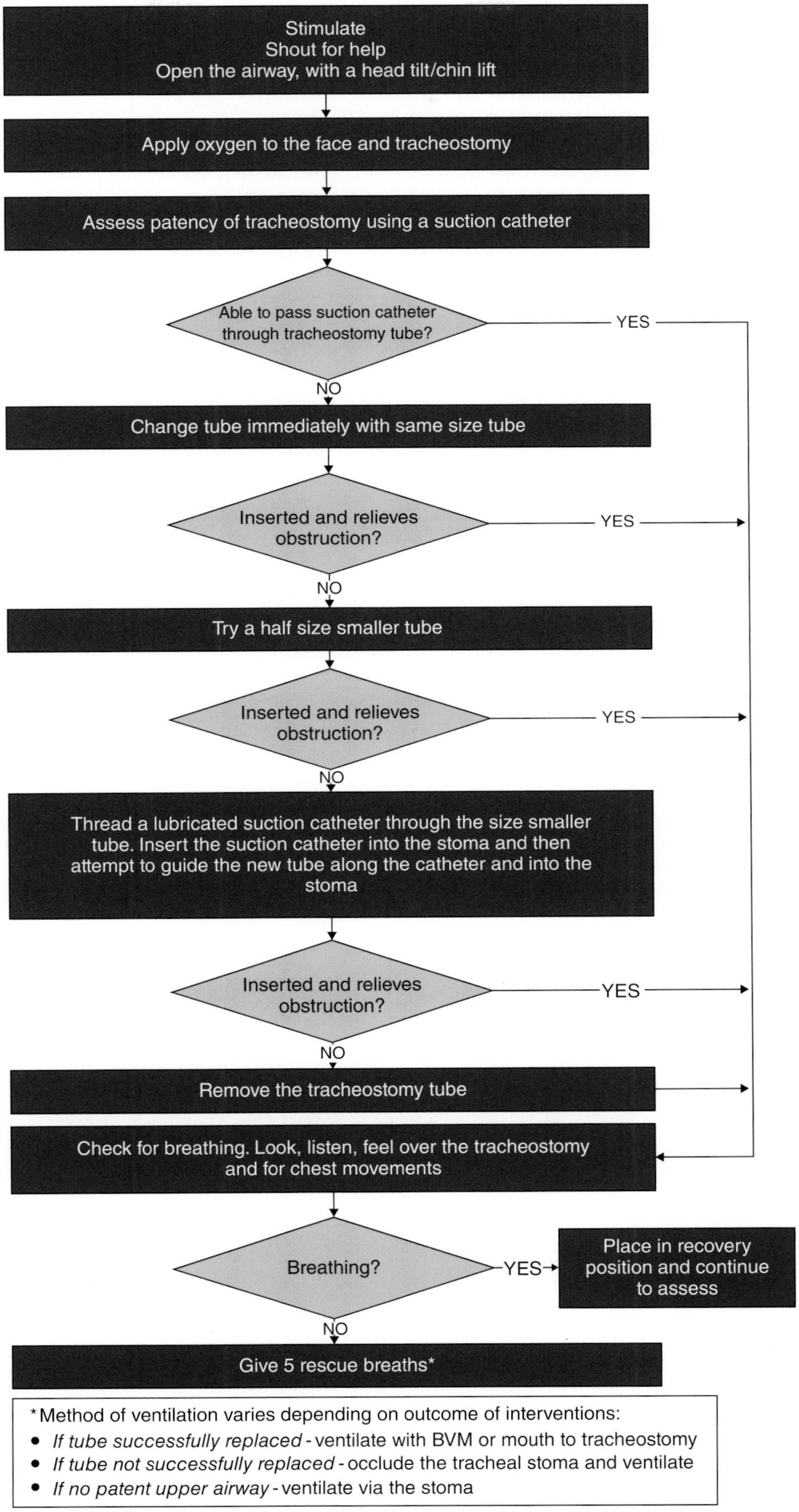

```
┌─────────────────────────────────────────────┐
│                 Stimulate                     │
│               Shout for help                  │
│   Open the airway, with a head tilt/chin lift │
└─────────────────────────────────────────────┘
                      │
                      ▼
┌─────────────────────────────────────────────┐
│      Apply oxygen to the face and tracheostomy│
└─────────────────────────────────────────────┘
                      │
                      ▼
┌─────────────────────────────────────────────┐
│  Assess patency of tracheostomy using a       │
│  suction catheter                             │
└─────────────────────────────────────────────┘
                      │
                      ▼
             ◇ Able to pass suction catheter ◇ ──── YES ──────┐
               through tracheostomy tube?                      │
                      │ NO                                     │
                      ▼                                        │
┌─────────────────────────────────────────────┐               │
│     Change tube immediately with same size    │               │
│     tube                                      │               │
└─────────────────────────────────────────────┘               │
                      │                                        │
                      ▼                                        │
             ◇ Inserted and relieves ◇ ──── YES ──────────────┤
               obstruction?                                    │
                      │ NO                                     │
                      ▼                                        │
┌─────────────────────────────────────────────┐               │
│         Try a half size smaller tube          │               │
└─────────────────────────────────────────────┘               │
                      │                                        │
                      ▼                                        │
             ◇ Inserted and relieves ◇ ──── YES ──────────────┤
               obstruction?                                    │
                      │ NO                                     │
                      ▼                                        │
┌─────────────────────────────────────────────┐               │
│ Thread a lubricated suction catheter through  │               │
│ the size smaller tube. Insert the suction     │               │
│ catheter into the stoma and then attempt to   │               │
│ guide the new tube along the catheter and     │               │
│ into the stoma                                │               │
└─────────────────────────────────────────────┘               │
                      │                                        │
                      ▼                                        │
             ◇ Inserted and relieves ◇ ──── YES ──────────────┤
               obstruction?                                    │
                      │ NO                                     │
                      ▼                                        │
┌─────────────────────────────────────────────┐               │
│        Remove the tracheostomy tube           │               │
└─────────────────────────────────────────────┘               │
                      │                                        │
                      ▼                                        │
┌─────────────────────────────────────────────┐               │
│ Check for breathing. Look, listen, feel over  │◄──────────────┘
│ the tracheostomy and for chest movements      │
└─────────────────────────────────────────────┘
                      │
                      ▼
             ◇ Breathing? ◇ ──── YES ──► ┌──────────────────┐
                      │ NO               │ Place in recovery │
                      ▼                  │ position and      │
┌─────────────────────────────────────┐ │ continue to assess│
│      Give 5 rescue breaths*          │ └──────────────────┘
└─────────────────────────────────────┘
```

┌───┐
│ *Method of ventilation varies depending on outcome of   │
│ interventions: │
│ • *If tube successfully replaced* - ventilate with BVM or   │
│   mouth to tracheostomy   │
│ • *If tube not successfully replaced* - occlude the tracheal   │
│   stoma and ventilate   │
│ • *If no patent upper airway* - ventilate via the stoma   │
└───┘

Figure 19.5 Management of a blocked tracheostomy. [BVM, bag–valve–mask]

Emergency equipment for tracheostomy change

- Usual size tracheostomy tube with tapes attached
- Half size smaller tracheostomy tube with tapes attached
- Suction catheter of appropriate size
- Resuscitation trolley: self-inflating bag and face masks, oxygen sources, simple airway adjuncts such as oropharyngeal airways, nasopharyngeal airways and laryngeal mask airways
- Scissors
- Spare tape
- Gauze swab
- Gloves

For more information see the UK National Tracheostomy Safety Project: www.tracheostomy.org.uk

Surgical airway: cricothyroidotomy cannulae and ventilation systems

Purpose-made cricothyroidotomy cannulae are available, usually in three sizes: 12 gauge for an adult, 14 gauge for a child and 18 gauge for a baby. They are less liable to kinking than intravenous cannulae and have a flange for suturing or securing to the neck.

In an emergency, an intravenous cannula can be inserted through the cricothyroid membrane and oxygen insufflated at 1 l/per year of age/min to provide some oxygenation (but no ventilation). A side hole can be cut in the oxygen tubing or a Y-connector can be placed between the cannula and the oxygen supply, to allow intermittent occlusion and achieve partial ventilation, as described in Chapter 21.

Needle crycothroidotomy is a technique of last resort to be used only in an emergency, and has a significant failure rate, as the cricothyroid membrane is difficult to feel in young patients. Many ENT surgeons, if present, will prefer an open tracheostomy (see Chapter 21).

19.11 Summary

Along with control of catastrophic haemorrhage, the management of airway and breathing has priority in the resuscitation of patients of all ages. The rate at which respiratory function can deteriorate in children is particularly high. Effective resuscitation techniques must be applied quickly and in order of priority.

You should now be able to:

- Describe how to respond to airway and breathing problems with a structured approach
- Recognise equipment that may be used to assess and support airway and breathing

CHAPTER 20
Management of cardiac arrest

Learning outcomes

After reading this chapter, you will be able to:
- Demonstrate how to assess the cardiac arrest rhythm and perform advanced life support

20.1 Introduction

Cardiac arrest has occurred when there is no effective cardiac output. Before any specific therapy is started, effective basic life support (BLS) must be established as described in Chapter 18. The cardiac arrest algorithm is shown in Figure 20.1.

Four cardiac arrest rhythms will be discussed in this chapter:

1. Asystole.
2. Pulseless electrical activity (including electromechanical dissociation).
3. Ventricular fibrillation.
4. Pulseless ventricular tachycardia.

The four are divided into two groups: two that do not require defibrillation (called 'non-shockable') and two that do require defibrillation ('shockable').

20.2 Non-shockable rhythms

This includes asystole and pulseless electrical activity (PEA).

Asystole

This is the most common arrest rhythm in children, because the response of the young heart to prolonged severe hypoxia and acidosis is progressive bradycardia leading to asystole (Figure 20.2). An ECG will distinguish asystole from ventricular fibrillation, ventricular tachycardia and PEA. The ECG appearance of ventricular asystole is an almost straight line; occasionally P-waves are seen. Check that the appearance is not caused by an artefact, e.g. a loose wire or disconnected electrode. Turn up the gain on the ECG monitor.

Pulseless electrical activity

This is the absence of signs of life or a palpable pulse despite the presence on the ECG monitor of recognisable complexes that normally produce perfusion (Figure 20.3). PEA is treated in the same way as asystole and is often a pre-asystolic state.

PEA may be due to an identifiable and reversible cause. In children the most common causes are hypovolaemia and hypoxia. Trauma is also most often associated with a reversible cause of PEA. This may be due to severe hypovolaemia, tension pneumothorax or pericardial tamponade. PEA is also seen in hypothermic patients and in patients with electrolyte abnormalities, including hypocalcaemia from calcium channel blocker overdose. Rarely in children, it may be seen after massive pulmonary thromboembolus.

Advanced Paediatric Life Support: A Practical Approach to Emergencies, Sixth Edition. Edited by Martin Samuels and Sue Wieteska.
© 2016 John Wiley & Sons, Ltd. Published 2016 by John Wiley & Sons, Ltd.

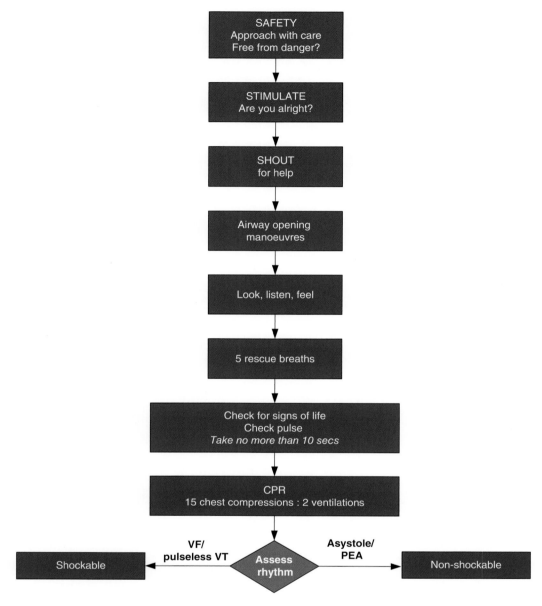

Figure 20.1 Cardiac arrest algorithm. [CPR, cardiopulmonary resuscitation; PEA, pulseless electrical activity; VF, ventricular fibrillation; VT, ventricular tachycardia]

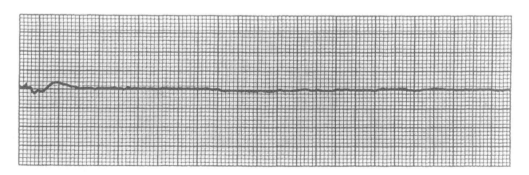

Figure 20.2 Asystole

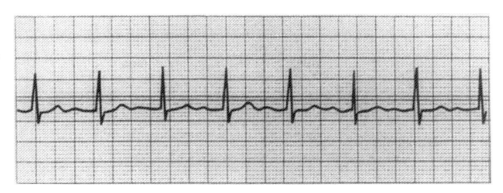

Figure 20.3 Pulseless electrical activity

Management of asystole/PEA

The first essential is to establish ventilations and chest compressions effectively. Ventilations are provided initially by bag-and-mask with high-concentration oxygen. Ensure a patent airway, initially using an airway manoeuvre to open the airway and stabilising it with an airway adjunct.

Provide effective chest compressions at a rate of 100–120 per minute with a compression : ventilation ratio of 15:2. The depth of compression should be at least one-third of the anteroposterior diameter of the chest (4 cm for infants, 5 cm for children). The child should have a cardiac monitor attached and the heart's rhythm assessed.

Although the procedures to stabilise the airway and gain circulatory access are now described sequentially, they should be undertaken simultaneously under the direction of a resuscitation team leader. The role of the team leader is to co-ordinate care and to anticipate problems in the sequence. If asystole or PEA is identified give adrenaline 10 micrograms/kg IV or IO. Adrenaline is the first line drug for asystole. Through α-adrenergic-mediated vasoconstriction, its action is to increase aortic diastolic pressure during chest compressions and thus coronary perfusion pressure and the delivery of oxygenated blood to the heart. It also enhances the contractile state of the heart and stimulates spontaneous contractions. The IV or IO dose is 10 micrograms/kg (0.1 ml/kg of 1:10 000 solution). Whenever venous access is not attainable within 1 minute, intraosseous access should be used. Central lines provide more secure long-term access, but compared to IO or peripheral IV access, offer no advantages. In each case the adrenaline is followed by a normal saline flush (2–5 ml).

As soon as is feasible a skilled and experienced operator should intubate the child's airway. This will both control and protect the airway and enable chest compressions to be given continuously, thus improving coronary perfusion. Both cuffed and uncuffed tracheal tubes are acceptable for infants and children undergoing emergency intubation (see Chapters 19 and 21). Once the child has been intubated and compressions are uninterrupted, the ventilation rate should be 10–12 per minute. It is important for the team leader to assess that the ventilations remain adequate when chest compressions are continuous. This is most proficiently done by the person doing the chest compressions who can feel the chest moving when ventilated. The protocol for asystole and PEA is shown in Figure 20.4.

During and following the administration of adrenaline, chest compressions and ventilations should continue. It is vital that chest compressions and ventilations continue uninterrupted during advanced life support as they form the basis of the resuscitative effort. The only reason to interrupt BLS is to shock the patient if needed and to check the rhythm. It may be necessary to briefly interrupt BLS during difficult intubation. Giving chest compressions is tiring for the operator so the team leader should change the operator every few minutes and continuously ensure that the compressions are achieving the recommended rate of 100–120 compressions per minute together with a depression of the chest wall by at least one-third of the anteroposterior diameter of the chest or by 4 cm for infants and 5 cm for children.

At intervals of 2 minutes briefly pause in the delivery of chest compressions to assess the rhythm on the monitor. If asystole remains, continue CPR while again checking the electrode position and contacts. If there is an organised rhythm, check for signs of life and for a pulse. If there a return of spontaneous circulation (ROSC), continue post-resuscitation care, increasing ventilations to 12–24 breaths per minute according to age. If there are no signs of life and no pulse continue the protocol. Give adrenaline every 4 minutes at a dose of 10 micrograms/kg.

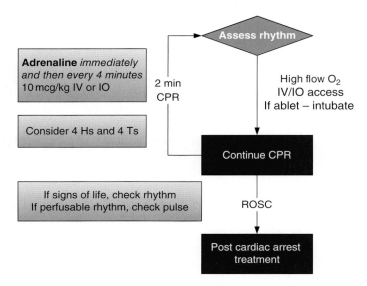

Figure 20.4 Protocol for asystole and pulseless electrical activity. [CPR, cardiopulmonary resuscitation; ROSC, return of spontaneous circulation]

Reversible causes

Continually during CPR consider and correct reversible causes of the cardiac arrest based on the history of the event, known underlying illness in the child and any clues that are found during resuscitation. The causes of cardiac arrest in infancy and childhood are multifactorial but the two commonest pathways are through hypoxia and hypovolaemia.

All factors are conveniently remembered as the **4Hs and 4Ts**:

- Hypoxia is a prime cause of cardiac arrest in childhood and is key to successful resuscitation.
- Hypovolaemia may be significant in arrests associated with trauma, anaphylaxis and sepsis and requires infusion of crystalloid (see Chapter 11).
- Hyperkalaemia, hypokalaemia, hypocalcaemia and other metabolic abnormalities may be suggested by the patient's underlying condition (e.g. renal failure), tests taken during the resuscitation or clues given in the ECG (see Appendices A and B). Intravenous calcium (0.3 ml/kg of 10% calcium gluconate) is indicated in hyperkalaemia, hypocalcaemia and calcium channel blocker overdose.
- Hypothermia is associated with drowning incidents and requires particular care: a low reading thermometer must be used to detect it (see Chapter 17).
- Tension pneumothorax and cardiac tamponade are especially associated with PEA and are found in trauma cases (see Chapter 12).
- Toxic substances either as a result of accidental or deliberate overdose or from an iatrogenic mistake may require specific antidotes (see Appendix E).
- Thromboembolic phenomena are rare events in children.

Adrenaline dosage

Adrenaline has been used for many years although its place has never been subjected to trial against placebo in children. In adults one prospective randomised study of drugs, including adrenaline, showed an improvement in ROSC but no increase in long-term neurologically intact survival. Another study with adrenaline against placebo showed similar results, but the number of patients was too low to make significant changes. The use of adrenaline is supported by animal studies and its known effects in improving relative coronary and cerebral perfusion. There was a trend to the use of higher doses of adrenaline in past years but evidence now links high dosage to poorer outcome, especially in asphyxial arrests.

Alkalising agents

Children with asystole will be acidotic as cardiac arrest has usually been preceded by respiratory arrest or shock. However, the routine use of alkalising agents has not been shown to be of benefit. Sodium bicarbonate therapy increases intracellular carbon dioxide levels so administration, if used at all, should follow assisted ventilation with oxygen and effective BLS. Once ventilation is ensured and adrenaline plus chest compressions are provided to maximise circulation, use of sodium bicarbonate may be considered for the patient with prolonged cardiac arrest. These agents should be administered only in cases where profound acidosis is likely to adversely affect the action of adrenaline. In addition, sodium bicarbonate is recommended in the treatment of patients with hyperkalaemia (see Appendix B) and tricyclic antidepressant overdose (see Appendix E).

In the arrested patient, arterial pH does not correlate well with tissue pH. Mixed venous or central venous pH should be used to guide any further alkalising therapy and it should always be remembered that good BLS is more effective than alkalising agents at raising myocardial pH.

Bicarbonate is the most common alkalising agent currently available, the dose being 1 mmol/kg (1 ml/kg of an 8.4% solution). If it must be used:

- Bicarbonate must not be given in the same intravenous line as calcium because precipitation will occur
- Sodium bicarbonate inactivates adrenaline and dopamine and therefore the line must be flushed with saline if these drugs are subsequently given

Calcium

In the past, calcium was recommended in the treatment of PEA and asystole, but there is no evidence for its efficacy and there is evidence for harmful effects as calcium is implicated in cytoplasmic calcium accumulation in the final common pathway of cell death. This results from calcium entering cells following ischaemia and during reperfusion of ischaemic organs. Administration of calcium in the resuscitation of asystolic patients is not recommended. Calcium is indicated only for treatment of documented hypocalcaemia and hyperkalaemia, and for the treatment of hypermagnesaemia and of calcium channel blocker overdose.

Atropine

Atropine has no place in the management of cardiac arrest. Its use is to combat excessive vagal tone causing bradycardia in the perfusing patient.

20.3 Shockable rhythms

This includes ventricular fibrillation (VF) and pulseless ventricular tachycardia (pVT). ECGs showing VF and pVT are shown in Figures 20.5 and 20.6, respectively.

These arrhythmias are less common in children but either may be expected in sudden collapse, in those suffering from hypothermia, in those poisoned by tricyclic antidepressants and in those with cardiac disease. The protocol for VF and pulseless VT is the same and is shown in Figure 20.7.

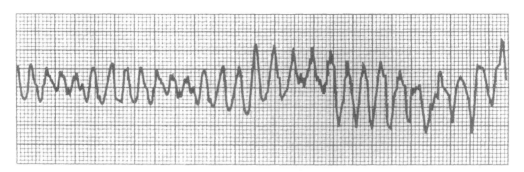

Figure 20.5 Ventricular fibrillation

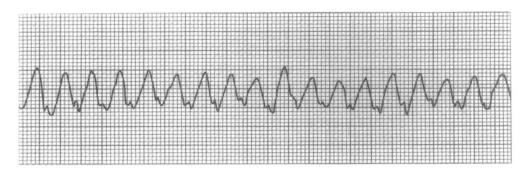

Figure 20.6 Pulseless ventricular tachycardia

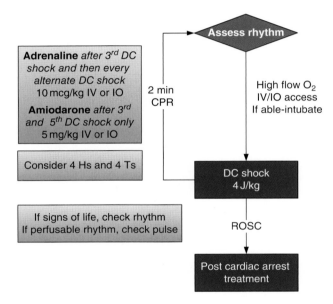

Figure 20.7 Protocol for ventricular fibrillation and ventricular tachycardia. [CPR, cardiopulmonary resuscitation; ROSC, return of spontaneous circulation]

There is little direct evidence for the best approach to cardiac arrest from VF/pVT in children. The guidance is based on that developed for adults, although it is recognised that the pathology causing VF/pVT arrest in children is both less common and more varied than that in adults. Recognised causes of VF/pVT in children include underlying cardiac disease, usually congenital, hypothermia and some drug overdoses. A sudden witnessed collapse is also suggestive of a VF/pVT episode.

The guidance here is for non-experts in paediatric cardiology. In the paediatric cardiac intensive care unit, theatre or catheter laboratory, patient treatment should be individualised appropriately. If the patient is being monitored, the rhythm can be identified before significant deterioration. With immediate identification of VF/pVT, asynchronous electrical defibrillation of 4 joules per kilogram (J/kg) should be carried out immediately and the protocol continued as below.

In unmonitored children, BLS will have been started in response to the collapse and the identification of VF/pVT will occur when the cardiac monitor is put in place. An asynchronous shock of 4 J/kg should be given immediately and CPR immediately resumed without reassessing the rhythm or feeling for a pulse. Immediate resumption of CPR is vital because there is a pause between successful defibrillation and the appearance of a rhythm on the monitor. Cessation of chest compressions will reduce the chance of a successful outcome if a further shock is needed. No harm accrues from 'unnecessary' compressions.

Appropriately sized adhesive defibrillation pads should be used. Recommended sizes are 4.5 cm for children <10 kg and 8–12 cm for children >10 kg. One pad is placed over the apex in the mid-axillary line, whilst the other is put immediately below the clavicle just to the right of the sternum. If only adult pads are available or your pads are too large for the infant/child, one should be placed on the upper back, below the left scapula, and the other on the front, to the left of the sternum. In the event of a neonate requiring defibrillation, commercially available paediatric pads are not sufficiently small enough and in a paediatric centre manual defibrillation paddles with paediatric attachments should be available.

Automated external defibrillators (AEDs) are now commonplace. If a manual defibrillator is not available use an AED with standard adult shock for children over 8 years. For children under 8 years, attenuated paediatric pads should be used with the AED.

For the infant of less than 1 year, a manual defibrillator that can be adjusted to give the correct shock is recommended. However, if an AED is the only defibrillator available, its use should be considered, preferably with paediatric attenuation pads. The order of decreasing preference for defibrillation in the under 1-year-olds is as follows:

1. Manual defibrillator.
2. AED with dose attenuator.
3. AED without dose attenuator.

Many AEDs can detect VF/pVT in children of all ages and differentiate 'shockable' from 'non-shockable' rhythms with a high degree of sensitivity and specificity.

If the shock fails to defibrillate, attention must revert to supporting coronary and cerebral perfusion as in asystole. Although the procedures to stabilise the airway and gain circulatory access are now described sequentially, they should be undertaken simultaneously under the direction of a resuscitation team leader.

The airway should be secured, the patient ventilated with high-flow oxygen and effective chest compressions continued at a rate of 100–120 per minute, a compression depth of at least one-third of the anteroposterior diameter of the chest or 4 cm for infants and by 5 cm for children and a ratio of 15 compressions to two ventilations. As soon as is feasible, a skilled and experienced operator should intubate the child's airway. This will both control and protect the airway and enable chest compressions to be given continuously, thus improving coronary perfusion. Once the child has been intubated and compressions are uninterrupted, the ventilation rate should be 10–12 per minute. It is important for the team leader to assess that the ventilations remain adequate when chest compressions are continuous. Gain circulatory access. Whenever venous access is not attainable within 1 minute, intraosseous access should be used as it is rapid and effective. Central lines provide more secure long-term access, but compared to IO or peripheral IV access, offer no advantages. In each case any drug is followed by a normal saline flush (2–5 ml).

Two minutes after the first shock, pause chest compressions briefly to check the monitor. If VF/pVT is still present, give a second shock of 4 J/kg and immediately resume CPR commencing with chest compressions. Consider and correct reversible causes (4Hs and 4Ts) while continuing CPR for a further 2 minutes. Pause briefly to check the monitor.

If the rhythm is still VF/pVT give a third shock of 4 J/kg. Resume chest compressions immediately and, once established, give adrenaline 10 micrograms/kg and amiodarone 5 mg/kg IV or IO, flushing after each drug. After completion of the 2 minutes of CPR, pause briefly to check the monitor and if the rhythm is still VF/pVT give an immediate fourth shock of 4 J/kg and resume CPR.

After a further 2 minutes of CPR, pause briefly to check the monitor and if the rhythm is still shockable, give an immediate fifth shock of 4 J/kg. Resume chest compressions immediately and, once established, give a second dose of adrenaline 10 micrograms/kg and a second dose of amiodarone 5 mg/kg intravenously or intraosseously. After completion of the 2 minutes of CPR, pause briefly before the next shock to check the monitor. Continue giving shocks every 2 minutes, minimising the pauses in CPR as much as possible. Give adrenaline after every alternate shock (i.e. every 4 minutes) and continue to seek and treat reversible causes.

Note: after each 2 minutes of uninterrupted CPR, pause briefly to assess the rhythm on the monitor. In addition, if at any time there are signs of life, such as regular respiratory effort, coughing, eye opening or a sudden increase in end tidal CO_2, stop CPR and check the monitor:

- If still VF/pVT, continue with the sequence as above
- If asystole, change to the asystole/PEA sequence
- If organised electrical activity is seen, check for signs of life and a pulse; if there is ROSC, continue post resuscitation care. If there is no pulse (or a pulse below 60 beats/min with no signs of circulation) and no other signs of life continue the asystole/PEA sequence

Antiarrhythmic drugs

Amiodarone is the treatment of choice in shock-resistant VF and pVT. This is based on evidence from adult cardiac arrest and experience with the use of amiodarone in children in the catheterisation laboratory setting. The dose of amiodarone for VF/pVT is 5 mg/kg via rapid intravenous bolus.

In VF/pVT caused by an overdose of an arrhythmogenic drug, the use of amiodarone should be omitted. Expert advice should be obtained from a poisons centre. Amiodarone is likely to be unhelpful in the setting of VF caused by hypothermia but may be used, nevertheless.

Lidocaine (lignocaine) is an alternative to amiodarone. The dose is 1 mg/kg IV or IO. It is the DC shock that converts the heart back to a perfusing rhythm, not the drug. The purpose of the antiarrhythmic drug is to stabilise the converted rhythm and the purpose of adrenaline is to improve myocardial oxygenation by increasing coronary perfusion pressure. Adrenaline also increases the vigour and intensity of ventricular fibrillation, which increases the success of defibrillation.

Magnesium 25–50 mg/kg (maximum of 2 g) is indicated in children with hypomagnesaemia or with polymorphic VT (torsades de pointes), regardless of cause.

Reversible causes

During CPR consider and correct reversible causes of the cardiac arrest based on the history of the event and any clues that are found during resuscitation. These factors are remembered as the 4Hs and 4Ts (see full list earlier in chapter).

If there is still resistance to defibrillation, different paddle positions or another defibrillator may be tried. In the infant in whom paediatric paddles have been used, larger paddles applied to the front and back of the chest may be an alternative.

If the rhythm initially converts and then deteriorates back to VF or pVT then the sequence should continue to cycle, omitting a further dose of amiodarone if two have already been given. If further amiodarone is thought necessary an infusion should be given of 300 micrograms/kg/h to a maximum of 1.5 mg/kg/h to a maximum of 1.2 g in 24 hours.

Automatic external defibrillators

The introduction of AEDs in the pre-hospital setting and especially for public access has significantly improved the outcome for VF/pVT cardiac arrest in adults in some situations. In the pre-hospital setting, AEDs are commonly used in adults to assess cardiac rhythm and to deliver defibrillation. Many AEDs can detect VF/pVT in children of all ages and differentiate 'shockable' from 'non-shockable' rhythms with a high degree of sensitivity and specificity. Thus, if an AED is the only defibrillator available, its use should be considered (preferably with the paediatric pads) as described earlier.

These devices have paediatric attenuation pads that decrease the energy to a level more appropriate for the child (1–8 years) or leads reducing the total energy to 50–80 joules. For the infant of less than 1 year, a manual defibrillator that can be adjusted to give the correct shock is recommended. However, if an AED is the only defibrillator available, its use should be considered, preferably with paediatric attenuation pads.

Modern defibrillators now use biphasic wave forms. Defibrillation appears to be as effective at lower energy doses as conventional wave forms in adults and the energy appears to cause less myocardial damage than monophasic shocks. Both monophasic and biphasic wave form defibrillators are acceptable for use in childhood.

Capnography

Monitoring of end-tidal CO_2 (ETCO$_2$) can be helpful in managing cardiac arrest as long as the operator appreciates that the absence of a waveform is more likely to be due to absent or very poor pulmonary perfusion than to tube misplacement. The presence of exhaled CO_2 during CPR is encouraging evidence of efficacy of the CPR or even ROSC. Adrenaline will decrease and bicarbonate increase the measured CO_2. Levels of less than 2 kPa (15 mmHg) should prompt attention to chest compression adequacy.

Oxygen use

While 100% oxygen, when available, remains the recommendation for use during the resuscitation process outside the delivery room, once there is ROSC this can be detrimental to recovering tissues from hyperoxia. Pulse oximetry should be used to monitor and adjust for oxygen requirement after a successful resuscitation. Saturations should then be maintained between 94% and 98%.

Therapeutic hypothermia

Recent data suggest that there is some evidence that post-arrest hypothermia (core temperatures of 32–34°C) may have beneficial effects on neurological recovery in adults and newborns. Current paediatric post arrest recommendations are either to cool to 32–34°C for at least 24 hours (mild hypothermia) or actively maintain normothermia (36–37.5°C). Conversely, increased core temperature increases metabolic demand by 10–13% for each degree centigrade increase in temperature above normal. Therefore, in the post-arrest patient, hyperthermia should be treated with active cooling to achieve a normal core temperature. Shivering should be prevented since it will increase metabolic demand. Sedation may be adequate to control shivering, but neuromuscular blockade may be needed. See also Chapter 17 on drowning.

Hypoglycaemia

All children, especially infants, can become hypoglycaemic when seriously ill. Blood glucose should be checked frequently and hypoglycaemia corrected carefully (see Chapter 6). It is important not to cause hyperglycaemia as this will promote an osmotic diuresis. Both hypoglycaemia and hyperglycaemia are associated with a worse neurological outcome in animal models of cardiac arrest.

Resuscitation of the newborn outside the delivery room

As there are some significant differences in the recommendations for resuscitation at birth and resuscitation of the infant and child, a dilemma presents itself to the clinician confronted with the collapsed neonate outside the delivery room. There is no research in this area, so current guidance is to recommend that providers use the resuscitation protocol with which they are familiar, i.e. the newborn protocol in the newborn intensive care unit (NICU) and the infant and child protocol in other areas (the PICU, emergency department, etc.). The exception is the neonate with a probable cardiac aetiology for the arrest who should be resuscitated using the infant and child protocol.

20.4 When to stop resuscitation

Resuscitation efforts are unlikely to be successful and cessation can be considered if there is no return of spontaneous circulation at any time with up to 20 minutes of cumulative life support and in the absence of recurring or refractory VF/pVT. Exceptions are patients with a history of poisoning or a primary hypothermic insult in whom prolonged attempts may occasionally be successful. Seek expert help from a toxicologist or paediatric intensivist. But importantly there is no single predictor for when to stop resuscitation.

20.5 Parental presence

In general, family members should be offered the opportunity to be present during the resuscitation of their child. Evidence also suggests that the presence of parents at the child's side during resuscitation enables them to gain a realistic understanding of the efforts made to save their child and they subsequently may show less anxiety and depression.

Important points:

- A staff member must be designated to be the parents' support and interpreter of events at all times
- The team leader, not the parents, decides when it is appropriate to stop the resuscitation. If the presence of the parents is impeding the progress of the resuscitation, they should sensitively be asked to leave
- After the resuscitation the team needs a debriefing session to support staff and reflect on practice

20.6 Summary

The teaching in this chapter is consistent with the International Liaison Committee on Resuscitation (ILCOR) guidelines, *Resuscitation 2015*, and there are an enormous number of references that have informed this process. These are available on the ALSG website (see details in the prelims).

PART 5
Practical application of APLS

CHAPTER 21

Practical procedures: airway and breathing

Learning outcomes

After reading this chapter, you will be able to identify the equipment for and describe the following procedures:
- Ventilation without intubation:
  - Mouth to mask
  - Bag and mask
- Oropharyngeal airway (Guedel) insertion
- Nasopharyngeal airway insertion
- Tracheal intubation and rapid sequence induction
- Laryngeal mask insertion
- Surgical airway:
  - Needle cricothyrotomy
  - Surgical cricothyrotomy
- Blocked tracheostomy

This chapter should be read in conjunction with Chapter 19. After all interventions, the patient should be reassessed to ascertain the success or otherwise of the intervention.

21.1 Ventilation without intubation

Mouth-to-mask ventilation

Procedure

1. Pocket masks and similar devices will need pushing into shape before use. A filter, if present, may be attached to the mask before use.
2. It is usual to use both hands to hold the mask. Apply the mask to the face, using a jaw thrust grip, the thumbs holding the mask. If using a shaped mask, it should be the right way up in children (Figure 21.1a) or upside down in infants (Figure 21.1b). Ensure a neutral head position in infants, and more extended in older children .
3. Ensure an adequate seal.
4. Blow into the mouth port, observing the resulting chest movement.
5. Ventilate at an initial 12–20 breaths/min, depending on the age of the child. If using the mask for CPR, then use two ventilations to 15 compressions.
6. Attach oxygen to the face mask if possible.

Advanced Paediatric Life Support: A Practical Approach to Emergencies, Sixth Edition. Edited by Martin Samuels and Sue Wieteska.
© 2016 John Wiley & Sons, Ltd. Published 2016 by John Wiley & Sons, Ltd.

(a)   (b)

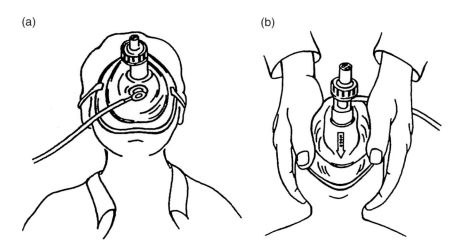

Figure 21.1 Mask position for mouth-to-mask ventilation in (a) a child and (b) an infant

Bag-and-mask ventilation

Bag-and-mask ventilation with a self-inflating bag is the core skill of emergency airway management. It is sometimes described as both simple and routine. In fact, it is a skill that takes practice and experience to acquire; this applies particularly to single-operator use.

Procedure

1. Apply the mask to the face. The thumb and first finger are placed on top of the mask; the third and fourth fingers perform a chin lift and the fifth finger a jaw thrust (Figure 21.2). The jaw and chin need to be pulled up to the mask to obtain a seal. Pushing the mask down into the face results in neck flexion and obstructs the airway.
2. Squeeze the bag, looking for chest movement, misting of the mask and end-tidal CO_2 if available. If the chest is not moving, consider: adjusting the head extension to one appropriate to the size of the patient; repositioning the mask; using an airway adjunct; or employing a two-person technique.
3. Ventilate at approximately 20 breaths/min or a ratio of two ventilations to 15 chest compression if performing CPR.
4. The bag should be connected to an oxygen supply at 15 l/min.
5. Continually reassess the efficacy of ventilation and oxygenation.

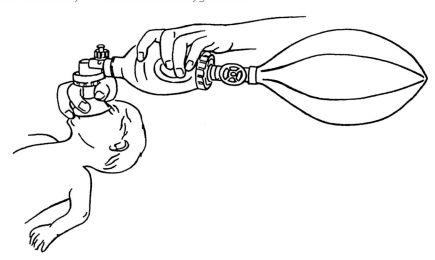

Figure 21.2 Bag-and-mask ventilation

A two-person technique (Figure 21.3) makes obtaining a seal around the mask easier, with both hands of one rescuer holding the mask. The thumbs are used on top of the mask and the first fingers used to perform a jaw thrust. The other rescuer supports and squeezes the bag. In conjunction with an oropharyngeal airway, this is an extremely effective method for airway management in an unconscious, apnoeic patient.

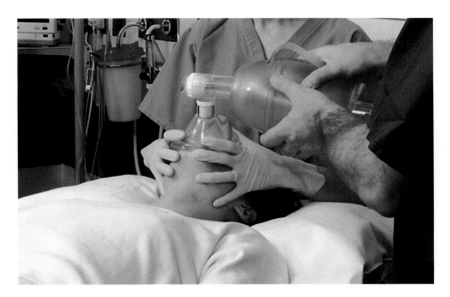

Figure 21.3 Two-person bag-and-mask ventilation

Overenthusiastic ventilation, with excessive tidal volumes or very rapid inspirations may force air into the stomach. The resulting gastric distension may inhibit ventilation, and also encourage regurgitation.

21.2 Oropharyngeal airway (Guedel) insertion

The Guedel airway prevents obstruction by the tongue. It is extremely effective but can only be used in unconscious or very obtunded patients with no gag reflex, due to the potential to provoke vomiting and laryngospasm.

Procedure

1. Select the appropriate size airway (see Chapter 19).
2. Extend the neck slightly if it safe to do so and open the mouth. In trauma patients open the mouth with a jaw thrust, avoiding excessive neck movement. (In most resuscitations, however, hypoxia is of greater risk to the patient than slight neck movement.)
3. The airway is usually inserted upside down and then rotated through 180° as it is passed over the tongue and soft palate, usually when the airway is approximately half way in.
4. It is sometimes easier to insert the airway the right way up, particularly for infants and for non-experts. Use of a tongue depressor or laryngoscope blade may aid insertion. When in position, the curve of the Guedel follows the natural curve of the tongue and pharynx (Figure 21.4), and the airway will sit naturally in place, with the flange just above the lip.
5. Be prepared to change to a different size if no airway improvement is achieved.

(a)   (b)   (c)

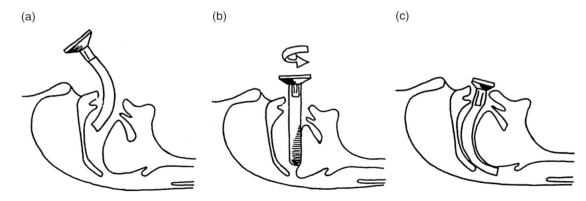

Figure 21.4 (a–c) Airway insertion using the rotational technique

21.3 Nasopharyngeal airway insertion

The nasopharyngeal airway can be useful to relieve airway obstruction in children who have a reduced level of consciousness but are not obtunded enough to tolerate a Guedel airway. It may be of use in a fitting child if the mouth is difficult to open. It is contraindicated when basal skull fracture is suspected. There is a risk of causing a nose bleed, which can seriously complicate airway management.

Procedure

1. Select an appropriate size airway (see Chapter 19).
2. Lubricate the airway with a water-soluble lubricant.
3. Insert the tip into the nostril and direct it posteriorly along the floor of the nose (not upwards).
4. Gently pass the airway past the turbinates with a slight rotating motion. As the tip advances into the pharynx, there should be a palpable 'give'.
5. Continue until the flange rests on the nostril.
6. If there is difficulty inserting the airway, consider using the other nostril or a smaller size from the original estimate. Do not use excessive force or have repeat attempts.
7. Reassess airway and breathing, provide oxygen and commence ventilation if necessary.

21.4 Tracheal intubation and rapid sequence induction

Intubation is performed only by appropriately trained and experienced practitioners. All children should be anaesthetised and paralysed before laryngoscopy. There are very few exceptions to this, although intubation may be performed without drugs during cardiopulmonary arrest and muscle relaxant may be omitted if gas induction is performed for upper airway obstruction.

The whole team should understand the steps involved in the process of induction of anaesthesia and intubation. Role allocation aided by the use of a checklist is helpful (Figure 21.5). Equipment and drugs must be organised, readily available and regularly checked in all areas of the hospital that may treat a critically ill child.

Laryngoscopy

There is a description of some of the equipment for laryngoscopy in Chapter 19. The priority is to see the vocal cords, pass an endotracheal tube into the trachea and to immediately recognise incorrect placement.

After intubation, inspection of chest wall movement, auscultation and expired CO_2 measurement (capnometry), if available, are mandatory components of confirming tracheal placement. Later, a chest X-ray will be performed to confirm tube tip placement in the mid-trachea at the level of T1, or the midpoint between the tip of the clavicles and the carina. An intubated patient should be constantly monitored, so that any problems are immediately recognised.

Rapid sequence induction

Traditionally, the delivery of emergency anaesthesia is in the form of a rapid sequence induction (RSI). It is a core skill for anaesthetists. It involves:

1. Pre-oxygenation with 100% oxygen for at least 3 minutes.
2. Induction of anaesthesia.
3. Application of cricoid pressure by a skilled assistant. The aim of cricoid pressure is to compress the oesophagus against the vertebral body behind, theoretically preventing passive regurgitation of gastric contents.
4. Administration of a rapid-acting muscle relaxant, normally suxamethonium or possibly a newer agent such as rocuronium.
5. Intubation of the trachea, followed by the release of cricoid pressure once correct intubation is confirmed.

This technique was intended to prevent aspiration of the gastric contents after induction and before intubation. There is little evidence that RSI reduces this small risk, however, and it is associated with a high incidence of hypoxia. This is because ventilation is not performed after induction of anaesthesia until the airway is secured, and the incidence of failed intubation is higher in the presence of cricoid pressure, which somewhat distorts the airway.

Hypoxia is a greater threat to children than aspiration during induction of anaesthesia, and for this reason classic RSI may be avoided. Ventilation should be maintained after induction and cricoid pressure omitted, although the intubator may use external laryngeal manipulation during laryngoscopy to improve the view of the vocal cords.

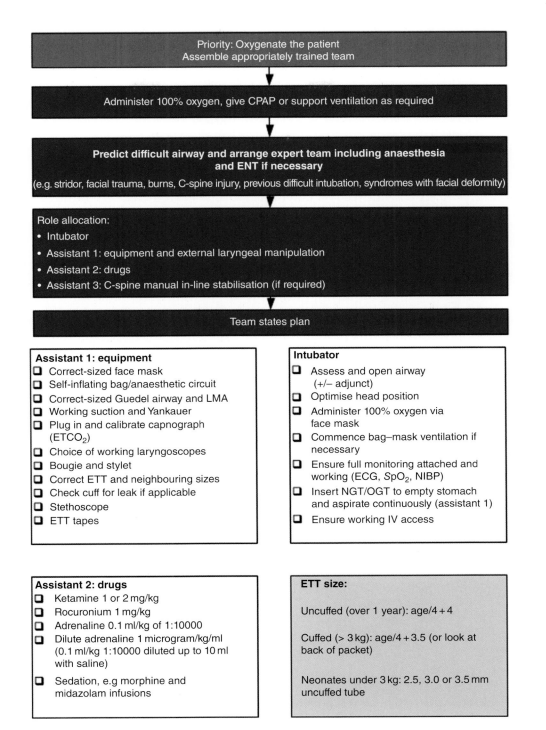

Figure 21.5 Intubation checklist. [CPAP, continuous positive airway pressure; ECG, electrocardiogram; ENT, ear, nose and throat; ETCO$_2$, end-tidal CO$_2$; ETT, endotracheal tube; LMA, laryngeal mask airway; NGT, nasogastric tube; NIBP, non-invasive blood pressure; OGT, orogastric tube]

Tracheal intubation

This is performed after pre-intubation checks have been performed, and the child is anaesthetised and paralysed.

Procedure

1. The head is normally positioned in a degree of extension, with the neck flexed. A pillow in older children, or shoulder roll in infants, may help achieve this and reduce head movement. A head ring is sometimes used for infants. If there are strong grounds to suspect cervical spine injury, then the neck should be manually immobilised by an assistant (this makes the vocal cords harder to visualise and a bougie or secondary intubation technique may be required). A cervical collar if present may need removing if it is impeding the process of intubation.

2. The laryngoscope should be held in the left hand and is inserted down the right side of the mouth, with the tongue to the left of the blade. The intubator will often hold the occiput with their right hand at this point, to control the head and apply the optimal degree of extension.

3. The tip of the blade is brought into the midline, and either rests in the vallecula or picks up the epiglottis. Failure to keep the blade in the midline is a common cause of difficulty in visualisation of the larynx.

4. The handle is then pulled forward rather than upwards to reveal the vocal cords, i.e. pulled in the direction of the laryngoscope handle (Figure 21.6). Inexperienced operators often lever the blade onto the top gum or teeth, which can cause trauma and should be avoided. In a baby, it is common to advance the laryngoscope blade well beyond the epiglottis and then slowly withdraw it until the vocal cords come into view

5. The tube should then be passed through the vocal cords. Most endotracheal tubes have a black line, which should rest at the level of the cords. The intubator should take a note of the tube length at the lips.

6. The tube position should be confirmed by inspecting the chest for bilateral movement and auscultation in both axillae for equal air entry, and over the stomach to confirm lack of air entry. The definitive test is measurement of expired CO_2 by capnometry, which must be used where it is available. If in doubt, remove the tube and reinstitute bag–mask ventilation. (NB These checks should also be performed when taking over the care of an intubated patient from another team.)

7. If intubation is not achieved quickly (less than 30 seconds) then oxygenation should be re-established before a further attempt. There should not usually be a fall in oxygen saturations during intubation.

8. Inflate the cuff (if present) to the appropriate pressure, sufficient to obtain a seal. (If cuff pressure is measured, this is usually 20 cmH$_2$O although it may need to be more if high ventilation pressures are required.)

9. Secure the tube at the correct length. Sticky tape may not be adequate if the face is wet with saliva, blood or vomit, in which case the tube should be tied with tape.

A chest X-ray is usually performed later to ensure the tip is appropriately positioned below the vocal cords but above the carina.

(a)   (b)

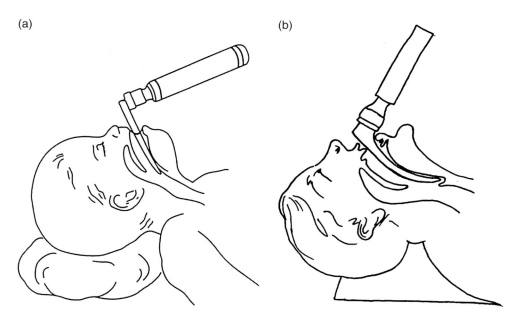

Figure 21.6 Technique using (a) a straight-blade laryngoscope, and (b) a curved-blade laryngoscope

21.5 Drugs

The following drugs may be used during intubation.

Ketamine is the induction agent of choice for anaesthesia in paediatric critical care. The dose is 1–2 mg/kg. The lower dose should be chosen when there is established circulatory shock. Ketamine causes the least cardiovascular instability of all induction agents due to stimulation of endogenous catecholamine release. Recent studies have shown that ketamine does not increase intracranial pressure as previously thought and can be used safely in head-injured patients. An induction dose of ketamine provides about 20 minutes of anaesthesia, which is useful time for ongoing resuscitation and vascular access before ongoing sedation needs to be commenced.

Propofol, thiopentone and volatile anaesthetic agents can all cause profound hypotension or even cardiac arrest in critically ill patients, especially if used at similar doses as induction for elective surgery. (Etomidate causes less hypotension but is rarely used because of the side effect of pituitary suppression.)

There are two situations when an alternative induction agent might be considered:

- **Thiopentone** is used to terminate a prolonged seizure, as described in the status epilepticus algorithm (see Chapter 9). Note that when a seizure is associated with cardiovascular compromise, ketamine is a better choice of induction agent and has anticonvulsant properties.
- **Gas induction** with sevoflurane or halothane might be preferred by anaesthetists managing the airway of a child with upper airway obstruction.

Muscle relaxant makes both bag–mask ventilation and intubation easier. Rapid acting agents are preferable in critical care scenarios. **Suxamethonium** (1–2 mg/kg) or **rocuronium** (1 mg/kg) are commonly used and both give excellent intubating conditions within approximately 1 minute. Suxamethonium depolarises muscle causing visible fasciculations to occur before the onset of paralysis. It is rapidly metabolised by plasma cholinesterase in most people and its effects last for just a few minutes. Suxamethonium is contraindicated after burns and spinal cord injury, when the serum potassium is high and when there is a personal or family history of malignant hyperthermia. Rocuronium is a non-depolarising muscle relaxant. A single dose will last for about 20–30 minutes. It has fewer side effects than suxamethonium and is often preferred.

Whichever drugs are used at induction, the team must be prepared for cardiovascular collapse, especially in shocked patients. Boluses of isotonic crystalloid should be prepared.

Dopamine can be infused peripherally at a low concentration and may be started for induction before central venous access is obtained. It is useful to have resuscitation doses of adrenaline (0.1 ml/kg of 1:10000) immediately available. According to local protocol, one of these adrenaline doses can be diluted in saline to a volume of 10 ml, giving a solution of 1 micrograms/kg/ml. Boluses of 1–2 ml can be given to treat significant hypotension before inotrope or vasopressor infusions are prepared and commenced. Morphine and/or midazolam infusions are commonly used for sedation.

21.6 Intubation algorithm

Anaesthetic induction and intubation may be a stressful part of the resuscitation, particularly in the critically ill or injured child. It is not unknown for paediatric intubations to be difficult even for experienced practitioners, but should difficulties occur, then all members of the team must be able to predict and prepare for the next steps. The presence of an intubation algorithm may help and inform non-anaesthetic members of the team. An example of an algorithm for a failed intubation is given in Figure 21.7.

In contrast to elective anaesthesia, in critical illness and injury there may not be an option to abandon intubation and wake the patient up. The steps in the intubation algorithm are moved through methodically until the airway is secured. Team-based simulation training improves performance managing these rare scenarios.

Complications of intubation and their recognition are discussed in Chapter 19.

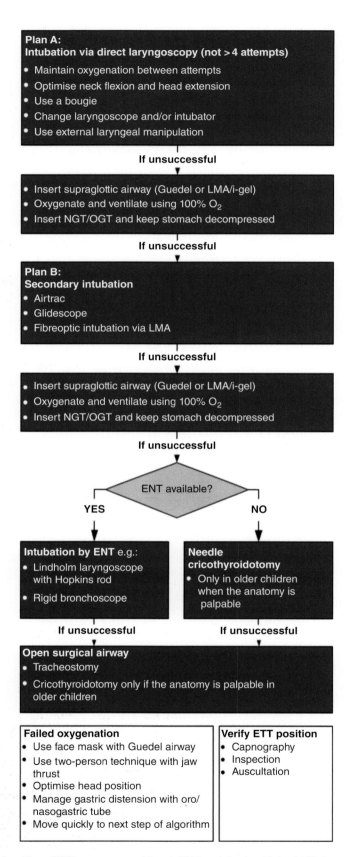

Figure 21.7 Failed intubation algorithm. [ENT, ear, nose and throat; ETT, endotracheal tube; LMA, laryngeal mask airway; NGT, nasogastric tube; OGT, orogastric tube]

21.7 Laryngeal mask airway

The LMA is a supraglottic airway (as is the similar i-gel). It is a popular choice for elective anaesthesia, to rescue the airway after failed intubation and sometimes as the airway of choice in pre-hospital care. They are relatively easy to insert but require some training and experience to know that they are sitting correctly. Once in position, placement should be confirmed in a similar way as an endotracheal tube (although of course endobronchial placement is not possible).

It is difficult to ventilate stiff lungs with an LMA, as there will be a leak around the cuff at pressures much above 20 cmH$_2$O. Intubation through an LMA, with or without a flexible bronchoscope is possible (see Chapter 19).

Insertion of the classic LMA

Insertion of LMAs is rapid, and blind (i.e. no laryngoscopy is required). LMAs can easily become displaced, however, and are not a definitive long-term airway. They do not protect completely from aspiration.

Equipment

- Appropriate size LMA (see Chapter 19)
- Syringe for LMA cuff inflation
- Water-soluble lubricant
- Stethoscope
- Tape to secure the LMA

Procedure

1. Whenever possible, administer 100% oxygen before inserting the LMA.
2. Check the LMA, in particular checking cuff inflation with no leak, and check the tube for blockage or loose objects; have lubricant and suction to hand.
3. Deflate the cuff and lightly lubricate the back and sides of the mask. Avoid excessive amounts of lubricant. In children, it may be preferred to have the cuff partially inflated for insertion.
4. Tilt the patient's head back (if safe to do so), open the mouth fully, and insert the tip of the mask along the hard palate with the open side facing, but not touching, the tongue (Figure 21.8a). A jaw thrust performed by an assistant may aid placement.
5. Slide the mask further, along the posterior pharyngeal wall, with your index finger initially providing support for the tube (Figure 21.8b). Eventually resistance is felt as the tip of the LMA lies at the upper end of the oesophagus (Figure 21.8c).
6. Fully inflate the cuff. The LMA should be allowed to rise up slightly as it is inflated.
7. Secure the LMA with adhesive tape and check its position during ventilation as for a tracheal tube: good equilateral chest rise, no leak, capnometry if available.

It is sometimes easier to insert an LMA rotated 90° or 180° from its final position. The mask is then quickly rotated into its natural position as it passes into position.

Complications of LMA use

- The epiglottis can get caught by the LMA and displaced over the larynx. This results in obstruction of the airway
- The tip of the LMA may fold over during insertion

If either of the above problems occurs, or if the airway is unsatisfactory for another reason, withdraw the LMA and reinsert.

- Rotation of LMAs may occur after insertion, more commonly with smaller LMAs and particularly while the breathing system or self-inflating bag is attached

I-gel insertion

The principles of insertion are broadly similar to the LMA.

The i-gel is supplied in a protective cradle. A small blob of water-soluble lubricant jelly can be placed onto the cradle to facilitate light lubrication of the back, sides and front of the gel cuff. The device is inserted into the mouth, sliding it backwards along the hard palate until a clear resistance is felt. It is not necessary to insert fingers into the patient's mouth during insertion. A jaw thrust by the assistant may aid insertion if early resistance is felt, or, alternatively, insertion 'upside down' followed by rotation may aid insertion.

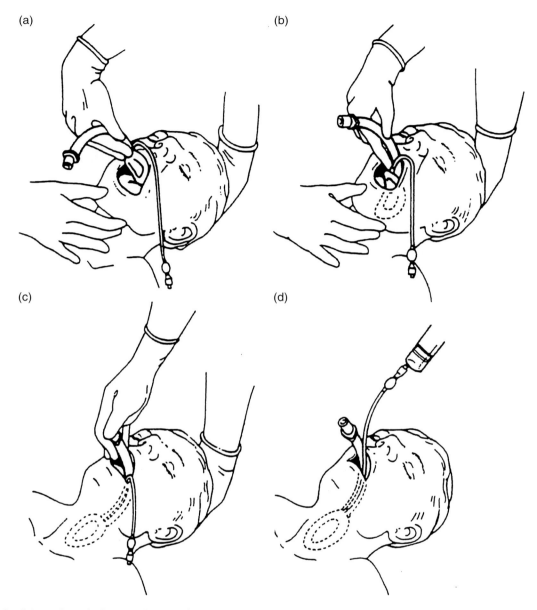

Figure 21.8 (a–d) Insertion of a laryngeal mask airway

With both LMA and i-gel insertion, the device is in place when definitive resistance is felt. Repeated to-and-fro pushing and pulling when this resistance is felt is not necessary.

21.8 Surgical airway

In an emergency 'cannot intubate, cannot ventilate' situation, it is necessary to perform a surgical airway. This is an absolute last resort but, when indicated, should be performed without delay. There is debate about which techniques are optimal for children; a national UK audit has reported that needle techniques do not have a high success rate even in adults.

The cricothyroid membrane is difficult to palpate in children under the age of 5, and nearly impossible to feel in infants. It is therefore recommended that needle techniques should not be considered the first line surgical airway in children under 5.

- Children up to 1 year of age should have an emergency tracheostomy, with direct visualisation of the tracheal wall
- Between the ages of 1 year and 5 years either emergency tracheostomy or a cricothyroidomy may be performed, the latter only if the cricothyroid membrane can be confidently identified

- In older children and adolescents (and adults), either the needle or surgical technique can be used but surgical techniques allow better protection of the airway. The relevant anatomy is shown in Figure 21.9

ENT specialists should be involved in the management of difficult airways as early as possible and are likely to be the most appropriately qualified team member to perform a surgical airway.

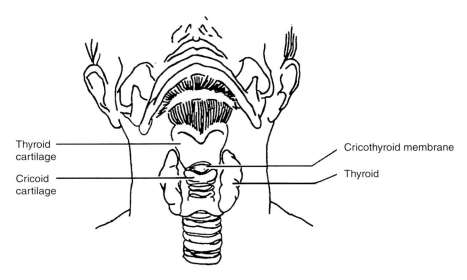

Thyroid cartilage

Cricoid cartilage

Cricothyroid membrane

Thyroid

Figure 21.9 Surgical airway anatomy

Needle cricothyroidotomy

Procedure

1. Consider extending the neck to improve access. (This technique is performed in a dire emergency: protection of the cervical spine is of secondary importance at this stage.)
2. Clean the skin with antiseptic.
3. Stabilise the larynx with the non-dominant hand, and with the other hand identify the cricothyroid membrane by palpation between the thyroid and cricoid cartilages.
4. Use a cricothyroidotomy cannula-over-needle (or 14 or 16 gauge intravenous cannula) attached to a 5 ml syringe and aim in a caudal direction, at an angle to the skin of about 45°, aspirating on the syringe while advancing (Figure 21.10). Always ensure the needle is advanced in the midline.
5. Confirm position by the aspiration of air, then advance the cannula over the needle.
6. Attach the hub of the cannula to either an oxygen flow meter via a Y-connector or an adjustable pressure-limiting device. (NB: the pressure relief valve on an anaesthetic machine means that the common gas outlet on the machine is unsuitable as the gas supply.)
7. Set the flow rate (starting flow in litres/min = age in years). If this is insufficient, cautiously increase the flow rate (in increments of 1 litre) or inflation pressure to achieve chest expansion using an inspiration time of 1 second. Observe the chest movements and auscultate to assess for adequate gas entry.
8. Maintain upper airway patency, allowing roughly 4 seconds for exhalation. NB: expiration occurs through the patient's upper airway, *not* through the cannula.
9. Constantly check the neck to exclude cannula misplacement, i.e. swelling from the injection of gas into the tissues rather than the trachea.
10. Secure the equipment to the patient's neck.
11. Arrange to proceed to a more definitive airway procedure, such as tracheostomy or intubation if more skilled help has arrived.

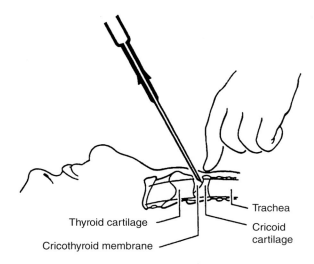

Thyroid cartilage

Cricothyroid membrane

Trachea

Cricoid cartilage

Figure 21.10 Needle cricothyroidotomy

Surgical cricothyroidotomy

Procedure

1. Place the patient in a supine position.
2. Consider extending the neck to improve access. Otherwise, maintain a neutral alignment.
3. Identify the cricothyroid membrane.
4. Prepare the skin and, if the patient is conscious, infiltrate with local anaesthetic.
5. Place your non-dominant hand on the neck to stabilise the cricothyroid membrane and to protect the lateral vascular structures from injury.
6. Make a vertical incision in the skin and press the lateral edges of the incision outwards, to minimise bleeding.
7. Make a transverse incision through the cricothyroid membrane, being careful not to damage the cricoid cartilage.
8. Insert a tracheal spreader, or use the handle of the scalpel by inserting it through the incision and twisting it through 90° to open the airway.
9. Insert an appropriately sized endotracheal or tracheostomy tube. It is advisable to use a slightly smaller size than would have been used for an oral or nasal tube.
10. Ventilate the patient and check that this is effective, and check correct tube position as for intubation.
11. Secure the tube to prevent dislodgement.

Emergency tracheostomy

Procedure

1. Place the patient in a supine position.
2. Consider extending the neck to improve access. Otherwise, maintain a neutral alignment if possible.
3. Palpate the trachea (the laryngeal cartilages are difficult to palpate in smaller children).
4. Place your left thumb and index finger firmly on the neck either side of the trachea from above to stabilise the trachea and to protect the lateral vascular structures from injury.
5. Make a low, vertical, midline incision in the skin, above the suprasternal notch, maintaining pressure and stabilising the trachea with your left hand thumb and index finger. Pressure and remaining in the midline will minimise bleeding and damage to lateral structures.
6. The incision should be midline through the strap muscles and thyroid isthmus (if encountered) and directly onto the tracheal wall.
7. Make a vertical incision through the tracheal rings (rings 3 to 5 if possible), being careful not to damage the cricoid cartilage or innominate artery (which may cross the trachea inferiorly).
8. Insert the tracheostomy tube with introducer. It is advisable to use a cuffed tube.
9. Ventilate the patient and check that this is effective.

10. Secure the tube to prevent dislodgement.

11. Having completed emergency airway management, stabilise the patient, transfer to theatres, address haemostasis and place lateral tracheal stay sutures.

Postoperative care

1. Perform a chest X-ray.

2. Check and monitor cuff pressure.

3. Inform staff how to use the stay sutures.

4. A tracheostomy tube care box should be kept at the bedside containing an introducer, spare tracheostomy tube of the same dimensions, one size smaller tracheostomy tube, suction catheters, tapes, non-adherent dressings, scissors and lubricant jelly.

5. A small artery clip or tracheal dilator should be available at the bedside.

Complications of tracheostomy or cricothyoroidotomy

- Subglottic oedema or stenosis.
- Haemorrhage.
- Pneumothorax or pneumomediastinum.
- Damage to lateral structures such as the recurrent laryngeal nerves, carotid sheath or oesophagus.
- Pulmonary oedema.
- Tracheostomy tube problems such as displacement and blockage.
- Subcutaneous emphysema.
- Swallowing difficulties.
- Local infection.
- Aspiration.
- False passage.

21.9 Management of a blocked tracheostomy

The equipment list, algorithm and checklist are detailed in Chapter 19.

CHAPTER 22
Practical procedures: circulation

Learning outcomes

After reading this chapter, you will be able to identify equipment for and describe the following procedures:
- Vascular access:
  - Intraosseous access
  - Peripheral venous access:
    upper and lower extremity veins
    scalp veins
    external jugular vein
    umbilical vein
    venous cut-down
  - Central venous access:
    femoral vein
    internal jugular vein
    external jugular vein
    subclavian vein
  - Arterial cannulation
- Defibrillation

22.1 Vascular access

Access to the circulation is a crucial step in delivering advanced paediatric life support. Many access routes are possible: intraosseous access, peripheral venous access, central venous access or arterial cannulation. The one chosen will reflect both clinical need and the skills of the operator.

If fluids are to be given, infusion pumps or paediatric infusion sets should be used. This avoids inadvertent overperfusion in small children.

Intraosseous infusion

Intraosseous access is indicated if other attempts at venous access fail, or if they will take longer than 1.0 minutes to carry out. It is the recommended technique for circulatory access in cardiac arrest.

Advanced Paediatric Life Support: A Practical Approach to Emergencies, Sixth Edition. Edited by Martin Samuels and Sue Wieteska.
© 2016 John Wiley & Sons, Ltd. Published 2016 by John Wiley & Sons, Ltd.

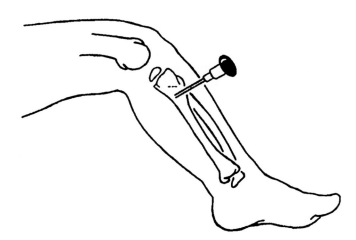

Figure 22.1 Tibial technique for intraosseous infusion

Equipment

- Alcohol swabs
- 18 or 15 gauge needle with trochar (at least 1.5 cm in length)
- Syringe: 5 ml
- Syringe: 20 ml
- Infusion fluid

Procedure

1. Identify the infusion site. Fractured bones should be avoided, as should limbs with fractures proximal to possible infusion sites. The landmarks for the upper tibial and lower femoral sites are shown in the box, and the tibial approach is illustrated in Figure 22.1.
2. This technique is comparable to central access – the more proximal the site the greater the efficacy of flow to the heart.
3. Clean the skin at the chosen site.
4. Insert the needle at 90° to the skin.
5. Continue to advance the needle until a 'give' is felt as the cortex is penetrated.
6. Attach the 5 ml syringe and aspirate – blood marrow may be used to check blood glucose and provide blood culture. Flush to confirm correct positioning.
7. Attach the filled 20 ml syringe and push in the infusion fluid in boluses.

Surface anatomy for intraosseous infusions

Tibial
Anterior surface, 2–3 cm below the tibial tuberosity

Femoral
Anterolateral surface, 3 cm above the lateral condyle

Other powered devices

The EZ-IO® drill is a powered device that enables rapid insertion of an intraosseous needle. The same landmarks are used as for manual insertion and the procedure is less painful for the conscious victim due to its rapidity. The option of using the proximal humerus as an access site for older children (>40 kg) can be utilised with the EZ-IO®. This provides optimum central access with extremely rapid uptake to the heart. The EZ-IO® needles come in three lengths (all 15 gauge): pink 3–39 kg, blue >3 kg and yellow >40 kg. The length of needle used will depend on the insertion site.

The procedure for insertion is as follows:

1. Universal precautions.
2. Clean site.
3. Choose appropriate size needle and attach to drill – it will fix magnetically – remove the needle cover.
4. Hold the drill and needle at 90° to the skin surface and push through the skin without drilling, until bone is felt and at least one 5 mm marker is visible above the skin – if not use the longer needle.

5. Push the drill button and drill continuously and push until there is loss of resistance – there is a palpable give as the needle breaches the cortex.
6. Remove the drill and unscrew the trochar.
7. Aspirate the marrow if possible – failure to aspirate marrow does not mean the insertion has failed.
8. Attach the pre-prepared connection tube.
9. There is an optional device to secure the needle but this is not essential.
10. Proceed with required therapy.
11. The device should be removed within 24 hours.

It should be noted that aspiration and infusion of fluid may be painful for the conscious patient and if this proves to be the case 0.5 mg/kg of 2% lidocaine may be infused slowly to combat this.

Other powered devices are available but have a less than ideal success rate in paediatrics hence are not described here.

Failed attempts at insertion can be identified by swelling around the insertion site and failure of fluids/drugs to flow. In this situation opposing limbs should be used with no further attempts on the failed side for 72 hours.

Complications of intraosseous infusion

- Compartment syndrome
- Infection
- Fracture

Peripheral venous access

Upper and lower extremity veins

Veins on the dorsum of the hand, the elbow, the dorsum of the feet and the saphenous vein at the ankle can be used for cannulation. Standard percutaneous techniques should be employed if possible. Topical or injected local anaesthetic should be used whenever time allows.

Scalp veins

The frontal superficial, temporal posterior, auricular, supraorbital and posterior facial veins can be used.

Equipment

- Skin-cleansing swabs
- Syringe and 0.9% saline
- Short piece of tubing or bandage

Procedure

1. Restrain the child.
2. Shave the appropriate area of the scalp.
3. Clean the skin.
4. Have an assistant distend the vein by holding a taut piece of tubing or bandaging perpendicular to it, proximal to the site of puncture.
5. Fill the syringe with 0.9% saline and flush the butterfly set.
6. Disconnect the syringe and leave the end of the tubing open.
7. Puncture the skin and enter the vein. Blood will flow back through the tubing.
8. Infuse a small quantity of fluid to see that the cannula is properly placed and then tape into position.

External jugular vein

Equipment

- Skin-cleansing swabs
- Appropriate cannula
- Tape

Procedure

1. Place child in a 15–30° head-down position (or with padding under the shoulders so that the head hangs lower than the shoulders).
2. Turn the head away from the site of puncture. Restrain the child as necessary in this position.
3. Clean the skin at the appropriate side of the neck.
4. Identify the external jugular vein, which can be seen passing over the sternocleidomastoid muscle at the junction of its middle and lower thirds (Figure 22.2).
5. Have an assistant place his or her finger at the lower end of the visible part of the vein just above the clavicle. This stabilises it and compresses it so that it remains distended.
6. Puncture the skin and enter the vein.
7. When a free flow of blood is obtained, ensure no air bubbles are present in the tubing and then attach a giving set.
8. Tape the cannula securely in position.

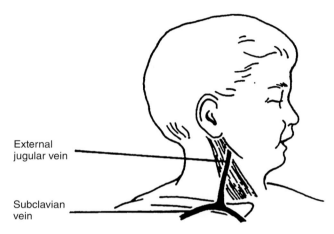

External
jugular vein

Subclavian
vein

Figure 22.2 The course of the external jugular vein

Umbilical vein

Venous access via the umbilical vein is a rapid and simple technique. It is used during resuscitation at birth.

Equipment

- Skin-cleansing swabs
- Umbilical tape
- Scalpel
- Syringe and 0.9% saline
- Catheter

Procedure

1. Loosely tie the umbilical tape around the cord.
2. Cut the cord with a scalpel, leaving a 1 cm strip distal to the tape.
3. If there is bleeding from the vein, gently tighten the tape to stop it.
4. Identify the umbilical vein. Three vessels will be seen in the stump: two will be small and contracted (the arteries sited inferiorly), and one at the head end will be dilated (the vein) (Figure 22.3).
5. Fill a 5 French gauge catheter with 0.9% saline.
6. Insert the catheter into the vein, and advance it approximately 5 cm.
7. Tighten the umbilical tape to secure the catheter. A purse-string suture may be used later to stitch the catheter in place.

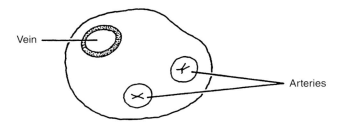

Figure 22.3 Umbilical cord cross-section

Venous cut-down

This technique may be useful in situations where intraosseous needles are not available.

Table 22.1 Surface anatomy of the brachial and long saphenous veins		
Child	Brachial vein	Saphenous vein (Figure 22.4)
Infant	One finger breadth lateral to the medial epicondyle of the humerus	Half a finger breadth superior and anterior to the medial malleolus
Small children	Two finger breadths lateral to the medial epicondyle of the humerus	One finger breadth superior and anterior to the medial malleolus
Older children	Three finger breadths lateral to the medial epicondyle of the humerus	Two finger breadths superior and anterior to the medial malleolus

Equipment

- Skin-cleansing swabs
- Lidocaine 1% for local anaesthetic with a 2 ml syringe and a 25 gauge needle
- Scalpel
- Curved haemostats
- Suture and ligature material
- Cannula

Procedure

1. Immobilise the appropriate limb.
2. Clean the skin.
3. Identify the surface landmarks for the relevant vein (Table 22.1).
4. If the child is responsive to pain, infiltrate the skin with 1% lidocaine.
5. Make an incision perpendicular to the course of the vein through the skin (Figure 22.4).
6. Using the curved haemostat tips, bluntly dissect the subcutaneous tissue.
7. Identify the vein and free 1–2 cm in length.
8. Pass a proximal and a distal ligature.
9. Tie off the distal end of the vein, keeping the ends of the tie long.

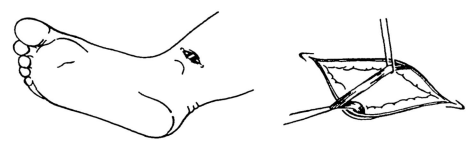

Figure 22.4 Site of a long saphenous cut-down and its technique

10. Make a small hole in the upper part of the exposed vein with a scalpel blade or fine-pointed scissors.
11. While holding the distal tie to stabilise the vein, insert the cannula.
12. Secure this in place with the upper ligature. Do not tie this too tightly; doing so would cause occlusion.
13. Attach a syringe filled with 0.9% saline to the cannula and ensure that fluid flows freely up the vein. If free flow does not occur, then either the tip of the cannula is against a venous valve or the cannula may be wrongly placed in the adventitia surrounding the vein. Withdrawing the catheter will improve flow in the former case.
14. Once fluid flows freely, tie the proximal ligature around the catheter to help immobilise it.
15. Close the incision site with interrupted sutures.
16. Fix the catheter or cannula to the skin and cover with a sterile dressing.

Central venous access

Central access can be obtained through the femoral, internal jugular, external jugular and (in older children) subclavian veins. The Seldinger technique is safe and effective. UK National Institute for Health and Care Excellence guidelines recommend ultrasound-guided insertion. The femoral vein is often used as it is relatively easy to cannulate away from the chest during CPR. Central venous access via the neck veins is not without dangers, and may be difficult in emergency situations. The course of the central veins of the neck is shown in Figure 22.5.

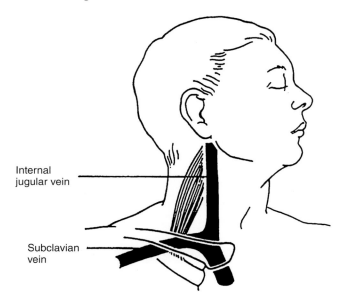

Internal jugular vein

Subclavian vein

Figure 22.5 The course of the central veins of the neck

Femoral vein

This procedure can be carried out with or without ultrasound guidance. The two techniques are described here.

Equipment

- Skin-cleansing swabs
- Lidocaine 1% for local anaesthetic with a 2 ml syringe and 23 gauge needle
- Syringe and 0.9% saline
- Seldinger cannulation set:
  - syringe
  - needle
  - Seldinger guide wire
  - cannula
- Suture material
- Prepared paediatric infusion set
- Tape

Procedure with ultrasound guidance

1. Place the child supine with the groin exposed and leg slightly abducted at the hip. Restrain the child's leg and body as necessary.
2. Clean the skin at the appropriate site.
3. Use a sterile probe cover or prep all around the probe once it is positioned, and use a sterile no-touch technique with the injecting hand.
4. Hold a 7–10 MHz linear probe in your non-dominant hand, placing it transversely, with the centre over the femoral artery pulse at the level of the groin skin crease (Figures 22.6 and 22.7). A cross-sectional view of the vessels and nerve will be obtained.
5. Identify the pulsating femoral artery and move the probe so that the artery is in the middle of the ultrasound view.
6. Identify the puncture site. The vein lies directly medial to the artery.
7. If the child is responsive to pain, infiltrate the area with 1% lidocaine.

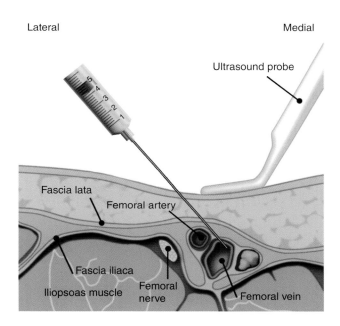

Figure 22.6 Ultrasound-guided needle approach

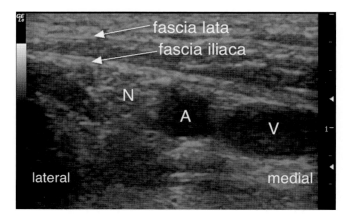

Figure 22.7 Ultrasound image of the femoral region. [A, artery; N, nerve; V, vein]

8. Attach the needle to the syringe.
9. Keeping one finger on the artery to mark its position, introduce the needle at a 45° angle pointing towards the patient's head directly over the femoral vein. Keep the syringe in line with the child's leg. Advance the needle, pulling back on the plunger of the syringe all the time.
10. As soon as blood flows back into the syringe, take the syringe off the needle. Immediately occlude the end of the needle to prevent blood loss.
11. If the vein is not found, withdraw the needle to the skin, locate the artery again and advance as in point 9 above.
12. Insert the Seldinger wire into the needle, and into the vein.
13. Withdraw the needle along the wire, ensuring that the wire is not dislodged from the vein.
14. Place the catheter over the wire and advance it through the skin, into the vein.
15. Suture the catheter in place.
16. Withdraw the wire, immediately occluding the end of the cannula to prevent blood loss.
17. Attach the infusion set.
18. Tape the infusion set tubing in place.

Procedure without ultrasound guidance

1. Place the child supine with the groin exposed and leg slightly abducted at the hip. Restrain the child's leg and body as necessary.
2. Clean the skin at the appropriate site.
3. Identify the puncture site. The femoral vein is found by palpating the femoral artery. The vein lies directly medial to the artery.
4. If the child is responsive to pain, infiltrate the area with 1% lidocaine.
5. Attach the needle to the syringe.
6. Keeping one finger on the artery to mark its position, introduce the needle at a 45° angle pointing towards the patient's head directly over the femoral vein. Keep the syringe in line with the child's leg. Advance the needle, pulling back on the plunger of the syringe all the time.
7. As soon as blood flows back into the syringe, take the syringe off the needle. Immediately occlude the end of the needle to prevent blood loss.
8. If the vein is not found, withdraw the needle to the skin, locate the artery again and advance as in point 9 above.
9. Insert the Seldinger wire into the needle, and into the vein.
10. Withdraw the needle along the wire, ensuring that the wire is not dislodged from the vein.
11. Place the catheter over the wire and advance it through the skin, into the vein.
12. Suture the catheter in place.
13. Withdraw the wire, immediately occluding the end of the cannula to prevent blood loss.
14. Attach the infusion set.
15. Tape the infusion set tubing in place.

Internal jugular vein

Equipment

- Skin-cleansing swabs
- Lidocaine 1% for local anaesthetic with a 2 ml syringe and 23 gauge needle
- Syringe and 0.9% saline
- Seldinger cannulation set:
  - syringe
  - needle
  - Seldinger guide wire
  - cannula
- Suture material
- Prepared paediatric infusion set
- Tape

Procedure

1. Place the child in a 15–30° head-down position.
2. Turn the head away from the side that is to be cannulated and restrain the child as necessary.
3. Clean the skin at the appropriate side of the neck.

4. Under ultrasound guidance (if available) identify the puncture site. This is found at the apex of the triangle formed by the two lower heads of the sternomastoid and the clavicle.
5. If the child is responsive to pain, infiltrate the area with 1% lidocaine.
6. Attach the needle to the syringe and puncture the skin at the appropriate place (see point 4 above).
7. Direct the needle downwards at 30° to the skin; advance the needle towards the nipple, pulling back on the plunger of the syringe all the time.
8. As soon as the blood flows back into the syringe, take the syringe off the needle. Immediately occlude the end of the needle to prevent air embolism.
9. If the vein is not found, withdraw the needle to the skin and advance it again some 5–10° laterally.
10. Insert the Seldinger wire into the needle, and into the vein.
11. Withdraw the needle along the wire, ensuring that the wire is not dislodged from the vein.
12. Place the catheter over the wire and advance it through the skin, into the vein.
13. Suture the catheter in place.
14. Withdraw the wire, immediately occluding the end of the cannula to prevent air embolism.
15. Attach the infusion set.
16. Tape the infusion set tubing in place.
17. Obtain a chest radiograph in order to see the position of the catheter and to exclude a pneumothorax.

External jugular vein

By using the Seldinger technique it is possible to obtain central venous access via the external jugular vein as described here. The anatomy is such that passage into the central veins can sometimes be more difficult compared with other approaches.

Equipment

- Skin-cleansing swabs
- Lidocaine 1% for local anaesthetic with a 2 ml syringe and 25 gauge needle
- Syringe and 0.9% saline
- Seldinger cannulation set:
  - syringe
  - needle
  - Seldinger guide wire (J wire)
  - cannula
- Suture material
- Prepared paediatric infusion set
- Tape

Procedure

1. Place the child in a 15–30° head-down position (or with padding under the shoulders so that the head hangs lower than the shoulders).
2. Turn the head away from the site of puncture. Restrain the child as necessary in this position.
3. Clean the skin at the appropriate side of the neck.
4. Identify the external jugular vein, which can be seen passing over the sternocleidomastoid muscle at the junction of its middle and lower thirds.
5. Have an assistant place his or her finger at the lower end of the visible part of the vein just above the clavicle. This stabilises it and compresses it so that it remains distended.
6. Attach the needle to the syringe and puncture the vein.
7. As soon as blood starts to flow freely, take off the syringe and occlude the end of the needle.
8. Insert a J wire into the needle and into the vein.
9. Advance the J wire. There may be some resistance as the wire reaches the valve at the proximal end of the vein. Gently advance and withdraw the wire until it passes this obstacle.
10. Gently advance the wire.
11. Withdraw the needle along the wire, ensuring that the wire is not dislodged from the vein.
12. Place the catheter over the wire and advance it through the skin, into the vein.
13. Suture the catheter in place.
14. Withdraw the wire, immediately occluding the end of the cannula to prevent air embolism.
15. Attach the infusion set.

16. Tape the infusion set tubing in place.
17. Obtain a chest radiograph in order to see the position of the catheter and to exclude a pneumothorax.

Subclavian vein

Equipment

- Skin-cleansing swabs
- Lidocaine 1% for local anaesthetic with a 2 ml syringe and 23 gauge needle
- Syringe and 0.9% saline
- Seldinger cannulation set:
  - syringe
  - needle
  - Seldinger guide wire
  - cannula
- Suture material
- Prepared paediatric infusion set
- Tape

Procedure

1. Place the child in a 15–30° head-down position.
2. Turn the head away from the site that is to be cannulated and restrain the child as necessary.
3. Clean the skin over the upper side of the chest to the clavicle.
4. Under ultrasound guidance (if available) identify the puncture site. This is 1 cm below the midpoint of the clavicle.
5. If the child is responsive to pain, infiltrate the area with 1% lidocaine.
6. Attach the needle to the syringe and puncture the skin at the appropriate place (see point 4 above).
7. Direct the needle under the clavicle, 'stepping down' off the bone.
8. Once under the clavicle, direct the needle towards the suprasternal notch. Advance the needle, pulling back on the plunger of the syringe all the time and staying as superficial as possible.
9. As soon as the blood flows back into the syringe, take the syringe off the needle. Immediately occlude the end of the needle to prevent air embolism.
10. If the vein is not found, slowly withdraw the needle, continuing to pull back on the plunger. If the vein has been crossed inadvertently, free flow will often be established during this manoeuvre.
11. If the vein is still not found repeat steps 7–10, aiming at a point a little higher in the sternal notch.
12. Insert the Seldinger wire into the needle, and into the vein.
13. Withdraw the needle along the wire, ensuring that the wire is not dislodged from the vein.
14. Place the catheter over the wire and advance it through the skin, into the vein.
15. Suture the catheter in place.
16. Withdraw the wire, immediately occluding the end of the cannula to prevent air embolism.
17. Attach the infusion set.
18. Tape the infusion set tubing in place.
19. Obtain a chest radiograph in order to see the position of the catheter and to exclude a pneumothorax.

Arterial cannulation

Arterial cannulation is used to monitor arterial blood pressure, guide dosage adjustments in shock and hypertensive crisis, obtain blood samples for respiratory and acid–base status, and calculate cerebral perfusion pressure. It should not be performed in sites where there is skin infection or interruption, or absent collateral circulation, and care should be taken in severe haemorrhagic sites. In children, the preferred sites include the radial, posterior tibial, dorsalis pedis, ulnar and femoral arteries. The site should remain visible and not prone to contamination.

Radial artery cannulation

Equipment

- Skin-cleansing swabs
- Lidocaine 1%

- Heparinised syringe
- Cannula:
  - pre-term: 24 gauge
  - infant/pre-school: 22 gauge
  - school-aged: 20–22 gauge
  - adolescent to adult: 18–20 gauge
- T-connector or three-way tap with extension
- Gauze, pad and tapes
- Transparent sterile dressing
- Flushed infusion set (saline 0.9% with heparin 0.5–1.0 U/ml) with pressure infusion bag or pump
- Pressure transducer and monitor

Procedure

1. Before using the radial artery check that the ulnar artery is present and patent. Occlude both arteries at the wrist and then release the pressure on the ulnar artery; circulation should return to the hand. (It will flush pink.) If this does not happen, do not proceed with a radial puncture on that side.
2. Keep the wrist hyperextended and restrained, and palpate the radial artery (usually located in the middle of the lateral third of the wrist).
3. Clean the skin, and infiltrate with local anaesthetic.
4. Insert the cannula over the artery at 45° to the skin and advance it slowly. When the artery is punctured, blood will be seen to pulsate into the syringe.
5. Advance the cannula over the needle and into the artery, and remove the needle whilst compressing the artery proximal to the position of the cannula tip.
6. Connect the T-connector or three-way tap with extension, ready flushed with 0.9% saline to test cannula patency.
7. Tape the cannula securely in place and cover with transparent dressing.
8. Connect the infusion set and calibrate the monitoring equipment.

Complications of cannulation

- Arteriospasm
- Haematoma
- Thrombosis
- Bacterial colonisation and sepsis

22.2 Defibrillation

In order to achieve the optimum outcome, defibrillation must be performed quickly and efficiently. This requires the following:

- Correct electrode pad/paddle selection
- Correct electrode pad/ paddle placement
- Good electrode pad /paddle contact
- Correct energy selection

Many defibrillators are available. Providers of advanced paediatric life support should make sure that they are familiar with those they may have to use.

Correct electrode pad/paddle selection

Defibrillators for paediatric use should be supplied with two sets of electrode pads – adult and paediatric. Adult electrode pads can be used for patients aged 8 years and above and paediatric electrode pads for the younger child. Children vary in size so there is some discretion. Ensure the electrode pads are at least 2 cm apart to prevent arcing. Electrode paddles are usually labelled pictorially to show placement positions.

Where there is a possibility that a neonate may be defibrillated, manual paddles with a 4.5 cm diameter should be available as paediatric electrode pads may not be of a sufficiently small diameter even for anterior posterior placement.

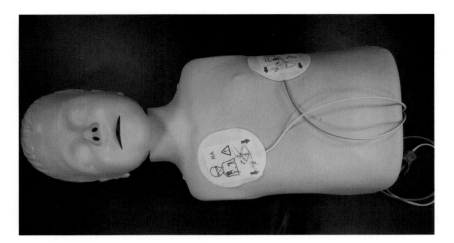

Figure 22.8 Standard anterolateral paddle placement

Correct electrode pad/paddle placement

Pads should be used in preference to paddles, because once placed they save time, resulting in less interruption to chest compressions and time to defibrillation and they are also safer. They promote charging during compressions which decreases hands-off chest time.

The usual placement is anterolateral. One paddle is put over the apex in the mid-axillary line (a finger breadth below the left nipple) and the other is placed just to the right of the sternum (a finger breadth below the right clavicle) (Figure 22.8).

If the anteroposterior placement is used, in a child one electrode pad/paddle is placed just to the left side of the lower part of the sternum and the other just below the tip of the left scapula. In an infant the pads will be placed as seen in Figure 22.9.

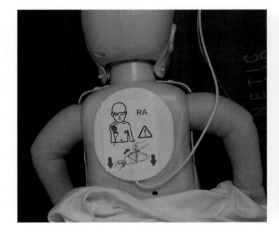
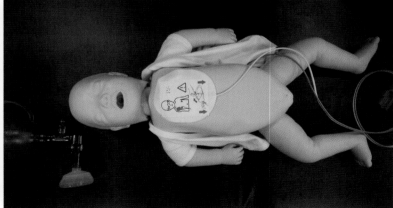

Figure 22.9 Anteroposterior paddle placement

Good electrode pad/paddle contact

Electrode pads should be placed on dry skin and smoothed on to ensure good contact to ensure effective energy delivery. Gel pads or electrode gel should always be used in conjunction with manual paddles (if the latter, care should be taken not to join the two areas of application). Firm pressure should be applied to the paddles.

Adult paddles are 13 cm diameter. If available, paddles of 4.5 cm diameter are for use in infants. The paediatric/infant paddles usually will be clipped over or hidden under the adult paddles.

Correct energy selection

The recommended levels are given in Chapters 20 and 22.

Automated external defibrillators (AEDs) are now commonplace. The standard adult shock is used for children over 8 years. For children under 8 years, attenuated paediatric paddles should be used with the AED. For the infant of less than 1 year, a manual defibrillator which can be adjusted to give the correct shock is recommended. However, if an AED is the only defibrillator available, its use should be considered, preferably with paediatric attenuation pads. The order of decreasing preference for defibrillation in the under 1-year-olds is as follows:

1. Manual defibrillator.
2. AED with dose attenuator.
3. AED without dose attenuator.

Many AEDs can detect ventricular fibrillation/ventricular tachycardia (VF/VT) in children of all ages and differentiate 'shockable' from 'non-shockable' rhythms with a high degree of sensitivity and specificity.

Safety

A defibrillator delivers enough current to cause cardiac arrest. The user must ensure that other rescuers are not in physical contact with the patient (or the trolley) at the moment the shock is delivered. When using paddles the defibrillator should only be charged when the paddles are either in contact with the child or replaced properly in their storage positions. When using electrode pads it is advisable to charge whilst compressions are ongoing.

In all cases disconnect the oxygen supply to the patient – even with closed ventilation circuits – as uncuffed tubes will leak oxygen around the axillary area.

Procedure: manual defibrillation

Basic life support should be interrupted for the shortest possible time (steps 4–9 below).

1. Apply gel pads or electrode gel.
2. Select the correct paddles.
3. Select the energy required.
4. Shout 'Stand back!'
5. Remove the paddles from the machine and place the paddles onto the gel pads, and apply firm pressure.
6. Shout 'Charging!' Press the charge button.
7. Wait until the defibrillator is charged.
8. Check that all other rescuers are clear.
9. Deliver the shock.
10. Recommence CPR.

Procedure: hands-free defibrillation

Basic life support should be interrupted for the shortest possible time (steps 8–10).

1. Apply adhesive monitoring electrodes to the correct positions whilst compressions continue.
2. Interrupt briefly to confirm VF then immediately recommence compressions.
3. Ensure all other personnel are clear and oxygen has been removed.
4. Select the energy required whilst compressions continue.
5. Shout 'Charging, continue compressions'.
6. Press the charge button whilst compressions continue.
7. Wait until the defibrillator is charged.
8. Shout 'Stop compressions, stand back!'
9. Check that team member performing compressions is clear.
10. Deliver the shock.
11. Recommence CPR.

CHAPTER 23
Practical procedures: trauma

Learning outcomes

After reading this chapter, you will be able to identify equipment for and describe the following procedures:
- Chest decompression:
  - Needle thoracocentesis
  - Chest drain placement
- Pericardiocentesis
- Femoral nerve block
- Cervical spine immobilisation:
  - Application of head blocks and straps
  - 20° tilt

23.1 Needle thoracocentesis

This procedure can be life saving and can be performed quickly with minimum equipment. It should be followed by chest drain placement.

Minimum equipment

- Alcohol swabs
- Large over-the-needle intravenous cannula (16 gauge or commercial devices are available for this procedure)
- Syringe: 20 ml

Procedure

1. Identify the second intercostal space in the mid-clavicular line on the side of the pneumothorax.
2. Swab the chest wall with surgical preparation solution or an alcohol swab.
3. Attach the syringe to the cannula. Fluid in the cannula will assist in the identification of air bubbles.
4. Insert the cannula vertically into the chest wall, just above the rib below, aspirating all the time (Figure 23.1).
5. If air is aspirated remove the needle, leaving the plastic cannula in place.
6. Tape the cannula in place and proceed to chest drain insertion as soon as possible.

Alternative method

1. Administer high-flow oxygen.
2. Attach a 10 ml syringe with 2 ml of saline to the rear of the cannula and needle.
3. Identify the fifth intercostal space in the mid-axillary line on the side of the suspected tension pneumothorax. This lateral approach provides a larger zone of safety than the anterior approach – but access may restrict its use.
4. Clean the skin and insert the cannula into the skin, just superior to the sixth rib. Once through the skin flush the needle with the saline – to expel any skin plug.
5. Remove the syringe plunger from the barrel of the syringe.

Advanced Paediatric Life Support: A Practical Approach to Emergencies, Sixth Edition. Edited by Martin Samuels and Sue Wieteska.
© 2016 John Wiley & Sons, Ltd. Published 2016 by John Wiley & Sons, Ltd.

6. Advance the needle and cannula to pierce the pleura; draining of saline out of the syringe suggests penetration of the pleura.
7. Bubbling in the syringe indicates the presence of a tension pneumothorax.
8. Advance the cannula over the needle into the pleural space.
9. The cannula or needle may need flushing due to occlusion with a skin plug.
10. Tape the cannula in place and proceed to chest drain insertion as soon as possible.
11. If needle thoracocentesis is attempted, and the patient does not have a tension pneumothorax, the risk of causing a pneumothorax is 10–20%. Patients who have had this procedure must have a chest radiograph, and will require chest drainage if ventilated.

A further alternative is to perform an immediate slit or finger thoracostomy rather than a needle thoracocentesis. This is a more reliable and definitive method of reducing a tension.

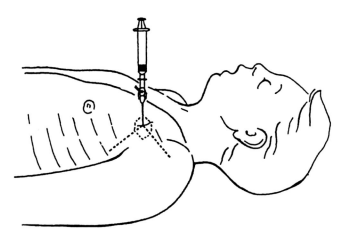

Figure 23.1 Needle thoracocentesis

23.2 Chest drain placement

Chest drain placement should be performed using the open technique described here. This minimises lung damage. In general, the largest size drain that will pass between the ribs should be used.

Minimum equipment

- Skin preparation and surgical drapes
- Scalpel
- Large clamps ×2
- Suture
- (Local anaesthetic)
- Scissors
- Chest drain tube

Procedure

1. Decide on the insertion site (usually the fifth intercostal space in the mid-axillary line) on the side with the pneumothorax (Figure 23.2).
2. Swab the chest wall with surgical preparation or an alcohol swab.
3. Use local anaesthetic if necessary.
4. Make a 2–3 cm skin incision along the line of the intercostal space, just above the rib below.
5. Bluntly dissect through the subcutaneous tissues just over the top of the rib below, and puncture the parietal pleura with the tip of the clamp.
6. Put a gloved finger into the incision and clear the path into the pleura (Figure 23.3). This will not be possible in small children.
7. Advance the chest drain tube into the pleural space during expiration.

8. Ensure the tube is in the pleural space by listening for air movement, and by looking for fogging of the tube during expiration.
9. Connect the chest drain tube to an underwater seal.
10. Suture the drain in place, and secure with tape.
11. Obtain a chest radiograph.

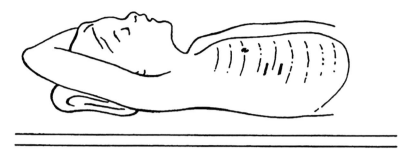

Figure 23.2 Chest drain insertion – landmarks

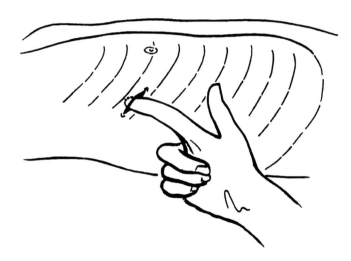

Figure 23.3 Chest drain insertion – clearing the path

23.3 Clamshell thoracotomy

This is a life-saving procedure and should be performed in children presenting in cardiac arrest after penetrating chest trauma. The definitive intervention should be performed within 10 minutes of loss of cardiac output. This technique should only be performed by those with expertise and therefore it is not described in detail within the practical procedures.

23.4 Pericardiocentesis

The removal of a small amount of fluid from the pericardial sac can be life saving. The procedure is not without risks and the ECG should be closely monitored throughout. An acute injury pattern (ST segment changes or a widened QRS) indicates ventricular damage by the needle. In traumatic cardiac arrest following penetrating injury, clamshell thoracotomy should be performed immediately.

Minimum equipment

- Skin preparation and surgical drapes
- ECG monitor
- (Local anaesthetic)
- Syringe: 20 ml
- Large over-the-needle cannula (16 or 18 gauge)

Procedure

1. Swab the xiphoid and subxiphoid areas with surgical preparation or an alcohol swab.
2. Use local anaesthetic if necessary
3. Assess the patient for any significant mediastinal shift if possible.
4. Attach the syringe to the needle.
5. Puncture the skin 1–2 cm inferior to the left side of the xiphoid junction at a 45° angle (Figure 23.4).
6. Advance the needle towards the tip of the left scapula, aspirating all the time (Figure 23.5).
7. Watch the ECG monitor for signs of myocardial injury.
8. Once fluid is withdrawn, aspirate as much as possible (unless it is possible to withdraw limitless amounts of blood, in which case a ventricle has probably been entered).
9. If the procedure is successful, remove the needle, leaving the cannula in the pericardial sac. Secure in place and seal with a three-way tap. This allows later repeat aspirations should tamponade recur.

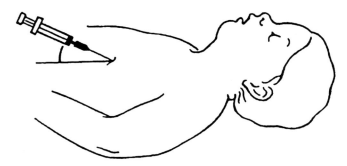

Figure 23.4 Needle pericardiocentesis – angle

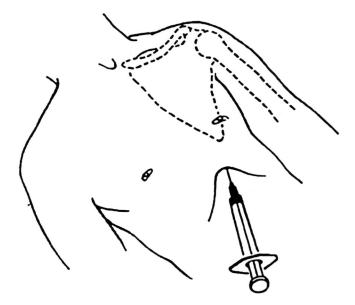

Figure 23.5 Needle pericardiocentesis – direction

23.5 Femoral nerve block

The femoral nerve supplies the femur with sensation, and a block is useful in cases of femoral fracture. The technique may also be of benefit when analgesic agents would interfere with the management or assessment of other injuries. A long-acting local anaesthetic agent should be used so that radiographs and splinting can be undertaken with minimal distress to the child.

Equipment

- Antiseptic swabs to clean
- Lidocaine 1%
- Syringe (2 ml) and a 25 gauge needle
- Syringe (5 or 10 ml) and a 21 gauge needle
- Bupivacaine 0.25%: 0.8 ml/kg of 0.25% (maximum 2 mg/kg)

Procedure

1. Move the fractured limb gently so that the femur lies in abduction and the ipsilateral groin is exposed.
2. Swab the groin clean with antiseptic solution.
3. Identify the femoral artery and keep one finger on it. The femoral nerve lies immediately lateral to the artery.
4. Using the 2 ml syringe filled with lidocaine and a 25 gauge needle, infiltrate the skin just lateral to the artery. Aspirate the syringe frequently to ensure that the needle is not in a vessel.
5. Inject the bupivacaine around the nerve using the 21 gauge needle, taking care not to puncture the artery or vein.
6. Wait until anaesthesia occurs (bupivacaine may take up to 20 minutes to have its full effect).

Femoral nerve block with ultrasound guidance

Sterile technique for ultrasound

Prepare the groin skin with antiseptic solution. Use a sterile probe cover or, for a single shot block, prep all around the probe once it is positioned, and use a sterile no-touch technique with the injecting hand.

Procedure

1. Hold a 7–10 MHz linear probe in your non-dominant hand, placing it transversely, with the centre over the femoral artery pulse at the level of the groin crease (Figure 23.6). A cross-sectional view of the vessels and nerve will be obtained.
2. Identify the pulsating femoral artery and move the probe so it is in the middle of the ultrasound view.
3. The femoral nerve is an oval, white, honeycomb-like structure, located lateral to the artery. A good ultrasound view of the nerve is dependent on angling the probe to ensure the beam transects the nerve at 90° (anisotropy). It may be extremely difficult to visualise the nerve if the probe is angled incorrectly. Tilt the probe towards the head and the feet until you optimise your view (Figure 23.7).
4. Sterile prep as above.

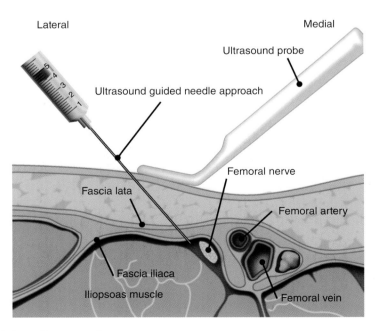

Figure 23.6 Ultrasound-guided needle approach

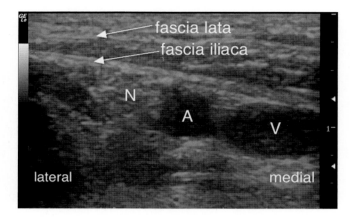

Figure 23.7 Ultrasound image of the femoral region. [A, artery; N, nerve; V, vein]

5. With your dominant hand insert a short bevel block needle, entering the skin at the lateral end of the probe (without touching it, to ensure sterility). Advance the needle slowly, keeping it parallel to and in the middle of the probe so the tip can be seen advancing towards the nerve, but stop just lateral to the nerve (to minimise the risk of intraneural injection). You may feel and see the needle breaching the fascia lata and the fascia iliaca (Figure 23.8).
6. Have an assistant inject the local anaesthetic, watching it surround the nerve, and reposition the needle if necessary to ensure good spread.

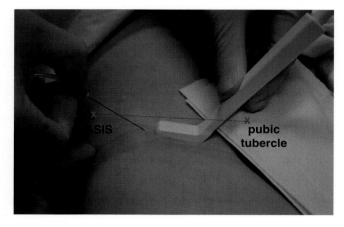

Figure 23.8 Ultrasound-guided block. [ASIS, anterior superior iliac spine]

23.6 Cervical spine immobilisation

All children with serious trauma must be treated as though they have a cervical spine injury. It is only when an adequate examination and history is taken or appropriate investigations have been performed that the decision to remove the cervical spine protection can be made and this should be as soon as possible. Specialist consultation may be needed prior to this decision. Manual in-line cervical stabilisation should be continued until the head blocks and tape has been applied or the cervical spine has been cleared clinically (Figure 23.9).

Once the head blocks are in place, the neck may be obscured. Before application of the head blocks, look for the following signs quickly and without moving the neck:

- Distended veins
- Tracheal deviation
- Wounds
- Laryngeal crepitus
- Subcutaneous emphysema

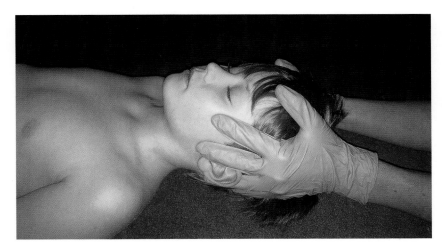

Figure 23.9 Manual in-line stabilisation (MILS)

Application of head blocks and tape

Equipment

- Two head blocks
- Attachment system

Procedure

1. Ensure in-line cervical stabilisation is maintained by a second person throughout.
2. Place a head block either side of the head.
3. Apply the forehead strap and attach it securely to trolley.
4. Apply the lower strap across the chin and attach it securely to the trolley.

Exceptions

An injured child may be uncooperative for many reasons including fear, pain and hypoxia. Manual immobilisation should be maintained and the contributing factors addressed. Overzealous immobilisation of the head and neck may paradoxically increase the leverage on the neck as the child struggles. Children with traumatic torticollis should be manually immobilised in their current position.

20° tilt

In order to minimise the chances of exacerbating unrecognised spinal cord injury and disruption of a clot in major abdominal trauma, non-essential movements of the spine must be avoided until adequate examination and investigations have excluded it. If manoeuvres that might cause spinal movement are essential (e.g. during examination of the back in the course of the secondary survey) or the child needs to be removed from a scoop stretcher, then the 20° tilt should be performed. The aim of the 20° tilt is to maintain the alignment of the spine during turning of the child. The basic requirements are an adequate number of carers and good control.

Procedure

1. Gather together enough staff to tilt the child. In larger children, four people will be required; three will be required in smaller children and infants (Figures 23.10 and 23.11)
2. Place the staff as shown in Table 23.1.
3. Ensure each member of staff knows what they are going to do, as shown in Table 23.2.
4. Carry out essential manoeuvres as quickly as possible.

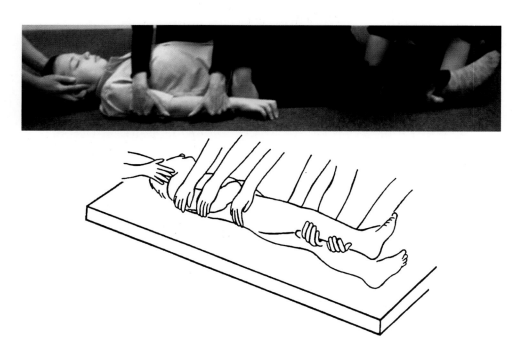

Figure 23.10 20° tilt (four-person technique)

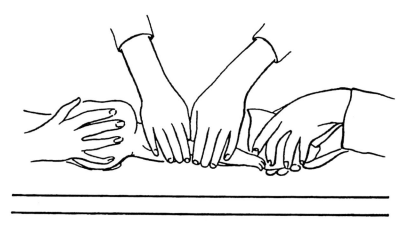

Figure 23.11 20° tilt (three-person technique)

	Position of staff for:	
Table 23.1 Position of staff for the 20° tilt		
Staff member no.	**Smaller child and infant**	**Larger child**
1	Head	Head
2	Chest	Chest
3	Legs and pelvis	Pelvis
4		Legs

Table 23.2 Tasks of individual members of staff

Staff member: position	Task
Head	Hold either side of the head (as for in-line cervical stabilisation) and maintain orientation of the head with the body in all planes during turning
	Control the 20° tilt by telling other staff when to roll and when to lay the child back onto the trolley
Chest	Reach over the child and carefully place both hands under the chest. When told to roll the child, support the weight of the chest and maintain stability. Watch the movement of the head at all times and roll the chest at the same rate
Legs and pelvis	This only applies to smaller children and infants. If it is not possible to control the pelvis and legs at the same time, get additional help immediately
	Place one hand either side of the pelvis over the iliac crests. Cradle the child's legs between the forearms. When told to roll the child, grip the pelvis and legs and move them together. Watch the movement of the head and chest at all times, and roll the pelvis and legs at the same rate
Pelvis	Place one hand over the pelvis on the iliac crest and the other under the top of the far leg. When told to roll the child, watch the movement of the head and chest at all times and roll the pelvis at the same rate
Legs	Support the weight of the far leg by placing both hands under it. When told to roll the child, watch the movement of the chest and pelvis and roll the leg at the same rate

CHAPTER 24
Imaging in trauma

24.1 Introduction

This chapter provides an overview of the use of emergency imaging in major trauma in children. It also provides an introduction to interpretation, as appropriate, for the clinician involved in managing paediatric trauma in the resuscitation room.

Radiological advice should be sought if there is any doubt about what to image and how, also in the interpretation of results. Discussing images with an experienced emergency physician or trauma, orthopaedic or neurosurgeon may also help. An experienced emergency radiographer (technician) is a valuable asset to any department and, if they consider a film is abnormal, their comments should be carefully noted. Reference should be made to the *Intercollegiate Guidelines on Imaging in Paediatric Major Trauma*.

All major trauma centres and trauma units should have in place 'hot reporting' by a senior radiologist such that images (whether plain film or CT) are reported on a primary survey report form within 5 minutes. This documents all potentially life-threatening problems. Fuller formal written reporting should occur within 60 minutes of the scan. A basic understanding of anatomy on the images is necessary but important clinical decisions about management will usually be made on the radiologist report.

The primary cause of death in trauma patients is bleeding. The modality of imaging for accurately detecting bleeding is CT. The use of CT in children has to weigh the benefits of finding injuries versus the real risks of ionising radiation in significant doses. The *routine use* of head to thigh polytrauma CTs in children is *not* appropriate.

> The principle is to keep radiation dose 'as low as reasonably achievable' – ALARA.

Whole body CT

The key investigation in the *critically injured* paediatric patient with multisystem trauma is likely to be a whole body CT. This usually means a head to symphysis pubis CT in fact. This incorporates all important body regions including the pelvis. National targets (for adults) state that this should be performed within 30 minutes of the patient's arrival in the emergency department. However, few paediatric patients meet the criteria of proper multisystem trauma so this approach cannot be justified as first line investigation.

Radiography of a seriously injured child is technically challenging as access is often limited and plain films are often taken with a mobile machine. Equipment such as sandbags may obscure bony landmarks, and the position in which the child is lying

Advanced Paediatric Life Support: A Practical Approach to Emergencies, Sixth Edition. Edited by Martin Samuels and Sue Wieteska.
© 2016 John Wiley & Sons, Ltd. Published 2016 by John Wiley & Sons, Ltd.

may cause difficulty in radiographic interpretation, e.g. the interpretation of a supine anteroposterior (AP) chest X-ray is more difficult than that of an erect posteroanterior (PA) film.

The radiology department is not a place to leave a sick or unstable patient without adequate clinical supervision. Plain films are taken by a radiographer, who will not be able to supervise an ill patient. Complex investigations including ultrasound scanning, CT and contrast studies take time, during which the child may deteriorate significantly without appropriate treatment. A core component of the trauma team should accompany the child on any transfer in the hospital and this includes to radiology.

Trauma is more likely to be blunt than penetrating, to be a fall (particularly from a low height) than a road traffic collision (RTC) and, therefore, significant bony injury to the cervical spine is rare and to the pelvis even rarer. TARN (Trauma Audit Research Network) data for the paediatric population (in 2012) shows that head injury is the commonest injury; followed by injuries to the extremities and then to the abdomen. A common combination is that all three areas are injured. However, data suggest that areas in between injury areas (e.g. the pelvis or cervical spine) are not commonly injured as part of the process and should not be routinely imaged just because they lie between two other body regions that are injured.

> In order to prevent unnecessary radiation only request CTs that will change management.

Do **not** request a CT chest in a patient who requires a CT head and CT abdomen (a common combination) simply because the chest lies between the two injured areas. This is inappropriate in children where multisystem trauma is the exception, not the rule.

Similarly, do **not** request a CT C-spine (200 × the radiation dose of a three-view C-spine X-ray is delivered to the developing thyroid gland) just because the head may require a CT scan.

Similarly, if a CT is required (e.g. CT head), it is **not** required to do a whole body CT in order to exclude other injury. This particularly applies to the C-spine which can be cleared by use of clinical assessment alone or in conjunction with X-rays.

> A primary survey routine ordering of C-spine, chest X-ray and pelvis X-ray **is no longer considered appropriate**.
>
> Recommended imaging in a primary survey is a chest X-ray, and a C-spine if the injury is unable to be cleared clinically and there is no up-front indication for C-spine CT.
>
> The need for pelvic X-rays should be considered carefully.

USS of the abdomen is 50% sensitive for free fluid and therefore while a USS of the chest may be a useful adjunct there is no role for the FAST (focused abdominal with sonography for trauma) scan in children. If there is suspicion of bleeding in the abdomen the imaging of choice is CT with contrast.

Much less useful are the lateral C-spine radiograph and pelvic radiograph. The lateral C-spine X-ray on its own it does not exclude bony injury and if the assessment of the child is difficult (due to depressed level of consciousness, alcohol or drugs) the cervical spine cannot be safely cleared.

Children rarely have significant pelvic ring disruption fractures (this excludes isolated pubic ramus fractures) and a routine pelvic X-ray is **not** required. Significant ring fractures should be clinically evident anyway and should be being treated, e.g. with fluids/blood and pelvic brace. While pubic rami fractures are relatively common they do not cause significant bleeding or threat to life, organ or limb. If there is strong clinical suspicion of pelvic ring injury then a pelvic X-ray is indicated in resuscitation with a chest X-ray.

Previously, all three provided a basic screen for major injuries. In fact most children do not sustain significant cervical spine injury and the lateral C-spine film is not the best investigation for excluding it. A routine lateral C-spine film is certainly not indicated. Assess the child first. If there is very strong clinical suspicion of injury, CT is the first line choice of imaging. Three views (AP, lateral and open mouth odontoid peg view (if possible)) are indicated for those where the index of suspicion is lower, but the high-dose radiation of CT is to be avoided. These images should only be taken after immediately life-threatening injuries have been identified and treated.

With all imaging, check that the image has:

- The name of the patient
- The date and time that the film was taken
- The orientation (side marker position)

24.2 Cervical spine imaging

Requesting

Cervical spine immobilisation should take place before any radiographs are performed. Cervical spine injuries should be imaged according to National Institute for Health and Care Excellence (NICE) guideline criteria. If sandbags rather than head blocks are used for immobilisation they may obscure bony landmarks.

Computed tomography of the cervical spine

If the plain films are unclear or abnormal or there is a high-risk mechanism of injury:

- Under 10 years: the recommendation is for CT of the upper cervical spine (from the occipital condyles and foramen magnum down to C3) – this covers the craniocervical junction. This is the most common site of fracture in this age group and it excludes the radiosensitive thyroid gland from the scan.
- Over 10 years: the recommendation is to image as adults – i.e. from the occipital condyles down to the C7/T1 junction.

Bony injury in itself is not the prime concern in spinal injury. The main risk is actual or potential injury to the cord. Any unstable fracture, if inadequately immobilised, may lead to progressive cord damage.

A lateral C-spine film is often requested to 'clear' the cervical spine, but a normal film may be falsely reassuring. The plain film only shows the position of the bones at the time the film was taken, and gives no idea of the magnitude of flexion and extension forces applied to the spine at the time of injury. The cord may be injured even in a child without any apparent radiographic abnormality. For this reason if there is strong clinical suspicion of significant cervical spine cord injury (paraesthesiae, neurological abnormalities) then MRI is the initial imaging modality of choice.

Unlike adult spines, most paediatric cervical spine injuries occur either through the discs and ligaments at the craniovertebral junction (C1, C2 and C3) or at C7/T1. The relatively large mass of the head, moving on a flexible neck with poorly supportive muscles, leads to injury in the higher cervical vertebrae. Children develop three patterns of spinal injury:

1. Subluxation or dislocation without fracture.
2. Fracture with or without subluxation or dislocation.
3. Spinal cord injury without radiographic abnormality (SCIWORA).

The last of these, SCIWORA, is said to have occurred when radiographic films are totally normal in the presence of significant cord injury. If the film is normal in a conscious child with clinical symptoms (such as pain, loss of function or paraesthesia in a limb) then neck protection measures should be continued and MRI should be obtained. In an unconscious child at high risk, a cord injury cannot be excluded until the patient is awake and has been assessed clinically, even in the presence of a normal C-spine film. Adequate spinal precautions should be continued until the child is well enough to be assessed clinically, or MRI has been carried out.

The most common site of a 'missed' spinal injury is where a flexible part of the spine meets the fixed part. In the neck these are the cervicocranial junction and the cervicothoracic junction.

Checking adequacy

The whole spine should be viewed from the lower clivus down to the upper body of the T1 vertebra. If the C7/T1 junction is not seen initially then gentle traction should be applied by pulling the arms down, holding them above the elbow joint. If the child is conscious they should be asked to relax their shoulders as traction is applied. If the child is on a spinal board then this must be stabilised by an assistant.

24.3 Chest radiograph

The most useful initial trauma film in terms of aiding immediate life-threatening problems in the emergency department is the chest radiograph. USS can help as it is actually more sensitive for the detection of air (pneumothorax) or fluid (haemothorax) than X-ray. X-rays can be done quickly via a portable machine in the resuscitation room. If this is abnormal, then CT can be requested for the chest. If normal, then CT chest is **not** required.

Checking the X-ray

Adequacy can be assessed by considering both penetration and depth of inspiration. The film should be sufficiently penetrated to just visualise the disc spaces of the lower thoracic vertebrae through the heart shadow. At least five anterior rib ends should be seen above the diaphragm on the right side. An expiratory film may mimic consolidation.

Alignment can be assessed by ensuring that the medial ends of both clavicles are equally spaced about the spinous processes of the upper thoracic vertebrae, as shown in Figure 24.1. Abnormal rotation may create apparent mediastinal shift. The trachea should be equally spaced between the clavicles.

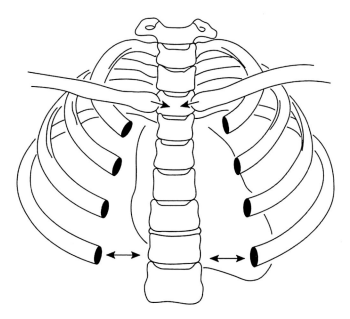

Figure 24.1 Assessing rotation – straight chest film

Check the position of any apparatus, including:

- Tracheal tube
- Central venous lines
- Chest drains

Misplacement of the endotracheal tube (ETT) should be evident clinically, but may be seen on a chest film if you look for it. Do this first when reviewing any chest X-ray on an intubated patient. Malposition of an ETT can result in reduced ventilation and hypoxia. The ideal position for an ETT is below the clavicles and at least 1 cm above the carina. To find the carina, identify the slope of the right and left main bronchi – the carina is where the two lines meet in the midline.

The posterior, lateral and anterior aspects of each rib must be examined in detail. This can be done by tracing out the upper and lower borders of the ribs from the posterior costochondral joint to where they join the anterior costal cartilage at the mid-clavicular line. The internal trabecular pattern can then be assessed.

The ribs in children are soft and pliable and only break when subjected to considerable force. Even greater force is required to fracture the first rib or to break multiple ribs. Consequently, the presence of these fractures should stimulate you to look for other sites of injury both inside and outside the chest.

Finish assessing the bones by inspecting the visible vertebrae, the clavicles, scapulae and proximal humeri.

Thoracic spine injuries may be overlooked on a chest radiograph. Abnormal flattening of the vertebral bodies, widening of the disc spaces or gaps between the spinous processes or pedicles may be seen. On AP views increased vertical or horizontal distances between the pedicles or spinous processes indicate an unstable fracture, as shown in Figure 24.2.

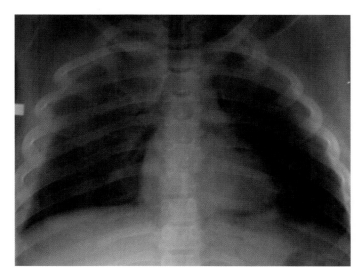

Figure 24.2 Vertical fracture of the thoracic spine

If there are rib fractures in the first three ribs, these may be associated with major spinal trauma and great vessel injury.

A suspected tension pneumothorax should be treated clinically in the emergency situation, without confirmatory X-ray. On a supine film, the air in a simple pneumothorax rises anteriorly and may only be evident from an abnormal blackness or 'sharpness' of the diaphragm or cardiac border. The standard appearances of a pneumothorax, where there is a sharp lung edge and the vessels fail to extend to the rib cage and the lung edges, may not occur in the supine film.

The cardiac outline should lie one-third to the right of midline and two-thirds to the left of midline. If the film is not rotated, then mediastinal shift is due to the heart being either pushed from one side or pulled from the other. For example, mediastinal shift to the left may be due either to a pneumothorax, air trapping or effusion on the right side, or to collapse of the left lung.

All trauma radiographs are taken in the supine position, often using portable X-ray machines. The tube is near to the patient and the heart is anterior with the film posterior. The heart in this situation appears abnormally magnified (widened) and the cardiothoracic ratio is difficult to assess on supine AP films.

The mediastinal cardiac outline should be clear on both sides. Any loss of definition suggests consolidation (de-aeration) of adjacent lungs. A 'globular' shape to the heart may suggest a pericardial effusion. Tamponade is managed clinically, not radiologically. A cardiac echo is useful in equivocal cases.

In the teenager, the mediastinum should appear as narrow as in an adult. In children under the age of 18 months, the normal thymus may simulate superior mediastinal widening (above the level of the carina). A normal thymus may touch the right chest wall, left chest wall, left diaphragm or right diaphragm, making it very difficult to exclude mediastinal pathology. Fortunately, mediastinal widening due to aortic dissection or spinal trauma is very rare in small children.

In cases of doubt, where there is a normal clinical examination, an opinion from a radiologist should be sought. In the older child involved in trauma, mediastinal widening may mean aortic dissection, or major vessel or spinal injury. Ultrasound, CT or angiography may be required to resolve this when the child is stable.

The cardiophrenic and costophrenic angles should be clear on both sides. The diaphragms should be clearly defined on both sides and the left diaphragm should be clearly visible behind the heart. Loss of definition of the left diaphragm behind the heart suggests left lower lobe collapse, an abnormal hump suggests diaphragmatic rupture, and an elevated diaphragm suggests effusion, lung collapse or nerve palsy.

At the end of the systematic review of the X-ray, check again in the key areas shown in the box.

> - Behind the heart (left lower lobe consolidation or collapse)
> - Apices for effusions, pneumothorax, rib fractures and collapse/consolidation
> - Costophrenic and cardiophrenic angles – fluid or pneumothorax
> - Horizontal fissure – fluid or elevation (upper lobe collapse)
> - Trachea for foreign body (and ETT)

24.4 The role of further imaging

Abdominal imaging

There is no place for FAST scanning in the emergency department resuscitation room in children. A formal radiologist USS of the abdomen can be helpful however. Most imaging of the abdomen will be by CT with contrast but only if specific criteria are met:

- Lap belt injury/bruising
- Abdominal wall bruising
- Abdominal tenderness in a conscious patient
- Abdominal distension
- Clinical evidence of persistent hypovolaemia
- Blood from the rectum or nasogastric tube
- Significant handle bar injuries

Head imaging

The NICE evidence is extrapolated from adult practice, as there are few studies to form a scientific basis for this guidance in the paediatric age group. CT brain scanning is the prime modality for excluding acute intracranial haemorrhage. A child with clinical suspicion of intracranial bleeding requires a CT scan, not a skull film, as intracranial bleeding in children often occurs without a skull fracture. Before the child is sent into the radiology department for a scan, he or she must be resuscitated, stabilised and supervised at all times by a doctor or appropriately trained senior nurse.

According to NICE guidelines if a child has an indication for a head CT and when there is strong clinical suspicion of a neck injury, then the cervical spine is included at the same time (see section on CT of the cervical spine).

24.5 Summary

- Radiological advice should be sought if there is any doubt about what to image and how, and also in the interpretation of results
- Only request CTs that will change management in order to prevent unnecessary radiation
- A primary survey routine ordering of C-spine, chest X-ray and pelvis X-ray **is no longer considered appropriate**
- The most useful initial trauma film in terms of aiding immediate life-threatening problems in the emergency department is the chest radiograph

CHAPTER 25
Structured approach to stabilisation and transfer

Learning outcomes

After reading this chapter, you will be able to:
- Describe a structured approach to the stabilisation of a seriously ill or injured child
- Describe a structured approach to the transfer of a seriously ill or injured child

25.1 Stabilisation of the child

After successful resuscitation of the seriously ill or injured child, frequent clinical reassessment must be carried out in order to detect any changes in the child's status. This is essential in order to provide the appropriate information to guide ongoing care. All patients should have the following monitored:

- Oxygen saturation
- CO_2 monitoring (if intubated)
- Pulse rate and rhythm
- Blood pressure (non-invasive)
- Urine output
- Core temperature
- Arterial pH and gases

Additionally, some patients will require:

- Invasive blood pressure monitoring
- Central venous pressure (CVP) monitoring
- Intracranial pressure (ICP) monitoring

The resources to measure some of these parameters may only be available in a static intensive care setting. The clinical team should carefully consider what surrogate signs they can consider where it is necessary to deviate from the ideal monitoring profile.

The investigations shown in the following box should be considered following successful resuscitation or during subsequent stabilisation:

Advanced Paediatric Life Support: A Practical Approach to Emergencies, Sixth Edition. Edited by Martin Samuels and Sue Wieteska.
© 2016 John Wiley & Sons, Ltd. Published 2016 by John Wiley & Sons, Ltd.

Post-resuscitation investigations

- Chest radiograph
- Arterial or central venous blood gasses
- Full blood count
- Group and save serum for cross-match
- Sodium, potassium, calcium, urea and creatinine
- Clotting screen
- Blood glucose
- Liver function tests
- Urinalysis, microscopy and culture
- Culture of blood and, if indicated, cerebrospinal fluid
- C-reactive protein or procalcitonin

Children who have been resuscitated from cardiorespiratory arrest may die hours or days later from multiple organ failure. In addition to the cellular and homeostatic abnormalities that occur during the preceding illness, and during the arrest itself, cellular damage continues after spontaneous circulation has been restored. This is called reperfusion injury and is caused by the following:

- Depletion of adenosine triphosphate (ATP)
- Entry of calcium into cells
- Free fatty acid metabolism activation
- Free-radical oxygen production

Similarly, children resuscitated with serious illness or injury may suffer multisystem dysfunction as a result of hypoxia or ischaemia. Ongoing activation of inflammatory mediators, as occurs in serious sepsis, also contributes to multisystem organ failure. Post-resuscitation management aims to achieve and maintain homeostasis in order to optimise the chances of recovery. Management should be directed in a systematic way.

Airway and breathing

Seriously ill children often exhibit an impaired conscious level and a depressed gag reflex. Intubation should always be considered and will usually have occurred during resuscitation. Any uncertainty regarding the indications for and against intubation should be discussed with a consultant intensivist or anaesthetist.

In many cases the process of intubating and ventilating a child, which converts physiological negative pressure ventilation to positive pressure ventilation, can lead to significant difficulty in ventilating (clearing CO_2) and oxygenating the child. The clinician managing the process should be ready for such an occurrence and be prepared to rapidly increase ventilator settings and ventilate by hand where necessary.

- The endotracheal tube should ideally, have a small leak. It should be secured according to local guidelines and ventilation should be monitored by continuous capnography. Endotracheal tubes should not be cut before a review of the chest radiograph by the receiving team to confirm the appropriate position. Even when the tube is well positioned it may be desirable to leave it uncut in order to allow heavy ventilator tubing/valves to be safety positioned provided there is no difficulty with ventilating the child.
- Ventilation settings should normally be maintained to keep blood gases normal (PCO_2 4.5–6.0 kPa (34–45 mmHg). Children with intracranial injuries should have their PCO_2 maintained as close to 4.5–5.0 kPa (34–38 mmHg) as possible. The rational for this is to minimise cerebral oedema and minimise any increase in ICP. If this is difficult because of airway or lung pathology, urgent advice should be obtained from a paediatric intensivist.
- Sufficient inspired oxygen should be given to maintain SpO_2 at between 94% and 98% except for children with cyanotic cardiac lesions and chronic lung disease. The latter group will normally target an SpO_2 of 88–92% (provided their normal saturations are not significantly higher). If anaemia or carbon monoxide poisoning is suspected, inspired oxygen should be delivered at the highest possible concentration irrespective of the SpO_2 value. Specialist advice regarding target saturations should be sought from a paediatric intensivist or cardiologist for all children where a cardiac abnormality or significant chronic lung disease is either known or suspected.

Circulation

If the child is intubated there may be a profound deterioration in cardiovascular function around the time of induction. This is due to the suppression of endogenous catecholamines, secondary to the induction agents used, and the physiological effect of positive pressure ventilation. A careful choice of induction agents can help reduce this risk.

Following resuscitation, there will often be a poor cardiac output, irrespective of the events around induction. This may be due to any combination of the following factors:

- An underlying cardiac abnormality
- The effects on the myocardium of hypoxia, acidosis and toxins, preceding and during any arrest
- Continuing acid–base or electrolyte disturbance
- Hypovolaemia

The following steps should be taken if there are signs of poor perfusion:

- Assess cardiac output clinically
- Infuse crystalloid or colloid in aliquots of 10 ml/kg and reassess cardiac output clinically
- Aim for a normal arterial pH (>7.3) and good oxygenation. This may require the use of inotropic drug support with or without further fluid boluses
- Monitor ventilation and intervene with support when inadequate
- Identify and correct hypoglycaemia. Start to correct other electrolyte abnormalities

A CVP line will give useful information about the preload to the heart. This may assist in decisions about fluid infusion and inotropic support. A target value for the CVP should be discussed and established with an expert team. The CVP may be best used in assessing the response to a fluid challenge. In hypovolaemic patients, CVP alters little with a fluid bolus, but in euvolaemia or hypervolaemia it usually shows a sustained rise. It is important to recognise that the maintenance of CVP should not be viewed as an isolated endpoint in itself; it must be interpreted and responded to within the overall clinical picture.

Drugs used to maintain perfusion following cardiac arrest or treatment of shock

There are no research data comparing one drug with another that show an advantage of any specific drug on outcome. In addition, the pharmacokinetics of these drugs vary from patient to patient and even from hour to hour in the same patient. Factors that influence, in an unmeasurable manner, the effects of these drugs include the child's age and maturity, the underlying disease process, metabolic state, acid–base balance, the patient's autonomic and endocrine response, and liver and renal function. Therefore, the recommended infusion doses are starting points; the infusions must always be adjusted according to patient response.

Wherever possible inotrope infusion should be administered via a central line. However, where this is not available because of pressure of time or non-availability of the skills to secure such access, then intraosseous or peripheral infusions may be used. When this option is used, the site of infusion must be easily accessed for regular inspection. If there is any evidence of extravasation or ischaemia an alternative should be sought as a matter of urgency. In all cases IO or peripheral inotrope infusions should be converted to central infusions at the earliest possible opportunity.

In the following text information is given on how to make up infusions customised to the child's weight. However, there is good evidence that fixed concentration infusions confer a greater safety profile and these should be used according to local protocol where available.

Dopamine

Dopamine is an endogenous catecholamine with complex cardiovascular effects. It is usually only used at infusion rates greater than 5 microgram/kg/min. Dopamine directly stimulates cardiac β-adrenergic receptors and releases noradrenaline from cardiac sympathetic nerves. Myocardial noradrenaline stores may be low in chronic congestive heart failure and in infants, so the drug may be less effective in these groups. It is generally used in preference to dobutamine in the treatment of circulatory shock following resuscitation.

Dopamine infusions may produce tachycardia, vasoconstriction and ventricular ectopy. Infiltration of dopamine into tissues can produce local tissue necrosis. Dopamine and other catecholamines are partially inactivated in alkaline solutions and therefore should not be mixed with sodium bicarbonate.

Infusion concentration: 15 mg/kg in 50 ml of 5% dextrose or normal saline to give 5 micrograms/kg/min if run at 1 ml/h. The infusion may then be run at 1–4 ml/h in order to deliver 5–20 micrograms/kg/min.

Dobutamine

Dobutamine increases the heart rate and myocardial contractility and has some vasodilating effect by decreasing peripheral vascular tone. The tachycardia induced is often significantly higher than dopamine at the same dose. It is potentially useful in the treatment of low cardiac output secondary to poor myocardial function. It is infused in a dose range of 5–20 micrograms/kg/min. Higher infusion rates often produce tachycardia or ventricular ectopy. Pharmacokinetics and clinical response vary widely, so the drug must be titrated according to individual patient response.

Infusion concentration: 15 mg/kg in 50 ml of 5% dextrose or normal saline will give 5 micrograms/kg/min if run at 1 ml/h. The infusion may then be run at 1–4 ml/h in order to deliver 5–20 micrograms/kg/min.

Adrenaline

An adrenaline infusion is a good first line treatment for shock with poor systemic perfusion from any cause that is unresponsive to fluid resuscitation. Adrenaline may be preferable to dopamine or dobutamine in patients with severe hypotensive shock; in very young infants in whom other inotropes may be ineffectual; or for speed if there is a rapid deterioration. The infusion is started at 0.05–0.1 micrograms/kg/min and may be incrementally increased to 2 micrograms/kg/min or higher depending on clinical response.

Infusion concentration: 0.3 mg/kg in 50 ml of 5% dextrose or normal saline will give 0.1 micrograms/kg/min if run at a rate of 1 ml/h. The infusion may then be run at 0.5–20 ml/h in order to deliver 0.05–2.0 micrograms/kg/min.

Kidneys

It is important both to maximise renal blood flow and to maintain renal tubular patency by maintaining urine flow. To achieve this, the following are necessary:

- Maintenance of an adequate blood pressure to drive renal perfusion
- Maintenance of adequate filling and a good cardiac output using inotropes and fluids as required
- Maintenance of good oxygenation
- Monitoring and normalisation of electrolytes (sodium, potassium, calcium, magnesium) and acid–base balance in blood should be undertaken as a supporting measure. Sodium bicarbonate should not be given without expert advice. Potassium should be given slowly and cautiously and only be given in small aliquots in oliguric or anuric patients

Liver

Hepatic cellular damage can become manifest up to 24 hours following an arrest. Coagulation factors can become depleted, and bleeding may be worsened by concomitant, ischaemia-induced intravascular coagulopathy. The patient's clotting profile and platelets should be monitored and corrected, as indicated, with fresh frozen plasma, cryoprecipitate or platelets.

Brain

The aim of therapy is to protect the brain from further (secondary) damage. To achieve this, the cerebral blood flow must be maintained, normal cellular homeostasis must be achieved and cerebral metabolic needs must be reduced.

When intracranial pathology is present, cerebral autoregulation may not function correctly. In these circumstances adequate cerebral blood flow may be achieved if the cerebral perfusion pressure (mean arterial pressure – intracranial pressure) is kept above 40–60 mmHg depending on age (lowest in infants). Maintenance of cellular homeostasis is helped by normalisation of the acid–base and electrolyte balances. Cerebral metabolic needs can be reduced by sedating and paralysing the child. Convulsions should prompt an investigation into their cause. They should be swiftly controlled and prophylactic medication, such as phenytoin, should be used if recurrent. Although a barbiturate coma reduces both cerebral metabolism and ICP, it has not been shown to improve neurological outcome.

Practical steps to minimise secondary brain injury are:

- Maintenance of good oxygenation
- Protection of cerebral perfusion through:
  - maintenance of adequate blood pressure using inotropes and fluids
  - intubation and maintenance of normal blood gases
  - nursing head-up at 20° and in midline
- Using osmotic agents for acutely raised ICP such as:
  - hypertonic (2.7) 3% saline 3 ml/kg IV over 15 minutes
  - mannitol 250–500 mg/kg IV over 15 minutes
- Control of blood glucose avoiding both hypoglycaemia and hyperglycaemia
- Maintenance of good analgesia, sedation and paralysis (where indicated)
- Monitoring and normalisation of electrolytes and acid–base balance
- Control of seizures
- Maintenance of normothermia

Although there is some evidence that post-arrest hypothermia (core temperatures of 32–34°C) has beneficial effects on neurological recovery in adults, the evidence does not support the use of hypothermia in children outside the newborn period. Harm may occur, however, with raised core temperature, which increases metabolic demand by 10–13% for each degree centigrade increase in temperature above normal. Therefore, in the post-arrest patient with compromised cardiac output, hyperthermia should be treated with active cooling to achieve a normal core temperature. Shivering should be prevented since it will increase metabolic demand. Sedation may be adequate to control shivering, but neuromuscular blockade is usually needed.

25.2 Assessment after stabilisation

After resuscitation and emergency treatment have been provided, consideration will need to be given to the best place to continue the child's care. This will usually involve a transfer to another unit, often another hospital. Critically ill children transferred by untrained personnel have been shown to be subjected to an excess of adverse events. These transfers have also been associated with a high incidence of serious transport-related adverse events. The impact of these events on long-term outcome is unknown. Nevertheless, international practice has focused on minimising adverse events during transfer. It should be noted that even when the child only needs to be transported from the emergency department to another department within the same hospital many of the same transfer risks are present and as such it should only be undertaken by appropriately trained staff.

In the UK, the Paediatric Intensive Care Society has set a standard of practice for the transport of critically ill children (www.picsociety.uk). Where possible, it is recommended that these are undertaken by specialised paediatric intensive care transfer teams. These teams can be contacted in the event of requests for the transfer of a child to a PICU or a specialised facility such as a neurosurgical or burns unit. *Neonatal, Adult and Paediatric Safe Transfer and Retrieval: the Practical Approach* (NAPSTaR) (ALSG, 2016) is a sister publication to this manual that supports a practical course of the same name. Although the interested reader should consider reviewing this text in detail, a summary of the principles described are detailed below.

25.3 Principles of safe transfer and retrieval

Transfers are undertaken to ensure that the child's care is of the highest possible standard at all times. To achieve this, the right child has to be taken at the right time, by the right people, to the right place, by the right form of transport, and receive the right care throughout. This requires a systematic approach that incorporates a high level of planning and preparation before the child is moved.

Differences between static and transport medicine

The medical care delivered on the move should, as far as possible, be identical to that delivered in the ward (static) environment. There are, however, limitations to this in that some therapies are not available in a mobile format and it is not always practical to take every piece of equipment that may be indicated even if it is suitable for the mobile environment. The team should also be aware of the additional challenges faced during transport. These may be summarised through the acronym SCRUMP.

S	Shared assessment
C	Clinical isolation
R	Resource limitation
U	Unfamiliar equipment
M	Movement and safety
P	Physical and physiological changes

A brief overview of these considerations will follow as the majority of these issues are covered in the detail of this chapter.

Shared assessment is included to highlight that in most instances of transfer, multiple teams are likely to be involved with the assessment and care of the child, at least one of which will be at a remote location. It is vital that each of these teams has access to all the key information they require in order to acquire and maintain their situation awareness. In practical terms this is achieved through fastidious, focused, closed-loop communication. This relies on all members of the team speaking up about information that they think is important and ensuring it is communicated to the other parties. It is also vital that team members are ready to speak up and request clarification on any aspect that is unclear to them because of confusing or incomplete information.

Clinical isolation is perhaps the most obvious difference when a team works outside their normal clinical area. When planning the transfer it is important to recognise that at the very least this manifests as physical isolation, with no additional supplies, equipment or personnel to hand, and at worst no support whatsoever if communication devices fail, separating the team from their expert support. The team must therefore be fully self-sufficient by the time they move from the ward – a lift, stuck between floors, is, in many respects, no less isolating than an aircraft or ambulance on the road.

Resource limitation occurs by virtue of the isolation described above. The team must ensure they carry sufficient consumables not only for the anticipated journey time, but also extra in case of delays. They must also pack appropriate supplies to address anticipated emergencies that might occur.

Unfamiliar equipment can present challenges at any time, but in the isolated environment of a transfer can present a major risk. Staff should never undertake transfers, however trivial, with equipment that they have not been trained to use.

Movement presents safety risks to the patient, the transfer team and potentially the public when out on the roads. 'Make haste, not speed' is an idiom well applied to the transfer process. The process of moving the child from their bed to a stretcher or pod is the time when tubes and lines are most likely to be displaced. Plan all such moves, and brief the team before undertaking them. A discussion of the speed of travel is included later in this chapter.

Physical and physiological changes occur due to movement, particularly acceleration and deceleration forces on the road. They may also occur due to changes in atmospheric pressure when using air transport. These should be anticipated and wherever possible mitigated against.

Detailed discussions of these issues may be found in the NAPSTaR text and course.

ACCEPT: the systematic approach to transfer of a child

One systematic approach to safe transfer and retrieval is the ACCEPT method, which is described in detail in the NAPSTaR text and course.

A	Assessment
C	Control
C	Communication
E	Evaluation
P	Preparation and packaging
T	Transportation

Assessment

When commencing the transfer process a formal (re)assessment of the situation must be undertaken. Sometimes the clinicians undertaking the transportation may have been involved in the care given up to that point. Increasingly, however, the transport team will have been brought in specifically for that purpose and will have no prior knowledge of the child's clinical history. The process of assessment and reassessment continues throughout the time of the transfer, continually monitoring for changes in the child's condition and taking remedial action where appropriate.

Control

Once the initial assessment is complete, the transport organiser needs to take control of the situation. This requires:

- Identification of the clinical and logistical team leader(s)
- Identification of the tasks to be carried out
- Allocation of tasks to individuals or teams

The lines of responsibility must be established promptly. In theory, ultimate responsibility is held jointly by the referring consultant clinician, the consultant clinician at the receiving centre and the transport personnel at different stages of the transport process. There should always be a clearly identified person with overall responsibility for organising the transport.

Communication

Moving ill children from one place to another requires cooperation and the involvement of many people. Key personnel need to be informed when transportation is being considered.

People who need to know about a transfer

Current (local) clinical team

- Consultant in charge
- Clinicians at bedside
- Referring doctor/nurse
- Lead nurse
- Child's family

Transfer team
The transfer coordinator should disperse information to:

- Consultant in charge
- Clinician(s) undertaking transfer
- Ambulance providers
- Child's family

Receiving team
The transfer coordinator or receiving unit coordinator should disperse information to:

- Consultant accepting referral
- Other consultants who will need to be involved in care (PICU, surgical and anaesthetic teams)
- Receiving doctors
- Receiving nursing staff
- Child's family

Communication may take a long time to complete if one person does it all. It is therefore advisable to share the tasks between appropriate people, taking into account expertise and local policies. In all cases it is important that information is passed on clearly and unambiguously. This is particularly the case when talking to people over the telephone. It is useful to plan what to say before telephoning and to use the systematic summary shown below. It is also useful in complex conversations to summarise the situation and repeat what you need from the listener at the end.

The content of all discussions should be documented in the child's notes. The person in overall charge can then assimilate this information so that a proper evaluation of the child's requirements for transportation can be made.

Key elements in any communication

- Who you are
- Contact details
- What the problem is (soundbite)
- What you need (from the listener)
- What you have done
- Effect of these actions
- Summarise agreed plans

Evaluation

The aim of evaluation is to confirm that transfer is appropriate for the child and, if so, what the clinical urgency is. Whilst evaluation is a dynamic process that starts from first contact with the child, it is usually only when the first phase of ACCEPT (that is, ACC) has been completed that enough information will have been gathered to fully evaluate the transport needs.

Is transport appropriate for this child?

Critically ill babies and children require transport because of the need for:

- Specialist treatment
- Specialist investigations that are unavailable in the referring hospital
- Specialist facilities that are unavailable in the referring hospital

The risks involved in transport must be balanced against the risks of staying and the benefits of care that can be given only by the receiving unit.

What clinical urgency does this child have?

Once it has been established that transfer is needed, the urgency must be evaluated. The degree of urgency for transfer and the severity of illness may be used to rank the child's transfer needs. This decision will determine both the personnel required and the mode and speed of transport.

Preparation and packaging

Both preparation and packaging have the aim of ensuring that transport proceeds uneventfully, with no deterioration in the child's condition. The first stage (preparation) involves the completion of stabilisation and preparation of transfer team personnel and equipment. The second stage (packaging) involves the final measures that need to be taken to ensure the security and safety of the child, equipment and staff during the transportation itself.

Child preparation

To reduce complications during any journey, meticulous resuscitation and stabilisation should be carried out before transfer. This may involve carrying out procedures requested by the receiving hospital or unit. The standard airway, breathing, circulation, disability, exposure and family (ABCDEF) approach should be followed. The airway must be cleared and secured and appropriate respiratory support established. Venous access is essential and should preferably include a minimum of two easily accessible cannulae or a sutured multilumen central line. Where this cannot be achieved an IO line may be substituted for one lumen of access. The child must have received adequate fluid resuscitation to ensure optimal tissue oxygenation. Hypovolaemic children tolerate the inertial forces of transportation very poorly. Children with a suspected spinal injury should be appropriately immobilised.

Occasionally, in time-critical situations such as an expanding intracranial lesion requiring neurosurgery, this process may not be fully completed before packing and transport. Decisions to transfer in these circumstances should be taken only by senior personnel.

Inadequate resuscitation or missed illnesses (and injuries) may result in instability during transfer and may adversely affect the child's outcome.

Equipment preparation

All equipment must be tested and have adequate power reserves. Supplies of drugs and fluids should be more than adequate for the whole of the intended journey. The essential items of equipment are shown in the box.

Paediatric transport equipment (*Continued overleaf*)

Airway

- Induction drugs for reintubation
- Oropharyngeal airways: sizes 000, 00, 0, 1, 2, 3 and 4
- Tracheal tubes: sizes 3.5–8.0 mm cuffed (in 0.5 mm steps) and 2.5–6.0 mm uncuffed
- Tracheal tube stylets
- Laryngeal masks sizes
- Laryngoscope handles ×2:
  - straight paediatric blades
  - curved blades
- Magill forceps
- Portable suction unit
- Yankauer suckers: paediatric and adult
- Soft suction catheters: sizes 6, 8, 10 and 12
- Humidity moisture exchange (HME) unit
- Needle cricothyroidotomy set

Breathing

- Oxygen masks with reservoir
- Self-inflating bags (with reservoir): sizes 240 ml (for pre-term infants only), 500 and 1600 ml
- Portable ventilator
- Face masks:
  - infant – circular 0, 01, 1, 2
  - child – anatomical 2, 3
  - adult – anatomical 4, 5
- Catheter mount and connectors
- Ayre's T-piece or Waters' circuit (Mapleson F and C, respectively), as appropriate for child's size.

Circulation

- ECG monitor – defibrillator (with paediatric pads)
- Invasive and non-invasive (oscillometric) blood pressure monitor (with appropriate-sized cuffs)
- Pulse oximeter (with infant- and child-sized probes)
- End-tidal CO_2 monitor

Usually the four monitors above will be combined within one monitoring device, which will also include temperature and pressure channels

- Intravenous access requirements:
  - intravenous cannulae (as available) 18–25 gauge
  - intraosseous infusion needles 16–18 gauge
  - graduated burette
  - intravenous giving sets
  - syringes: 1–50 ml
  - three-way taps, Luer-locking T-extensions, etc.

- Intravenous drip monitoring device/syringe pumps
- Central (or umbilical for newborns) and arterial line sets

Fluids

- Plasma-Lyte 148, Hartmann's solution or Ringers lactate
- 0.9% saline
- 0.45% saline and 5% dextrose
- 10% dextrose
- Colloid

Drugs

- Adrenaline 1:10 000
- Adrenaline 1:1000
- Atropine 600 micrograms/ml or 1 mg/ml
- Sodium bicarbonate 4.2%
- Dopamine 40 mg/ml
- Lidocaine 1%
- Amiodarone
- Calcium chloride 10%
- Furosemide (frusemide) 20 mg/ml
- Mannitol 10% or 20%
- Antibiotics: penicillin, gentamicin, ampicillin, cefotaxime and cefuroxime
- Morphine, benzodiazepine and paralysing agent, made up as infusions

Miscellaneous

- Battery-operated suction device
- Nasogastric tubes: sizes 6, 8 and 10
- Chest drain set
- Stick test for glucose
- Sharps disposal box

Particular care should be taken with supplies of oxygen, inotropes, sedative drugs and batteries for portable electronic equipment. An example oxygen calculation is shown below:

Calculate the amount of oxygen required for the journey using the following:

$$\text{Number of cylinders} = \frac{2 \times \text{duration of journey} \times \text{flow}\ [l/min]}{\text{cylinder capacity}\ [litres]}$$

For example, if oxygen is provided at 10 l/min for a journey intended to take 120 minutes, this would need four size E cylinders, each containing 600 litres. This allows for at least twice as much oxygen as the estimated journey time requires. Always take more than one cylinder in case of leakage or failure.

A member of the team should be allocated the task of ensuring that all of the child's documents, including case notes, investigations, radiographs, reports and a transfer form, accompany the child. The team should carry a mobile phone together with contact names and numbers to enable direct communication with both the receiving and base units. In addition, all personnel need appropriate clothing, food if the journey is long and enough money to enable them to get home independently if needed.

Personnel preparation

The number and nature of staff accompanying children during transport will depend on their transfer category. All staff must practise within their competences. Whatever the category of the child, all personnel should be familiar with the relevant transfer procedures and the equipment that is to be used, as well as the details of the child's clinical condition. The team should be covered with accident insurance with adequate provision for personal injury or death sustained during the transfer.

Packaging

All lines and drains must be secured to the child, the child must be secured to the trolley and the trolley must be secured to the transport vehicle. This is especially important in neonatal transfers using a transport system that typically weighs over 100 kg. In an ambulance, all equipment fastenings should be CEN compliant (http://www.dft.gov.uk/vca/vehicletype/ambulances.asp). Chest drains should be secured and unclamped, with any underwater seal devices replaced by an appropriate flutter valve system. A special kit should be prepared to enable chest drain insertion or replacement en route if necessary. The child should be adequately covered to prevent heat loss. Care must be taken to ensure that coverings are arranged to permit ready access to the child, lines and drains during transfer.

Transportation

Mode of transport

The choice of transport needs to take into account several factors.

Road ambulances are by far the most common means of transport. They have a low overall cost and rapid mobilisation time, and are not generally affected by weather conditions. They also give rise to less physiological disturbance. Air transfer may be preferred for journeys of more than 80 km or 2 hours in duration, or if road access is difficult. The speed of the journey itself has to be balanced against organisational delays and also the need for inter-vehicle transfer at the start and end of the journey. Staff undertaking air transfers should have received specific training with regard to safety and flight physiology. They should not undertake such transfers without supervised experience.

Factors affecting mode of transfer

- Nature of illness
- Urgency of transfer
- Mobilisation time
- Geographical factors
- Weather
- Traffic conditions
- Cost

Care during transport

Destabilisation may occur during transportation and may arise from the effects of the transport environment on the vulnerable physiology of the child. Careful preparation can minimise the deleterious effects of inertial forces, such as tipping, acceleration and deceleration, as well as changes in temperature and barometric pressure.

The standard of care and the level of monitoring carried out before transfer needs to be continued, as far as possible, during the transfer. Monitoring should include:

- Oxygen saturation
- ECG and heart rate
- Continuous intra-arterial pressure
- End-tidal CO_2 in all intubated children and neonates
- Core and ambulance temperature

The child should be well covered and kept warm during the transfer.

Road speed decisions depend on clinical urgency. Although blue lights and sirens may be appropriate in order to get through heavy traffic, excessive speed is very rarely indicated. It is a risk to the child, the transfer team and the general public, and should be the exception rather than the rule.

With adequate preparation, the transportation phase is usually incident-free. However, untoward events do occur. Should this be the case, the child needs to be reassessed using the ABC approach and appropriate corrective measures then instituted. If the transport team need to release their seatbelts, the ambulance must slow down immediately, and then stop at the first available safe place. If a major deterioration occurs, transfer to the nearest hospital for further stabilisation and support may be appropriate. The benefits of intervention should always be weighed against the risks of delaying arrival at the receiving hospital with its better facilities. Following any untoward events, communication with the receiving unit is important. This should follow the systematic summary described earlier.

Handover

At the end of the transfer direct contact with the receiving team must be established. A succinct, systematic summary of the child and transfer should be provided *before* transferring the child on to the local bed/cot. It must be accompanied by a written record of the child's history, vital signs, therapy and significant clinical events during transfer. All the other documents that have been taken with the child should also be handed over. Once verbal handover has been completed, the child may be moved with monitoring and ventilator from the transport trolley to the receiving unit's cot or bed. The team can then retrieve all of their equipment and personnel and make their way back to their home unit.

25.4 Summary

Meticulous attention to initial assessment and resuscitation together with appropriate emergency treatment will reduce the risk of transport-related morbidity and mortality. Where possible, a specialised paediatric transport team should transfer critically ill and injured children to minimise the risk of adverse events. Irrespective of the origin of the transferring team, a useful checklist is shown in the box.

Checklist prior to transporting a child

1. Is the airway protected and is ventilation satisfactory? (Substantiated by blood gases, pulse oximetry and capnography if possible)
2. Is the neck appropriately immobilised?
3. Is there sufficient oxygen (and air) available for the journey?
4. Is vascular access secure and will the pumps in use during transport work by battery?
5. Have adequate fluids been given prior to transport?
6. Is the child receiving adequate sedation, analgesia and, if used, paralysis?
7. Are fractured limbs appropriately splinted and immobilised?
8. Are appropriate monitors in use?
9. Will the child/baby be sufficiently warm during the journey – ambulance heater, head coverings for patient, etc.?
10. Is documentation available? Include:
    - child's name
    - age and date of birth
    - known or estimated weight
    - clinical notes
    - observation charts, including neurological charts
    - time and route of all drugs given
    - fluid charts
    - ventilator records
    - results of investigations, including blood, urine, X-rays and scans
    - names and contacts of medical and nursing staff involved in referral, receipt and during transport
11. Is the necessary resuscitation equipment available?
12. Is appropriate treatment available for managing anticipated emergencies, e.g. rising ICP?
13. Has the case been discussed with the receiving team directly?
14. Has the receiving unit been advised of an estimated time of arrival?
15. Have plans been discussed with the parents, including issues of consent?

PART 6
Appendices

APPENDIX A
Acid–base balance

Learning outcomes

After reading this appendix, you will be able to:
- Describe the approach to acid–base balance in the seriously ill or injured child

---

A.1 Introduction

Acid–base problems may be respiratory or metabolic in origin, or a combination of the two. Impairments to respiration and metabolism usually lead to an accumulation of acid, although respiratory and metabolic alkaloses are sometimes also encountered.

Respiratory When alveolar ventilation is inadequate, either due to inadequate breathing or inadequate artificial ventilation, carbon dioxide accumulates, and blood PCO_2 rises. The carbon dioxide combines with water to form carbonic acid, which contributes to an acid (low) pH.

Hence this is called a respiratory acidosis. The treatment is to lower the CO_2 by treating the respiratory problem, or adjusting the ventilator settings, to increase alveolar ventilation.

Metabolic Impairment of normal metabolism may occur, for example in shock when a reduced supply of oxygenated blood reduces oxidative metabolism. In this case lactic acid forms, and it is this that contributes to an acid pH, which is described as a metabolic acidosis. In a pure metabolic acidosis the PCO_2 is normal or may be low.

The terms acidosis and acidaemia are sometimes loosely used interchangeably. However acidaemia and alkalaemia represent acidity of the blood that is outside the normal range. The terms acidosis and alkalosis refer to the underlying processes that lead to the acidaemia/alkalaemia, if severe enough to drive the pH or [H+] out of the normal range. For example, diabetic ketoacidosis (DKA) starts gradually and the acidaemia only occurs after it has been progressing for a period of time long enough to change the pH/[H+] significantly. The DKA still exists early on, yet the pH remains within the 'normal range' as various buffers in the blood act to inhibit pH changes. In DKA and all other acid–base abnormalities, it is important to identify and treat the underlying process, which is the driver of the pH/[H+] change, not simply attempt to normalise pH/[H+].

A.2 Hydrogen ion concentration, acidity and pH

Many chemical reactions in our cells are rate dependent on the appropriate temperature and acidity. The concentration of many chemicals in the blood is measured in millimoles (mmol; thousandth of a mole). For example, a sodium concentration [Na+] may be expressed as 140 mmol/l. Acidity is determined by hydrogen ions, whose concentration [H+] is very much lower in the blood and is expressed in nanomoles (nmol; thousand-**millionth** of a mole).

Advanced Paediatric Life Support: A Practical Approach to Emergencies, Sixth Edition. Edited by Martin Samuels and Sue Wieteska.
© 2016 John Wiley & Sons, Ltd. Published 2016 by John Wiley & Sons, Ltd.

Acidity could be simply expressed as a value of the hydrogen ion concentration in nanomoles. Indeed, it has been argued that blood acidity could and should be expressed directly as the hydrogen ion concentration in nanomoles; however, it remains the case that pH is far more widely used.

Because of the enormous variation in hydrogen ion concentrations that may be encountered in general (Table A.1), the pH scale was devised. In the pH scale, [H⁺] is expressed as the negative logarithm of [H⁺]. The lower the pH, the greater the acidity; quite small differences in the numerical pH reflect large differences in hydrogen ion concentration (Figure A.1 and Table A.1). A whole integer change in pH reflects a 10-fold change in [H⁺], so that [H⁺] is 10 nmol at pH 8, 100 nmol at pH 7 and 1000 nmol at pH 6.

Table A.1 The pH scale		
Concentration of hydrogen ions compared with distilled water	**Approx. pH**	**Examples of solutions of this pH**
10 000 000	pH = 0	Battery acid
100 000	pH = 2	Vinegar
1000	pH = 4	Tomato juice, acid rain
1	pH = 7	'Pure' water at 25°C
0.01	pH = 9	Baking soda
0.0001	pH = 11	Ammonia solution
0.0000001	pH = 14	Liquid drain cleaner

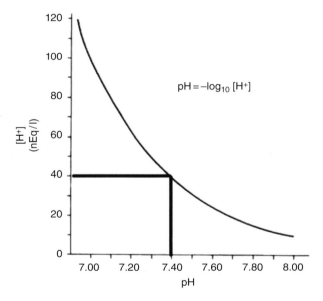

$$pH = -\log_{10} [H^+]$$

Figure A.1 Relationship between hydrogen ion concentration and pH. As can be seen a pH of 7.4 relates to a hydrogen ion concentration of 40 nmol/l (0.000040 mmol/l)

Thus at a normal blood pH of 7.4, [H⁺] is 40 nmol/l, whereas at pH 7.0 it is 100 nmol/l. Although the concentrations of hydrogen ions may vary widely in proportionate terms, their absolute concentrations in nanomoles are very low compared with other ions in millimoles. Thus we control the absolute concentration of hydrogen ions much more precisely than sodium ions (measured in millimoles). On the other hand, we may survive a 2.5× increase in [H⁺] from 40 nmol/l to 100 nmol/l whereas we may not survive a 2.5× increase in [Na⁺] from say 140 mmol/l to 350 mmol/l.

Strictly speaking we should refer to hydrogen ion activity, not concentration, as ions may interact with each other and reduce their effective concentration. However, at the low levels found in the body (Table A.2), this is not a significant consideration.

Table A.2 pH in different parts of the body

Site	pH	Hydrogen ion concentration (mmol/l)	Hydrogen ion concentration (nmol/l)
Stomach, maximum acidity	0.8	150	150 000 000
Urine, maximum acidity	4.5	0.03	30 000
Plasma:			
Severe acidosis	7.0	0.0001	100
Normal	7.4	0.00004	40
Severe alkalosis	7.7	0.00002	20

A.3 Carbonic acid reaction

The chemical relationship between CO_2 and water (the 'carbonic acid reaction') shown below in equation 3 is important. It shows how CO_2 can be carried in the blood, as HCO_3^-, and be released in the lungs to allow ventilation to remove this end product of cellular respiration.

$$CO_2 + H_2O \rightleftharpoons H_2CO_3 \rightleftharpoons H^+ + HCO_3^-$$

Equation 1

CO_2 and H_2O can combine to form H_2CO_3 (carbonic acid), which in turn can dissociate into H^+ and HCO_3^-. The $[H^+]$ will depend on the ratio between the PCO_2 and the bicarbonate concentration ($[HCO_3^-]$, and this is expressed in equation 2, where K is the dissociation constant:

$$\left[H^+\right] = K \times \left(\left[CO_2\right] / \left[HCO_3^-\right]\right)$$

Equation 2

which can then be expressed logarithmically as the Henderson–Hasselbalch equation:

$$pH = pK + \log\left(\left[HCO_3^-\right] / PCO_2\right)$$

Equation 3

(The pK is approximately 6.1.)

Importantly, pH is thus dependant on the ratio between $[HCO_3^-]$ and PCO_2, which are not independent of each other (see equation 3).

As we breathe, we exhale CO_2 produced as a metabolic waste product (the PCO_2 thus being determined by the balance between CO_2 production in the body, and the rate at which we exhale CO_2). The rate at which we exhale CO_2 is directly related to alveolar ventilation. In ventilated patients the PCO_2 is determined by the ventilator strategy, while in spontaneously breathing patients the PCO_2 is determined by their respiratory centre.

One of the major stimuli to breathing is the pH of the cerebrospinal fluid (CSF). If the CSF becomes acidotic, then there is increased respiratory drive to exhale CO_2; if the CSF becomes alkalotic, then the reverse is true. Bicarbonate does not cross the blood–brain barrier, but is secreted in the CSF as it is produced in the choroid plexus (CSF bicarbonate levels thus approximate serum levels some hours previously). CO_2 does cross the blood–brain barrier easily, with CSF PCO_2 being essentially equivalent to current serum PCO_2.

The CSF pH is thus affected by the underlying bicarbonate levels and the current PCO_2 (remembering that the pH depends on the ratio between the two, which means that if the bicarbonate levels are low, a low PCO_2 is required for a normal pH and if bicarbonate levels are high, the reverse is true). The consequence of this system is that a rise in PCO_2 in the blood will usually be followed by an increase in ventilatory effort from increased respiratory drive.

Thus short-term control of pH happens via the brain and the respiratory system. However, over the longer term the kidneys can produce bicarbonate by excreting H^+ ions. If pH levels are persistently low, the kidneys will respond by increased excretion of acid and thus increased production of HCO_3^-, which will tend to compensate for the acidosis. This is a relatively slow process, taking place over several hours or days. On the other hand, ventilatory changes can rapidly alter blood PCO_2. Hence in an acute respiratory illness PCO_2 may be raised with a normal HCO_3^-, whereas in a chronic respiratory illness PCO_2 may be raised alongside a raised, 'compensatory' HCO_3^-.

A.4 Standard bicarbonate

Blood gas analysers measure pH, PCO_2 and PO_2, and use the Henderson–Hasselbalch equation to calculate the HCO_3^- levels; other parameters such as base excess (BE) are in turn derived. As PCO_2 and HCO_3^- are not independent of each other, the concept of 'standard bicarbonate' has been established. The standard bicarbonate (SBC) is 'what the HCO_3^- would have been if the PCO_2 were normal'. In the past this was measured by exposing the blood in an analyser to a gas mixture with a PCO_2 of 5.3 kPa (40 mmHg in the units then used). Now it is calculated by blood gas analysers using data from *in vitro* studies.

SBC and BE have been researched in an attempt to provide some insight into whether abnormalities in acid–base balance are related to respiratory or metabolic factors. If acidosis is related to a respiratory problem, then the SBC will be normal or high, with a base excess; if it is related to a metabolic problem, then the SBC will be low and there will be a base deficit. The reverse is true for alkalosis.

A.5 Stewart's strong ion theory

For many years acid–base balance in the body was seen primarily in terms of the carbonic acid reaction. It is still the case that for many acid–base disturbances the 'traditional' approach to acid–base balance outlined above is of the most practical use, and for the clinician the three measures of pH, PCO_2 and SBC or BE are of the most use.

However, there are some problems with this approach as the carbonic acid system is not the only relationship between pH, anion⁻ and acid in the body, and it is not possible to identify and fully understand the causes of metabolic and respiratory acidosis or alkalosis from the carbonic acid reaction alone. There are other pH and anion relationships, including the phosphate systems and the protein system (where albumen is normally the predominant protein). In addition, [H⁺] is affected by factors such as the need for electrical neutrality in the body.

In 1981, Stewart proposed his 'strong ion theory'. According to that proposal, there are six 'dependent' ion concentrations, whose concentrations are determined by concentrations of other ions and molecules. These are [H⁺], [OH⁻], [HCO_3^-], [CO_3^-], [HA] and [A⁻] (weak, or poorly dissociated, acids and ions). The concentration of each of the 'dependent variables' is dependent on three 'independent variables'. The three independent variables that affect the pH in the body are:

- PCO_2 as discussed in the carbonic acid reaction section
- SID, the 'strong ion difference', which is the charge difference between negatively charged ions or anions (e.g. chloride) and positively charged cations (e.g. sodium) in the plasma
- [A_{TOT}], the total concentration of all the non-volatile weak acids in the body (this includes phosphates and proteins, of which albumin is usually the dominant factor)

The important consideration is that the variables that actually control pH are PCO_2, SID and [A_{TOT}]. All other variable are dependent on these factors. Thus acidosis or alkalosis is the consequence of a combination of changes in these three parameters. Calculating the effect of the three independent variables is complicated, however, involving six complex simultaneous equations. This is a major shortcoming of the direct clinical application of Stewart's ideas, which have, however, made significant contributions to our understanding of acid–base physiology.

Total weak acids

These non-volatile weak acids are albumin and other plasma proteins, and phosphate. Phosphate levels are usually low. Albumin and other proteins are weak acids; hence albumin infusions may contribute to acidaemia.

Strong ion difference

Stewart pointed out that acid base–balance is profoundly affected by strong ions (which are ions that exist mostly in ionic form, rather than in combined form as molecules). One over-riding principle is that electrical neutrality has to be maintained in a system. The strong ions in the extracellular fluid include the positively charged ions, or cations, Na⁺, K⁺, Ca²⁺ and Mg²⁺, and the negatively charged ions, or anions, HCO_3^-, Alb⁻, phosphate²⁻, lactate⁻ and Cl⁻.

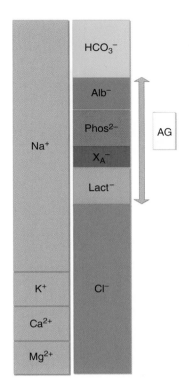

Figure A.2 Ions and their charges in extracellular fluid.
[AG, anion gap; X_A^-, unmeasured weak acids]

As can be seen in Figure A.2, Na^+ and Cl^- make up the majority of the cations and anions, respectively, and changes in their concentrations (and ratios) will be expected to have the most impact on the $[HCO_3^-]$, while changes in Ca^{2+}, Mg^{2+} or phosphate will have little effect. Under normal circumstances, lactate concentration would also be very low, with minimal effect, although this will change as levels rise. The H^+ concentration is so tiny that in electrical terms it is irrelevant to this balance. HCO_3^- is, in fact, an electrical buffer (not just a 'biochemical' one) and its function is to 'flex up and down' to accommodate other electrolyte changes (and charges). Hence the value of HCO_3^- depends on all the other (metabolic) values in the figure, i.e. HCO_3^- is a dependent variable, dependent on metabolic values. The $[HCO_3^-]$ in this context is largely dependent on the need to maintain electrical neutrality.

Hyperchloraemic acidosis

The consequence of this concept is that an increase in $[Cl^-]$ relative to $[Na^+]$ would have the effect of decreasing the $[HCO_3^-]$ and thus create an acidosis. As an example, an infusion of 0.9% saline (154 mmol/l of both Na^+ and Cl^- in a ratio of 1:1) would increase the ratio of $[Cl^-]$ relative to $[Na^+]$ (as the normal ratio $[Na^+]:[Cl^-]$ in the extracellular fluid is <0.8) and create an acidosis. Similarly, an infusion of a weak acid such as albumen would result in a decrease in $[HCO_3^-]$ and create an acidosis.

Conversely, an increase in $[Na^+]$ relative to $[Cl^-]$ would have the effect of increasing $[HCO_3^-]$ and thus create alkalosis. A typical example is what happens when patients are given loop diuretics. The diuretic therapy increases Cl^- losses relative to Na^+ and this will create an increase in $[HCO_3^-]$ with metabolic alkalosis.

The important issue to note is that changes in $[HCO_3^-]$ are not the primary cause of changes in acid–base status of the patient but that this is the consequence of other changes. This is true when considering both metabolic and respiratory acidosis or alkalosis.

Figure A.2 represents the ions and their charges in extracellular fluid. The left hand column contains cations (positive charge) and the right hand column anions (negative charge). **Positive and negative charges must be balanced at all times (electroneutrality).** A change in charge will be balanced by an increase or decrease in HCO_3^- and H^+. The unmeasured weak acids (X_A^-) would include acids such as may be present in ketoacidosis (diabetic, starvation or alcoholic);

renal failure (residual acids are normally renally eliminated); poisons (e.g. methanol, ethanol, ethylene glycol or aspirin; organic acidaemia (including methylmalonic acidaemia, propionic acidaemia, isovaleric acidaemia and maple syrup urine disease).

The anion gap is defined as $(Na^+ + K^+) - (Cl^- + HCO_3^-)$. It incorporates all the other anions and/or cations for which measurements are not usually available (sometimes termed unmeasured anions or cations). Strictly speaking the anion gap should calculated by the formula $(Alb^- + Phosph^{2-} + X_A^- + Lact^-) - (Ca^{2+} + Mg^{2+})$, but since Ca^{2+} and Mg^{2+} concentrations are small and vary minimally, we can ignore these ions and so simplify the anion gap as meaning simply the remaining anions after removing $(Cl^- + HCO_3^-)$. Hence $AG = (Alb^- + Phosph^{2-} + X_A^- + Lact^-)$.

The anion gap

The anion gap (AG) is a useful concept. It is calculated by the formula:

$$AG = \left(Na^+ + K^+\right) - \left(Cl^- + HCO_3^-\right)$$

As can be seen from Figure A.2 (and expanded in Figure A.3), a large component of the normal anion gap is made up of the albumin. As albumin frequently changes dramatically in acute illness or injury and this might then mask the severity of an acidotic process, it is sometimes useful to use the corrected anion gap in order to take those changes into account.

$$AG_c = \left(Na^+ + K^+\right) - \left(Cl^- + HCO_3^-\right) + 0.25 \times \left(42 - Alb\right)$$

Albumin is only slightly charged (about a quarter of a unit of charge per molecule, compared with 1 or 2 units of charge for most of the strong ions Na^+ and $Phosph^{2-}$) so we add a quarter of the albumin deficit to the normal, raw, uncorrected AG.

In Figure A.3 the left column shows normal anion values and a normal AG (grey arrow) in a normal patient. The middle column shows results from a patient with raised lactic acid and hence an increased AG (bigger grey arrow) and a fall in HCO_3^-. In the patient shown in the right column, the high lactate has been offset by the fall in albumin, so the AG is apparently normal, hiding the underlying pathology, a lactic acidosis. This would be highlighted by recalculating the albumin-corrected anion gap, which would be abnormal.

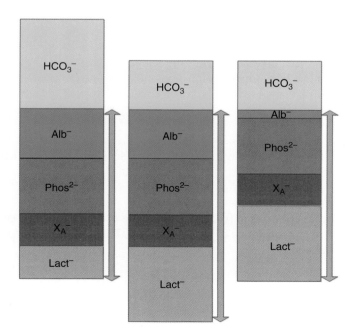

Figure A.3 Expansion of the components of the anion gap

Causes of a raised anion gap

- Lactic acidosis
- Other acids (X_A^-):
  - Ketoacidosis (diabetic, starvation, alcoholic)
  - Renal failure (residual acids are normally renally eliminated)
  - Rhabdomyolysis
  - Medications – isoniazid intoxication
  - Poisons – methanol, ethanol, ethylene glycol, propylene glycol, aspirin

- Organic acidaemia:
  methylmalonic acidaemia
  propionic acidaemia
  isovaleric acidaemia
  maple syrup urine disease

A.6 Applying this in practice

Changes in acid–base homeostasis may be caused by respiratory or metabolic processes or a combination of the two (Figure A.4). In the Henderson–Hasselbalch equation pH is related to the ratio of the metabolic (HCO_3^-) components to the respiratory (PCO_2) components.

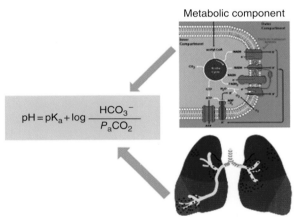

Metabolic component

$$pH = pK_a + \log \frac{HCO_3^-}{P_aCO_2}$$

Respiratory component

Figure A.4 Changes in acid–base homeostasis

Primary respiratory abnormalities

Respiratory acidosis

In respiratory failure there is an increase in PCO_2. If this happens rapidly, there will be a drop in pH (see the Henderson–Hasselbalch equation). However, if this happens gradually, or is persistent, there will be an increase in HCO_3^- production in the kidneys with 'compensation' or correction of the pH (Figure A.5). The SBC will tend to rise as the compensation occurs.

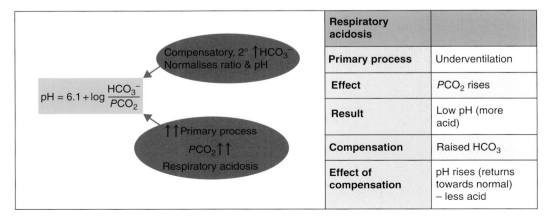

Respiratory acidosis	
Primary process	Underventilation
Effect	PCO_2 rises
Result	Low pH (more acid)
Compensation	Raised HCO_3
Effect of compensation	pH rises (returns towards normal) – less acid

Figure A.5 Primary and compensatory changes in respiratory acidosis. Note the direction of changes in the numerator (HCO_3^-) and denominator (PCO_2) are in the same direction (arrows) – to normalise the ratio

Respiratory alkalosis

A primary increase in ventilation beyond that needed to keep PCO_2 normal drives the PCO_2 down. This reduces the denominator and hence increases pH. The respiratory alkalosis (a fall in PCO_2) moves the carbonic acid equilibrium to reduce HCO_3^- immediately, to a small degree, but over many hours and up to 2 days, the HCO_3^- value falls (with a drop in SBC). This reduces the numerator, tending to normalise the ratio of HCO_3^- to PCO_2, thus reducing the impact on pH change and bringing pH back towards normal (metabolic compensation) (Figure A.6).

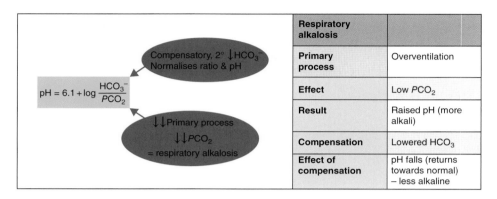

Respiratory alkalosis	
Primary process	Overventilation
Effect	Low PCO_2
Result	Raised pH (more alkali)
Compensation	Lowered HCO_3
Effect of compensation	pH falls (returns towards normal) – less alkaline

Figure A.6 Primary and compensatory changes in respiratory alkalosis. Note the direction of changes in the numerator (HCO_3^-) and denominator (PCO_2) are in the same direction (arrows) – to normalise the ratio

It is important to note that HCO_3^- moves in response to primary changes in PCO_2. Therefore, the value of HCO_3^- is **dependent** on the value of PCO_2, which is dependent on changes in the respiratory system, i.e. ventilation. Below we will see that whilst HCO_3^- represents the metabolic component, paradoxically, it is **dependent** on metabolic issues too!

Primary metabolic abnormalities

A variety of metabolic processes can lead to primary acid–base abnormalities. When using the Henderson–Hasselbalch equation this is indicated by change in HCO_3^-. A reduction in HCO_3^- reduces the numerator and therefore reduces pH (see Figure A.2). An increase in HCO_3^- has the opposite effect. In a spontaneously breathing patient with intact feedback mechanisms, primary metabolic changes can be partially or fully compensated by adjustments of alveolar ventilation and therefore PCO_2. When HCO_3^- is decreased (metabolic acidosis) a resulting drop in pH can be moved back towards normal by increasing ventilation and reducing PCO_2. During a primary metabolic alkalosis (increased HCO_3^-) ventilation slows down, PCO_2 rises and pH is moved back towards normal.

It is important to note that HCO_3^- is only useful as a 'marker' as it is not in itself part of the underlying cause. It is an entirely **dependent** variable – its value changes in response to other (causative) metabolic processes. This provides some explanation of why the administration of sodium bicarbonate may not be helpful in the context of metabolic acidosis. The low bicarbonate is not actually the cause of the problem, it is merely a consequence of the problem and the focus needs to be on what is creating the situation.

Bicarbonate can be calculated from the Henderson–Hasselbalch equation, but it can also be calculated from the SID and $[A_{TOT}]$, where:

$$\left[HCO_3^-\right] = SID - \left[A_{TOT}\right]$$
Equation 4

SID is the difference between the positive strong ions and the negative strong ions (a strong ion is one that exists mostly in the ionic rather than the associated, un-ionised form). Thus:

$$SID = \left(\left[Na^+\right] + \left[K^+\right] + \left[Ca^{2+}\right] + \left[Mg^{2+}\right]\right) - \left(\left[Cl^-\right] + \left[Lact^-\right]\right)$$
Equation 5

As $[K^+] + [Ca^{2+}] + [Mg^{2+}]$ are always small numbers that do not vary much, this formula can be simplified to:

$$SID = \left[Na^+\right] - \left(\left[Cl^-\right] + \left[Lact^-\right]\right)$$
Equation 6

and

$$\left[A_{TOT}\right] = \left(Alb^- + Phos^{2-} + XA^-\right)$$
Equation 7

Thus:

$$pH = pK + \log\left\{Na^+ - \left(Cl^- + Lact^- + Alb^- + Phos^{2-} + XA^-\right)\right\} / PCO_2$$
Equation 8

Thus from a metabolic perspective anything that increases the numerator in the formula (or increases the HCO_3^-) will increase the pH. This would include an increase in sodium or a drop in chloride, albumen or weak acids. Conversely a fall in sodium, or an increase in chloride, albumin or weak acids, would drop the pH.

Quantifying the aetiology of the metabolic acidosis

A metabolic acidosis produces a fall in HCO_3^-. This is mirrored by a fall in base excess, i.e. it becomes more negative (to put it another way, the base deficit increases). Base excess is the amount of acid or base that needs to be added to a blood sample in order to return the pH to 7.40 at a temperature of 37°C at a PCO_2 of 5.3 kPa (this is calculated using the standard bicarbonate as mentioned above).

Base excess eliminates any respiratory contributions and allows us to quantify the metabolic components of the acid–base abnormality. Both HCO_3^- and base excess are useful indicators of the magnitude of the problem and run in parallel.

Each of the numerator components contributes to the overall base excess on its own. We can identify and quantify the effects of the contributions of each of the numerator components to the overall net base excess (and overall acid–base balance) by using some simple rules. Note that the total base excess is the sum of base excess changes arising from each component in the numerator:

- BE change due to sodium and chloride relationship $= (Na^+ - Cl^-) - 38$
- BE change due to the lactate present $= 2 - lactate$
- BE change due to albumin $= 0.25 \times (42 - albumin)$
- BE change due to other acids (XA^-) $=$ total base excess – sum of the others

Some examples may help.

Patient 1: Post-surgery, intraoperative arterial blood gas after administration of a significant volume of 0.9% saline

	Normal values	Patient 1
pH	7.35–7.45	7.28
H+	45–35	52.5
PO_2	13	13
PCO_2	5	3.3
Stanadard bicarbonate	24–25	17.8
BE	0 ± 2	−6.7
Saturation	>90	99
Lactate	2	1.5
Glucose	5	5
Na+	140	142
K+	4.5	4.2
Cl−	95–100	115
Albumin	42	28
Urea	<7	5
Creatinine	< 0	90
(1) Na − Cl − 38 BE	(Na − Cl) − 38 =	−11
(2) Lactate BE	2 − lactate =	0.5
(3) Albumin BE	0.25 × (42 − alb) =	3.5
(4) Residue (XA BE)	BE − (1) − (2) − (3) =	0.3

- The pH has fallen, base excess is −6.7
- Using formulae 1, 2, 3 and 4 above, it becomes clear that the main contributor is the hyperchloraemia caused by the saline, which alone would generate a base excess of −11
- This is offset by the dilution effect on the albumin, which generates a metabolic alkalosis, giving a base excess change of +3.5. Lactate contributes minimally as it is normal and residual base excess is minimal

Patient 2: A sick patient in the emergency department with abdominal pain, 4 hours after treatment has begun

	Normal values	Patient 2
pH	7.35–7.45	6.799
H+	45–35	159
PO_2	13	18.3
PCO_2	5	1.68
Standard bicarbonate	24–25	4.3
BE	0 ± 2	−35.2
Saturation	>90	96.6
Lactate	2	1
Glucose	5	35
Na+	140	127
K+	4.5	3.8
Cl−	95–100	106
Albumin	42	41
Urea	<7	9.7
Creatinine	<90	98
(1) Na − Cl − 38 BE	(Na − Cl) − 38 =	−17
(2) Lactate BE	2 − lactate =	1
(3) Albumin BE	0.25 × (42 − alb) =	0.25
(4) Residue (XA BE)	BE − (1) − (2) − (3) =	−19.45

- The pH has fallen, base excess −35.2!
- Using formulae 1, 2, 3 and 4 above, the base excess change is partially due to the hyponatraemia and hyperchloraemia and partially due to other acids
- The other acids here are ketones of DKA – note the glucose of 35
- Note that the low pH stimulates respiration, hence Kussmaul breathing, and the low PCO_2, respiratory compensation for the metabolic acidosis
- This is a common scenario, where the DKA itself and the treatment with normal saline produce changes in electrolyte status. The metabolic acidosis (and here profound metabolic acidaemia) is initially due to DKA but, as treatment continues, there is a phase of profound (sodium chloride induced) metabolic acidosis

Patient 3: A sick patient on the ward with fever, hypotension and confusion

	Normal values	Patient 3
pH	7.35–7.45	6.83
H^+	45–35	145.7
PO_2	13	8.6
PCO_2	5	6.8
Standard bicarbonate	24–25	6.7
BE	0 ± 2	−22.9
Saturation	>90	80
Lactate	2	15
Glucose	5	3
Na^+	140	133
K^+	4.5	6.6
Cl^-	95–100	104
Albumin	42	8
Urea	<7	17
Creatinine	<90	204
(1) Na − Cl − 38 BE	(Na − Cl) − 38 =	−9
(2) Lactate BE	2 − lactate =	−13
(3) Albumin BE	0.25 × (42 − alb) =	8.5
(4) Residue (XA BE)	BE − (1) − (2) − (3) =	−9.4

- The pH has fallen, base excess is −22.9
- Using formulae 1, 2, 3 and 4 above, the base excess changes can be quantified. There is some sodium to chloride (strong ion) imbalance (contributing −9 to base excess), a profound lactic acidosis (contributing −13 to total base excess), the low albumin produces a metabolic alkalosis (+8.5 contribution to overall base excess), and there is acute kidney injury (contributing −9 to overall base excess)
- This is a mixed picture of severe sepsis with all components of the numerator contributing somewhat to the overall picture

A.7 Summary

Acid–base theory has developed with an increased understanding of chemistry and electrostatic considerations. H^+ can be generated from water and this equilibrium is influenced by strong ions (dissociated charged particles), weak acids and CO_2.

H^+ is involved many reactions. $[H^+]$ depends on the log of the ratio of HCO_3^- to PCO_2. Since PCO_2 isin the denominator, a rise in PCO_2 causes an acidosis and a fall causes an alkalosis.

HCO_3^- is in the numerator so rises and falls in HCO_3^- are seen in metabolic alkalosis and acidosis, respectively. A change in concentration and net charge in one negatively charged component has to be matched by electro-neutrality and hence a change in HCO_3^-. This is the role of HCO_3^-, to provide both electrical and biochemical buffering to maintain electro-neutrality.

Some simple rules allow quantification of these components and hence identification of the cause of the problem.

APPENDIX B
Fluid and electrolyte management

Learning outcomes

After reading this appendix, you will be able to:
- Describe the approach to the management of fluid and electrolytes in the seriously ill or injured child

---

B.1 Introduction

At birth, approximately 80% of a child's body weight is water. This percentage falls gradually during childhood, reaching 60% water by adulthood. Total body water is distributed between the intracellular, interstitial and intravascular spaces, moving from one compartment to another depending on various pressure and osmotic gradients. In illness and injury these fluid shifts may be rapid, with significant clinical consequences.

B.2 Fluid balance

Normally fluid balance is tightly controlled by thirst, hormonal responses and renal function: the quantities in Table B.1 provide a guideline to appropriate fluid intake. These formulae are based on an assumption of 100 kcal/kg/day of caloric intake, 3 ml/kg/hour of urine output and normal stool output.

For example:

- A 6 kg infant would require 600 ml/day
- A 14 kg child would require 1000 + 200 = 1200 ml/day
- A 25 kg child would require 1000 + 500 + 100 = 1600 ml/day

In critical illness or injury some or all of these mechanisms may be profoundly disrupted, and fluid therapy has to be tailored to the needs of the specific child. In the presence of anuria due to acute renal failure, fluid requirements may fall below 30 ml/kg/day, while in high-output diarrhoea requirements may be as high as 400 ml/kg/day.

Fluid intake is required to replace fluid losses and to enable the excretion of various waste products through the urine. Insensible losses (via respiration and sweat) generally amount to between 10 and 30 ml/kg/day. The actual volume of insensible fluid loss is related to the caloric content of the feeds, ambient temperature, humidity of inspired air, presence of pyrexia and quality of the skin. Insensible losses from a child on a ventilator in a cool environment with minimal caloric intake may be minimal. Usually between 0 and 10 ml/kg/day are lost in the stool (this will increase markedly in diarrhoea, where losses in excess of 300 ml/kg/day are not uncommon). Urinary losses are between 1 and 2 ml/kg/h (i.e. approximately 30 ml/kg/day).

Advanced Paediatric Life Support: A Practical Approach to Emergencies, Sixth Edition. Edited by Martin Samuels and Sue Wieteska.
© 2016 John Wiley & Sons, Ltd. Published 2016 by John Wiley & Sons, Ltd.

Table B.1 Fluid requirements in well, normal children

Body weight	Fluid requirement per day (ml/kg)	Fluid requirement per hour (ml/kg)
First 10 kg	100	4
Second 10 kg	50	2
Subsequent kilograms	20	1

Dehydration and shock

Concepts

- Dehydration does not cause death, shock does. Shock may occur with the loss of 20 ml/kg from the intravascular space, while clinical dehydration is only evident after total losses of >25 ml/kg
- As a guide, the child with dehydration and no shock can be assumed to be 5% dehydrated; if shock is present, then 10% dehydration or greater has occurred
- The treatment of shock requires the rapid administration of an intravascular volume of fluid that approximates in electrolyte content to plasma
- The treatment of dehydration requires a gradual replacement of fluids with an electrolyte content that relates to the electrolyte losses, or to the total body electrolyte content
- Pathology from electrolyte changes is related to either extreme levels, or rapid rates of change
- Administration of sodium bicarbonate is rarely indicated
- Overhydration is potentially as dangerous as dehydration

The intravascular volume of an infant is c. 80 ml/kg, and of an older child 70 ml/kg. A rapid loss of 25% of this volume (i.e. 20 ml/kg) will cause shock unless that volume is replaced from the interstitial fluid at a similar rate. Clinical signs of dehydration (Table B.2) are only detectable when the patient is 2.5–5% dehydrated. Five per cent dehydration implies that the body has lost 5 g per 100 g body weight, i.e. 50 ml/kg. Clearly, shock may occur in the absence of dehydration, dehydration may occur in the absence of shock, or both may occur together – all dependent on the rate of fluid loss and the rate of fluid shifts.

Table B.2 Signs and symptoms of dehydration and shock (adapted from NICE, 2009)

No clinically detectable dehydration	Clinical dehydration	Clinical shock
Appears well	Appears to be 'unwell'	Pale, lethargic or mottled
Normal breathing pattern	Normal or tachypnoea	Tachypnoea
Normal heart rate	Normal or tachycardia	Tachycardia
Normal peripheral pulses	Normal peripheral pulses	Weak peripheral pulses
Normal capillary refill time	Normal or mildly prolonged capillary refill time	Prolonged capillary refill time
Normal blood pressure	Normal blood pressure	Hypotension
Normal skin turgor	Reduced skin turgor	
Normal urine output	Decreased urine output	Decreased urine output
Alert and responsive	Altered responsiveness (e.g. irritable, lethargic)	Decreased level of consciousness
Eyes not sunken	Sunken eyes	
	Depressed fontanelle*	
Moist mucous membranes (except after a drink)	Dry mucous membranes (except for 'mouth breathers')	
Warm extremities	Warm extremities	Cold extremities

*Only useful in an infant if still patent and in the absence of disorders such as meningitis.

The priorities of management are to identify shock and treat it effectively and rapidly (see Chapter 6), identify dehydration and institute a treatment programme that will enable effective rehydration over 24–48 hours, identify the presence and aetiology of acid–base problems and correct these where necessary, and identify the presence and aetiology of electrolyte abnormalities and correct these gradually without precipitating complications.

One factor remains unknown at the initiation of therapy, namely the ongoing fluid losses that will occur during therapy. Thus any plan of fluid management represents a starting point, and this will have to be modified in the light of data from constant monitoring.

The critical clinical questions are therefore:

- Is the patient shocked?
- Is the patient dehydrated?
- Does the patient have a significant acid–base abnormality?
- Are there significant electrolyte problems?

Shock

The treatment of hypovolaemic shock secondary to fluid loss (after securing the airway and providing high-flow oxygen) is the rapid administration of crystalloid. The starting volume is 20 ml/kg, and this can be repeated if there is inadequate clinical response (with no evidence of intravascular overload). The fluids used should approximate in electrolyte concentrations to those of serum (options include 0.9% saline and Hartmann's solution, however the latter should be used with care in renal impairment as it contains potassium). The presence of hyper- or hyponatraemia does not affect the choice of fluids during this phase of resuscitation.

In the context of severe sepsis there is some concern about the use of fluid boluses for resuscitation. It seems reasonable to continue with fluid bolus administration with careful monitoring of the patient's response. Unless there is evidence of cardiac dysrhythmia or neurological abnormality, electrolyte abnormalities should be corrected gradually.

Once shock has been adequately treated, attention can turn to management of hydration. Frequent reassessment remains necessary as the patient may well become shocked again if the underlying cause of the fluid shifts (e.g. gastroenteritis) is ongoing.

Dehydration

Many clinical signs of dehydration are individually unreliable (Table B.2) and have poor interobserver reproducibility, but taken together they provide a reasonable estimate of total body fluid losses. Weight is the only clinically available objective measure of total body fluid changes, and enables an accurate assessment of fluid balance over time (unfortunately initial fluid therapy must usually be based on a clinical assessment of hydration because the pre-sickness weight is not often available).

The measured weight loss or percentage dehydration:

> 5% dehydration = loss of 5 ml of fluid per 100 g body weight, or 50 ml / kg
>
> 10% dehydrated = loss of 10 ml of fluid per 100 g body weight, or 100 ml / kg

Management of dehydration consists of the administration of calculated daily maintenance fluids in addition to calculated replacement fluids over a 24-hour period. Therapy should be monitored at 3–4-hourly intervals using weight as an objective measure, to ensure that the patient is gaining weight at an appropriate rate. If the calculated fluid administration rate is too slow or too fast, then the rate should be modified appropriately. See Table B.3 for the commonly available crystalloid fluids.

When the gut is functioning, oral rehydration using standard solutions is preferred (the World Health Organisation (WHO) formulation provides 75 mmol sodium, 20 mmol potassium, 65 mmol chloride, 10 mmol citrate and 75 mmol glucose per litre; the formulations recommended in the UK have lower sodium concentrations of 50–60 mmol/l). This fluid should be administered frequently in small volumes (a cup and spoon works very well for this process). Generally, normal feeds should be administered in addition to the rehydration fluid, particularly if the infant is breast-fed.

Table B.3 Commonly available crystalloid fluids

Fluid	Na$^+$ (mmol/l)	K$^+$ (mmol/l)	Cl$^-$ (mmol/l)	Energy (kcal/l)	Other
Sodium chloride 0.9%	150	0	150	0	0
Sodium chloride 0.45%, dextrose 5%	75	0	75	200	0
Hartmann's solution	131	5	111	0	Lactate
Dextrose 5%	0	0	0	200	0
Dextrose 10%	0	0	0	400	0

When there is excessive vomiting or there are signs of damaged bowel, fluid therapy should be given intravenously. Unless there is bowel damage, attempt early and gradual introduction of oral rehydration therapy during intravenous fluid therapy. If tolerated, stop intravenous fluids and complete rehydration with oral rehydration therapy.

Example

A 6 kg child is clinically shocked and 10% dehydrated as a result of gastroenteritis.

Initial therapy
20 ml/kg for shock = 6 × 20 = 120 ml of 0.9% saline given as a rapid intravenous bolus

Estimated fluid therapy over the next 24 hours
100 ml/kg for 10% dehydration = 100 × 6 = 600 ml

100 ml/kg for daily maintenance fluid = 100 × 6 = 600 ml

Rehydration + maintenance = 1200 ml

Therefore start with an infusion of 1200/24 = 50 ml/h

Application of fluid therapy
Reassess clinical status and weight at 4–6 hours, and if satisfactory continue. If the child is losing weight increase the fluid rate, and if the weight gain is excessive decrease the fluid rate. Start giving more of the maintenance fluid as oral feeds if the child is tolerating the fluids.

Fluid overload and overhydration

In the same way that fluid losses may cause shock, dehydration or both, excessive fluid administration can cause intravascular fluid overload, overhydration or both.

In the patient with nephrotic syndrome, fluid has leaked out of the intravascular space and into the tissues because of a low serum albumin. Such children may be grossly overhydrated, with diffuse severe oedema. However, many patients with nephrotic syndrome have a contracted intravascular space, and attempts to diurese these patients without first expanding the intravascular space with albumin may result in shock.

By contrast the patient with myocardial dysfunction may have an intravascular compartment that is grossly overfilled. The clinical signs of intravascular overload may be present, and yet the patient (particularly if they have been on diuretics) may actually be total body fluid depleted and may appear dehydrated.

Children with renal impairment may present with a combination of intravascular and total body fluid overload. Administration of further fluid can worsen fluid overload leading to pulmonary oedema.

The treatment of fluid overload can be complex and the non-specialist should seek expert advice.

Electrolyte abnormalities

Table B.4 shows the normal electrolyte requirements.

Body weight	Water (ml/kg/day)	Sodium (mmol/kg/day)	Potassium (mmol/kg/day)	Energy (kcal/day)	Protein (g/day)
Table B.4 Water, electrolyte and energy requirements in well, normal children					
First 10 kg	100	2–4	1.5–2.5	110	3.0
Second 10 kg	50	1–2	0.5–1.5	75	1.5
Subsequent kilograms	20	0.5–1	0.2–0.7	30	0.75

Sodium

Both low and high sodium levels are potentially dangerous. Severe hypernatraemia may be associated with brain damage, because brain tissue shrinks as a result of intracellular dehydration and blood vessels may tear or clot up. Too rapid correction of hypernatraemia may lead to cerebral oedema and convulsions. Similarly, rapid correction of hyponatraemia may also be associated with demyelination and permanent brain injury.

The electrolyte losses during dehydration depend on the reason for dehydration. In gastroenteritis, sodium losses in diarrhoea stool range from approximately 50 mmol/l (rotavirus) to approximately 80 mmol/l (cholera and enteropathogenic *Escherichia coli*). In renal dysfunction sodium losses may be minimal (diabetes insipidus) or high (renal tubular dysfunction).

Hypernatraemia

Hypernatraemia in the dehydrated patient may be the end result of excessive loss of water (e.g. diabetes insipidus, diarrhoea), excessive intake of sodium (e.g. iatrogenic poisoning, non-accidental injury), or a combination of both (e.g. children with gastroenteritis given excessive sodium in rehydration fluid).

The electrolyte content of the replacement solution depends on the cause of the dehydration. Previously, 0.45% NaCl, containing 75 mmol/L NaCl, was considered a safe starting solution for intravenous rehydration. This was based largely on the electrolyte content of stool in diarrhoea. By contrast, patients with rare renal tubular dysfunction who lose excessive sodium and water through their kidneys may require 0.9% NaCl to replace the renal losses of sodium. Measurement of the sodium content of urine and stool may help direct replacement therapy. More recently, consensus guidelines have recommended starting with an isotonic solution such as 0.9% NaCl, or 0.9% NaCl with 5% glucose, for fluid-deficit replacement and maintenance for hypernatraemic dehydration due to a number of children developing a rapid fall in sodium with hypotonic solutions.

The principles in the treatment of hypernatraemia are:

1. Treat shock first.
2. Calculate the maintenance fluid and estimate the fluid deficit carefully.
3. Aim to lower the serum sodium at a rate of no more than 0.5 mmol/h.
4. Check other electrolyte levels such as calcium and glucose.
5. Monitor the electrolytes frequently – obtain expert advice if correction is not improving.
6. Clinically assess hydration and weigh frequently.

Hyponatraemia

Hyponatraemia may be due to excessive water intake or retention, excessive sodium losses, or a combination of both.

If the child is fitting from hyponatraemia, partial rapid correction of the serum sodium level will be necessary to stop the fitting. Administration of 4 ml/kg of 3% NaCl solution over 15 minutes will raise the serum sodium by approximately 3 mmol and will usually stop the seizures.

If hyponatraemia is due to excessive water intake or retention, and the patient is not symptomatic, the restriction of fluid intake to 50% of normal estimated requirements may be adequate therapy. If dehydrated and intravenous fluids are required then 0.9% NaCl is an appropriate fluid.

The principles in the treatment of hyponatraemia are:

1. Treat the child's seizures with hypertonic 3% NaCl (seizure control should happen simultaneously).
2. Calculate the maintenance fluid and estimate the fluid deficit carefully.
3. Aim to raise the serum sodium at a rate of no more than 0.5 mmol/h.
4. Check other electrolyte levels such as calcium and glucose.
5. Monitor the electrolytes frequently – obtain expert advice if correction is not improving.
6. Clinically assess hydration and weigh frequently.

Potassium

Unlike sodium, potassium is mainly an intracellular ion and the small quantities measurable in the serum and extracellular fluid represent only a fraction of the total body potassium. The intracellular potassium acts as a large buffer to maintain the serum value within a narrow normal range. Cardiac arrhythmias can occur at values outside this range. Thus hypokalaemia is usually only manifest after significant total body depletion has occurred. Similarly, hyperkalaemia represents significant total body overload, beyond the ability of the kidney to compensate, or massive break down of blood cells resulting in the release of potassium. The causes of hyper- and hypokalaemia are given in Table B.5.

Table B.5 Causes of hypo- and hyperkalaemia

Hypokalaemia	Hyperkalaemia
Diarrhoea	Renal failure
Alkalosis	Acidosis
Volume depletion	Adrenal insufficiency
Primary hyperaldosteronism	Cell lysis
Diuretic abuse	Excessive potassium intake
	In the critically ill neonate, inadequate cardiac output must always be excluded as a cause

Hypokalaemia

Hypokalaemia is rarely an emergency and is usually the result of excessive potassium losses from acute diarrhoeal illnesses. As total body depletion will have occurred, large amounts are required to return the serum potassium to normal. Oral supplementation is the preferred route. In cases where this is not suitable, intravenous supplements are required. However, strong potassium solutions are highly irritant and can precipitate cardiac arrhythmias, thus the concentration of potassium in intravenous solutions ought not to exceed 40 mmol/l except when given centrally with close cardiac monitoring.

Patients who are alkalotic or are receiving insulin or salbutamol will have high intracellular potassium stores. The hypokalaemia in these cases is the result of a redistribution of potassium into cells rather than potassium deficiency, and management of the underlying causes is indicated.

Hyperkalaemia

Hyperkalaemia is a dangerous condition. Although the normal range extends up to 5.5 mmol/l, it is rare to get arrhythmias below 7.5 mmol/l. Precise blood taking is critical as a squeezed sample lyses blood cells, raising potassium level spuriously. The most common cause of hyperkalaemia is renal failure – either acute or chronic. Hyperkalaemia can also result from potassium overload, loss of potassium from cells due to acidosis or cell lysis, or endocrine causes such as hypoaldosteronism and hypoadrenalism.

The immediate treatment of hyperkalaemia is shown schematically in Figure B.1. If there is no immediate threat to the patient's life because of an arrhythmia then a logical sequence of investigation and treatment can be followed. Beta-2 stimulants, such as salbutamol, are the immediate treatment of choice. They rapidly act within 30 minutes by stimulating the cell wall pumping mechanism and promoting cellular potassium uptake. They are easily administered by a nebuliser. The serum potassium will fall by about 1 mmol/l with these dosages.

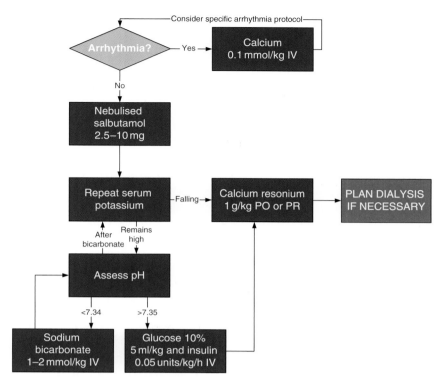

Figure B.1 Algorithm for the management of hyperkalaemia

Summary of emergency management of hyperkalaemia in children (*Continued overleaf*)

Basics	Definition: K$^+$ significantly above upper end of normal for age and/or rising ABC
	Monitoring: continuous ECG (first signs are tented T-waves then loss of P-waves), SaO_2, blood pressure, urine output, weight
	Recheck urea and electrolytes urgently – hours may have elapsed since last sample. Sample may have haemolysed
	Consider the cause: high K$^+$ intake, high production or low output
Stop K$^+$ intake	Stop any potassium in diet and in any fluids being infused
	Stop drugs that can cause hyperkalaemia, e.g. angiotensin-converting enzyme inhibitor (ACE inhibitor), angiotensin II blockers and β-blockers
Stabilise myocardium	10% calcium gluconate
	0.5–1 ml/kg IV over 5 min, max. 20 ml; give undiluted
	Give if ECG changes or K$^+$ significantly above upper end of normal for age or rising
	Effect occurs within minutes. Duration of action approx. 1 h, repeat within 5–10 min as necessary
Shift K$^+$ into cells	Nebulised salbutamol
	<2 year: 2.5 mg or ≥2 years: 5 mg; repeat 2-hourly as necessary
	Onset of action: within 30 min, max. effect at 60–90 min

Seek specialist advice
The following strategies can be used depending on clinical situation:

Shift K$^+$ into cells	Sodium bicarbonate 1–2 mmol/kg IV over 30 min
	(1 mmol = 1 ml of 8.4% $NaHCO_3$, dilute 1:5 in 5% dextrose)

Glucose (± insulin):
> peripheral access: 10% glucose 5–10 ml/kg/h
> central access: 20% glucose 2.5–5 ml/kg/h

Maintain blood glucose at 10–15 mmol/l. Physiological homeostasis should increase endogenous insulin production

Add insulin after an hour if blood sugar >15 mmol/l

Make up a syringe of 50 units insulin in 50 ml 0.9% NaCl (=1 unit/ml); commence infusion at 0.05 ml/kg/h

Maintain blood glucose at 10–15 mmol/l by adjusting infusion rate in 0.05 ml/kg/h steps

Can cause severe hypoglycaemia. Measure blood sugar frequently (15 min after commencing or increase in dose, then every 30 min until stable)

Remove K$^+$ from body — Calcium resonium:
> by rectum: 250 mg/kg (max. 15 g) 6-hourly, repeat if expelled within 30 min
> by mouth: 250 mg/kg (max. 15 g) 6-hourly

Limited role for oral route as it is unpalatable. Takes 4 h for full effect

Dialysis — In specialist environment

Sodium bicarbonate is also effective at rapidly promoting intracellular potassium uptake. The effect is much greater in the acidotic patient (in whom the hyperkalaemia is likely to be secondary to movement of potassium out of the cells). The dosage is the same as that used for treating acidosis, and 1–2 ml/kg of 8.4% $NaHCO_3$ is usually effective. It is important to also check the serum calcium because hyperkalaemia can be accompanied by marked hypocalcaemia, particularly in patients with profound sepsis or renal failure. The use of bicarbonate in these situations can provoke a crisis by lowering the ionised calcium fraction rapidly, precipitating tetany, convulsions or hypotension and arrhythmias, so frequent blood monitoring is required.

Insulin and glucose are the classic treatment for hyperkalaemia. They are not, however, without risk, and the use of salbutamol has reduced the requirement for such therapy. It is easy to precipitate hypoglycaemia if monitoring is not adequate. Large volumes of fluid are often used as a medium for the dextrose and, particularly in the patient with renal failure fluid overload, can then be a problem. Many children are quite capable of significantly increasing endogenous insulin production in response to a glucose load, and this endogenous insulin is just as capable of promoting intracellular potassium uptake. It thus makes sense to start treatment with just an intravenous glucose load and then to add insulin as the blood sugar rises.

The above treatments are the fastest means of securing a fall in the serum potassium, but all work through a redistribution of the potassium into cells. Thus the problem is merely delayed rather than treated in the patient with potassium overload. The only ways of removing potassium from the body are with dialysis or ion exchange resins such as calcium resonium administrated via the gut. Dialysis can only be started when the patient is in an appropriate nephrology or critical care setting, but will be the most effective and rapid means of lowering the potassium.

In an emergency situation where there is an arrhythmia (heart block or ventricular arrhythmia) the treatment of choice is intravenous calcium. This will stabilise the myocardium temporarily but will have no effect on the serum potassium. Thus the treatments discussed above will still be necessary.

Calcium

Some mention of disorders of calcium metabolism is relevant because both hyper- and hypocalcaemia can produce profound clinical pictures.

Hypocalcaemia

Hypocalcaemia can be a part of any severe illness, particularly septicaemia. Other specific conditions that may give rise to hypocalcaemia are severe rickets, hypoparathyroidism, pancreatitis or rhabdomyolysis, and citrate infusion (in massive blood transfusions). Acute and chronic renal failure can also present with severe hypocalcaemia. In all cases, hypocalcaemia can produce weakness, tetany, convulsions, hypotension and arrhythmias. Treatment is that of the underlying condition. In the emergency situation, however, intravenous calcium can be administered. As most of the above conditions are associated with a total body depletion of calcium and because the total body pool is so large, acute doses will often only have a transient effect on the serum calcium. Continuous infusions will also often be required, and most appropriately given through a central venous line as calcium is irritant to peripheral veins. In renal failure, high serum phosphate levels may prevent the serum calcium from rising. The use of oral phosphate binders or dialysis may be necessary in these circumstances.

Hypercalcaemia

Hypercalcaemia usually presents as long-standing anorexia, malaise, weight loss, failure to thrive or vomiting. Causes include hyperparathyroidism, hypervitaminosis D or A, idiopathic hypercalcaemia of infancy, malignancy, thiazide diuretic abuse and skeletal disorders. Initial treatment is with volume expansion with normal saline and furosemide diuretic. Following this, investigation and specific treatment are indicated.

B.3 Diabetic ketoacidosis

Diabetic ketoacidosis (DKA) is a condition in which a relative or absolute lack of insulin leads to an inability to metabolise glucose. This leads to hyperglycaemia and an osmotic diuresis. Once urine output exceeds the ability of the patient to drink, dehydration occurs. In addition, without insulin, fat is used as a source of energy, leading to the production of large quantities of ketones and metabolic acidosis. There is initial compensation for the acidosis by hyperventilation and a respiratory alkalosis but, as the condition progresses, the combination of acidosis, hyperosmolality and dehydration leads to coma. DKA is often the first presentation of diabetes; it can also be a problem in known diabetics who have decompensated through illness, infection or non-adherence to their treatment regimes.

History

The history is usually of weight loss, abdominal pain, vomiting, polyuria and polydipsia, although symptoms may be much less specific in under 5-year-olds who also have an increased tendency to ketoacidosis.

Examination

Children may be dehydrated with deep and rapid (Kussmaul) respiration. They may also be drowsy with the smell of ketones on their breath. Salicylate poisoning and uraemia are differential diagnoses that should be excluded. Whilst rare, infection often precipitates decompensation in both new and known diabetics. Fever is not part of DKA. Suspect sepsis in the presence of fever, hypothermia, hypotension and a refractory acidosis or lactic acidosis.

Management

- Assess:
  - Airway
  - Breathing
  - Circulation
- Give 100% oxygen and place on a cardiac monitor
- Place on a cardiac monitor (observe for peaked T-waves from hyperkalaemia)
- Consider placement of a nasogastric tube
- Take blood for:
  - Blood gases
  - Urea and electrolytes, creatinine
  - Glucose
  - Ketones
- Take urine for:
  - Sugar
- Take other investigations only if indicated:
  - Full blood count (leucocytosis commonly occurs in DKA and is not necessarily a sign of infection)
  - Chest X-ray
  - Blood culture
  - CSF
  - Throat swab
  - Urinalysis, culture and sensitivity

The principles of management of diabetic ketoacidosis are:

1. Fluid boluses are only to be given in DKA to reverse signs of shock and should be given slowly in 10 ml/kg aliquots. If there are no signs of shock, do not routinely give a fluid bolus. If a second saline bolus is needed, specialist advice should be sought.
2. To rehydrate after signs of shock have been reversed with 48 hours of replacement fluid.
3. The first 20 ml/kg of fluid resuscitation are given in addition to replacement fluid calculations and should not be subtracted from the calculations for the fluids for the next 48 hours. Resuscitation volumes over 20 ml/kg should be subtracted from the fluid volume calculated for the 48-hour replacement.
4. Discuss the use of inotropes with a paediatric intensive care specialist if a child in DKA has signs of hypotensive shock.

- When calculating the fluid requirement for children and young people with DKA, assume a 5% fluid deficit in mild to moderate DKA (indicated by a blood pH of 7.1 or above) or a 10% fluid deficit in severe DKA (indicated by a blood pH below 7.1). Replace this deficit over 48 hours
- Calculate the maintenance fluid requirement for children and young people with DKA using the following 'reduced volume' rules:
  - if they weigh less than 10 kg, give 2 ml/kg/h
  - if they weigh between 10 and 40 kg, give 1 ml/kg/h
  - if they weigh more than 40 kg, give a fixed volume of 40 ml/h
- These are lower than standard fluid maintenance volumes because large fluid volumes are associated with an increased risk of cerebral oedema
- The total replacement fluid to be given over 48 hours is calculated as follows:

Hourly rate = (deficit/48 hours) + maintenance per hour

5. To replace insulin; start an intravenous insulin infusion 1–2 hours after beginning intravenous fluid therapy. Use a soluble insulin infusion at a dosage between 0.05 and 0.1 units/kg/h.
6. To return the glucose level to that approaching normal.
7. To avoid hypokalaemia, hypoglycaemia and rapid changes in serum osmolarity.
8. To treat the underlying precipitating cause of the DKA.

The detailed management of DKA is complex. Advice should be sought from experienced local practitioners and published guidelines.

Complications

All of the complications in the box require intensive monitoring on an intensive care unit.

Major complications of diabetic ketoacidosis	
Cerebral oedema	Most important cause of death and poor neurological outcome. Attempt to avoid by slow normalisation of osmolarity with attention to glucose and sodium levels, and hydration over 48 h
	Monitor for headache, recurrence of vomiting, irritability, Glasgow Coma Scale score, inappropriate slowing of heart rate and rising blood pressure
	Treat with hypertonic (3%) saline 3 ml/kg or mannitol infusion (250–500 mg/kg over 20 min), or alternatively hypertonic saline may be used
	Hyperventilation has been associated with worse outcomes
Cardiac dysrhythmias	Usually secondary to electrolyte disturbances, particularly potassium
Pulmonary oedema	Careful fluid replacement may limit the occurrence of pulmonary oedema
Acute renal failure	Uncommon because of high osmotic urine flow

B.4 Summary

You should now be able to:

- Describe the approach to the management of fluid and electrolytes in the seriously ill or injured child

APPENDIX C
Child abuse and neglect

Learning outcomes

After reading this appendix, you will be able to:
- Recognise child abuse and neglect as a potential differential diagnosis
- Describe your approach to a child where abuse and neglect may be suspected
- Identify your role and that of other agencies

C.1 Introduction

The United Nations Convention on the Rights of the Child 1989 provides a set of principles and standards to ensure that, among other things, children are protected. These apply to the practice of children's healthcare for all children and young people up to the age of 18 years.

Article 3 provides that any decision or action affecting children either as individuals or as a group should be taken with 'their best interest' as the most important consideration.

Article 9 holds that children have a right not to be separated from their parents or carers unless it is judged to be in their child's best interest.

Article 12 obliges health professionals to seek a child's opinion before taking decisions that affect her or his future.

Article 19 states that legislative, administrative, social and educational measures should be taken to protect children from all forms of physical and mental violence, injury and abuse (including sexual abuse) and negligent treatment.

Article 37 states that no child shall be subjected to torture or other cruel, inhuman or degrading treatment or punishment.

In 2012, World Health Organisation data showed that 54 581 children died from intentional injuries globally – this is the equivalent of 150 children every day. Child abuse is a universal occurrence. This appendix focuses on generic principles associated with managing child abuse and neglect in the acute situation including recognition, urgent interventions and referral. Health professionals should seek guidance and legal details specific to their setting from national sources.

- Safeguarding is everyone's responsibility. If you have concerns that a child is being/has been abused you have an obligation to refer
- Abuse should always be considered as a potential differential diagnosis (it can often be rapidly excluded but if it is not thought about it will be missed)

Advanced Paediatric Life Support: A Practical Approach to Emergencies, Sixth Edition. Edited by Martin Samuels and Sue Wieteska.
© 2016 John Wiley & Sons, Ltd. Published 2016 by John Wiley & Sons, Ltd.

Healthcare workers will come into contact with:

- Children who have been abused by adults or by other children
- Children who have abused other children
- Adults who were abused as children

Present classifications are shown in Table C.1.

Table C.1 Classification of child abuse	
Neglect	The persistent failure to meet a child's basic physical and/or psychological needs, likely to result in the serious impairment of the child's health or development. Neglect may occur during pregnancy as a result of maternal substance abuse. Once a child is born, neglect may involve a parent or carer failing to: • provide adequate food, clothing and shelter (including exclusion from home or abandonment) • protect a child from physical and emotional harm or danger • ensure adequate supervision (including the use of inadequate care-givers) • ensure access to appropriate medical care or treatment It may also include neglect of, or unresponsiveness to, a child's basic emotional needs
Physical abuse	A form of abuse that may involve hitting, shaking, throwing, poisoning, burning or scalding, drowning, suffocating or otherwise causing physical harm to a child. Physical harm may also be caused when a parent or carer fabricates the symptoms of, or deliberately induces, illness in a child
Sexual abuse	Involves forcing or enticing a child or young person to take part in sexual activities, not necessarily involving a high level of violence, whether or not the child is aware of what is happening. The activities may involve physical contact, including assault by penetration (e.g. rape or oral sex) or non-penetrative acts such as masturbation, kissing, rubbing and touching outside of clothing. They may also include non-contact activities, such as involving children in looking at, or in the production of, sexual images, watching sexual activities, encouraging children to behave in sexually inappropriate ways, or grooming a child in preparation for abuse (including via the internet). Sexual abuse is not solely perpetrated by adult males. Women can also commit acts of sexual abuse, as can other children
Emotional abuse	The persistent emotional maltreatment of a child such as to cause severe and persistent adverse effects on the child's emotional development. It may involve conveying to a child that they are worthless or unloved, inadequate or valued only insofar as they meet the needs of another person. It may include not giving the child opportunities to express their views, deliberately silencing them or 'making fun' of what they say or how they communicate. It may feature age or developmentally inappropriate expectations being imposed on children. These may include interactions that are beyond a child's developmental capability, as well as overprotection and limitation of exploration and learning, or preventing the child participating in normal social interaction. It may involve seeing or hearing the ill treatment of another. It may involve serious bullying (including cyber bullying), causing children frequently to feel frightened or in danger, or the exploitation or corruption of children. Some level of emotional abuse is involved in all types of maltreatment of a child, although it may occur alone

Susceptibility to abuse

The possibility of child ill treatment or abuse must be considered in the differential diagnosis of all children who have suffered injury. Child abuse/ill treatment occurs in all social classes. However, the possible features of parenting known to be associated with child ill treatment or abuse include:

- Where the relationship between the parent and child does not appear loving and caring
- Where one or both parents have been abused themselves as children
- Parents who are young, single, unsupportive or substitutive
- Parents with learning difficulties
- Parents who have a poor or unstable relationship
- Situations where there is domestic violence or drug or alcohol dependence
- Parents who have mental illness or personality disorders

Factors in the child that make them vulnerable to abuse and ill treatment include:

- Prematurity
- Separation and impaired bonding in the neonatal period
- Physical or mental handicap
- Behavioural problems
- Difficult temperament or personality
- Soiling and wetting past developmental age
- Hyperactivity and attention deficit
- Screaming or crying interminably and inconsolably

C.2 Recognition of child abuse and neglect

As highlighted above, abuse should always be considered as a potential differential diagnosis. It can often be rapidly excluded but if it is not thought about it will be missed. In emergency paediatrics consider the following key areas:

- Asphyxial event: suffocation, hanging
- Subdural haemorrhage
- Poisoning and other induced illness (e.g. septicaemia)
- Ruptured abdominal viscus
- Cervical spine injury
- Rib cage and long bone fractures
- Drowning
- Burns

The following boxes list presentations where you may have a higher index of suspicion.

Presentations of physical abuse

- Head injuries – fractures, intracranial injury. These may present as an acute life-threatening event with breathing difficulty or apnoea, or with raised intracranial pressure including symptoms or signs of poor feeding, vomiting, drowsiness and seizures
- Fractures of long bones: single fracture with multiple bruises, multiple fractures in different stages of healing, possibly with no bruises or soft tissue injury, or metaphyseal or epiphyseal injuries (often multiple)
- Fractured ribs and spinal injuries
- Internal damage, e.g. rupture of bowel
- Burns and scalds – 'glove and stocking' appearance for scalds, implement imprints for contact burns
- Cold injury – hypothermia, frostbite
- Poisoning – drugs or household substances
- Suffocation
- Cuts and bruises – imprints of hands, sticks, whips, belts, bites, etc. may be present
- Bruising in a non-mobile infant

Presentations of sexual abuse (*Continued overleaf*)

- Disclosure by child
- Disclosure by witness
- Suspicion by third party because of the behaviour of the child, especially changes in behaviour. These include insecurity; fear of men; sleep disorders; mood changes, tantrums and aggression at home; anxiety, despair, withdrawal and secretiveness; poor peer relationships; lying, stealing or arson; school failure; eating disorders like anorexia and compulsive overeating; running away and truancy; suicide attempts, self-poisoning, self-mutilation and abuse of drugs, solvents and alcohol; unexplained acquisition of money; sexualised behaviour such as drawings with a sexual content; knowledge of adult sexual behaviour shown in speech, play or drawing; apparent sexual approaches; and promiscuity
- Symptoms such as a sore bottom, vaginal discharge, bleeding per vagina in a pre-pubertal child, bleeding per rectum, or inflamed penis that the care-giver believes is due to sexual abuse.
- Symptoms as above and/or signs (e.g. unexplained perineal tear and/or bruising, torn hymen or perineal warts), but the doctor is the first person to suspect abuse
- Faecal soiling or relapse of enuresis

- Sexually transmitted disease
- Pregnancy where the girl refuses to name the putative father or even indicate the category, e.g. boyfriend, casual acquaintance
- Sexual intercourse with a child younger than 13 years is unlawful and therefore pregnancy in such a child means the child has been maltreated
- Female genital mutilation (FGM)

Presentations of neglect

- Severe and persistent infestations, such as scabies or head lice
- A child's clothing or footwear is consistently inappropriate (e.g. for the weather or the child's size)
- A child is persistently smelly and dirty, especially if seen at times of the day when it is unlikely that they would have had an opportunity to become dirty or smelly (e.g. early morning)
- Repeated observation or reports of the home environment being of a poor standard of hygiene that affects a child's health
- The home environment is unsuitable for the child's stage of development and impacts on the child's safety or well-being
- It may be difficult to distinguish between neglect and material poverty. However, care should be taken to balance recognition of the constraints on the parents' or carers' ability to meet their children's needs for food, clothing and shelter with an appreciation of how people in similar circumstances have been able to meet those needs
- Child abandonment
- Non-organic failure to thrive
- Repeated non-attendances at appointments that are necessary for the child's health and well-being
- Parents or carers fail to administer essential prescribed treatment for their child
- Parents or carers fail to seek medical advice for their child to the extent that the child's health and well-being is compromised
- Poor/inadequate supervision which may lead/has led to injury

The following box lists some other pointers to be aware of during history taking and examination.

- There is delay in seeking medical help or medical help is not sought at all
- The story of the 'accident' is vague, is lacking in detail and may vary with each telling and from person to person. Innocent accidents tend to have vivid accounts that ring true
- The account of the accident is not compatible with the injury observed
- The injury is not compatible with the child's level of development or of the level of development of another child alleged to have caused the injury
- The parents' affect is abnormal. Note anything that appears abnormal to you in this regard
- The parents' behaviour gives cause for concern. They may become hostile, rebut accusations that have not been made or leave before the consultant arrives
- The child's appearance and his interaction with his parents are abnormal. He may look sad, withdrawn or frightened. There may be visible evidence of failure to thrive. Full-blown frozen watchfulness is a late stage and results from repetitive physical and emotional abuse over a period of time

---

C.3 Assessment

The assessment of all children should follow the standard ABCDE procedure and full medical assessment approach.

Consent for examination is mandatory in all cases unless a serious life-threatening injury is suspected. This needs to be given by an adult with parental responsibility or the child if competent. Social care may need to get a court order if appropriate consent is not available or refused. This is also an aspect that will be subject to national laws, policies and procedures and you should familiarise yourself with those relevant to your practice using national guidance.

Details of medical assessment

History

A full history should be taken as in any medical assessment. There are some specific issues to consider if child abuse and neglect is on your list of differential diagnoses.

- Full details of the history of the incident(s) should be obtained from the child and the caregivers. If social workers and police officers have previously talked to the child, then taking this history from them may be appropriate, especially for alleged sexual offences. Frequent repetition of the details can be very disturbing to the child and can jeopardise evidence
- In history related to the gastrointestinal tract remember to ask about soiling, constipation, rectal pain and rectal bleeding
- In history related to the urogenital system remember to ask about wetting, vaginal bleeding, vaginal discharge and, when appropriate, menarche, cycle, sanitary protection and previous sexual intercourse
- Personal history must start with pregnancy, birth, the neonatal period and subsequent developmental milestones. Then details of immunisations, drug history (including alcohol and street drugs) and allergies are obtained. Information on the child's performance at nursery or school should include social factors
- Enquiries are made about previous illnesses and injuries, with dates of attendance at hospital or the surgery of the family doctor. Past records should be obtained and relevant information should be extracted
- The traditional family history should include details of the natural parents, all co-habitees and any other people who regularly care for the child, e.g. relatives and childminders
- Parental illness should be discussed, particularly psychiatric illness
- The presence of domestic abuse should be explored
- Then the names, ages and medical histories of all siblings and half-siblings are obtained. Any miscarriages, stillbirths or deaths of siblings are discussed sensitively
- Familial illnesses that are particularly important are inherited skin or blood disorders

Remember to remain objective and show professional sensitivity. Document who is present and their relationship to the child. Use open questions and avoid leading questions. Full contemporaneous notes are essential. If the child has been video-interviewed you may be able to obtain the transcript of this prior to examination to avoid unnecessary repetition.

Examination

Ensure an appropriate chaperone is present. The general examination starts while the history is being taken. During that time the doctor observes the affect of the child, the relationships between the child, mother, father and others present, and any behavioural problems. If the child is reluctant to be examined, then playing with toys or the doctor's stethoscope often breaks the ice. No child should be examined against his or her will as this constitutes an assault. Examination under anaesthesia is rarely required.

General examination

- Full head-to-toe examination
- Plot growth on growth chart including head circumference in younger children
- Comment on general level of hygiene, clothing, etc.
- Document any injuries on a body map
- Comment on developmental level and interaction with carers

Sexual abuse examination

- This should be undertaken by a doctor with the necessary competences
- Best practice is to use a colposcope for magnification and to take digital images
- If there has been acute assault, then forensic examination taking forensic swabs will be needed – often this is as a joint examination with the paediatrician/forensic medical examiner
- Need to consider post-coital contraception or screening for sexually transmitted infections

Investigations

The investigations are dependent on the initial presentation and injuries.

Young babies presenting with concerns about physical abuse all need:

- Full blood count and clotting
- Neuro-imaging

- Fundoscopy
- Skeletal survey – which should include a repeat chest X-ray 10–14 days later to exclude rib fractures

Blood investigations to exclude differential diagnosis will also depend on clinical presentation and may include:

- Blood cultures
- Metabolic investigations
- Renal and bone profile
- Extended clotting studies

C.4 Initial management

Medical treatment is the priority, especially if the child has serious or life-threatening injuries. At the end of the medical assessment the diagnosis may be clear. More often, there is a differential diagnosis that includes abuse.

For paediatric trauma, ask the following questions:

- Does the story of the mechanism fit with the injury pattern seen? (e.g. a 'fall down the stairs' with bruising on the abdomen)
- Do the injuries fit with what is reasonable for this child's developmental age? (e.g. a 1-month-old baby who 'rolled off the bed')
- Could the parents or carers have done anything in advance to prevent the accident happening? (e.g. a burn injury in an unsupervised toddler)
- Could the parents or carers have done anything after the accident to improve medical care? (e.g. an injury that has not had prompt care)

When the diagnosis or differential diagnosis is one of child abuse then the decisions to be made on management are the following:

- Does the child need admission for treatment of the injuries?
- Will the child be safe if returned home?
- If the child needs protection from an abuser who is in his or her own home, how can this be done?
- What support/protection is needed for the rest of the family, including siblings?

Significant harm and thresholds for intervention

In addition to the areas listed above, also consider the following.

Grave concern

This is described in children whose situations do not currently fit the above categories, but where social and medical assessments indicate that they are at significant risk of abuse. These could include situations where another child in the household has been harmed or the household contains a known abuser, including situations where an adult is the subject of domestic abuse.

Organised abuse

This characteristically involves multiple perpetrators, involves multiple victims and is a form of organised crime. There are three subsections. The first is paedophile and/or pornographic rings. The second is cult-based ritualistic abuse in which the abuse has spiritual or social objectives. The third is pseudo-ritualistic abuse in which the degradation of children is the end rather than the means. The details of management of these many facets require a referral and a multiagency response.

C.5 Referral

Where there are concerns of child abuse and neglect, discussion takes place among the social workers, healthcare workers and police officers, who have information about the family, to balance the probabilities of abuse having occurred. Approaches to this will vary from country to country, but in all cases should include a decision about whether it may be necessary to arrange for the child to be taken to a place of safety.

If abuse and neglect are likely then a multiagency assessment involving social care, health and the police will be required. As a separate, parallel process, police will consider whether criminal investigation is appropriate or necessary; in many cases a full criminal investigation will not take place. The approach to this will vary according to national laws, policies and procedures.

All child protection work is based on cooperation between families, social workers, police officers, healthcare workers and educationalists. This multiagency approach is to ensure that all aspects of the care of the family are considered when decisions are being made. Certain decisions in management must be made by a professional, e.g. only a doctor can decide on the treatment required for a fracture and only a police officer can decide the charge that is appropriate for the alleged offence. However, whenever possible, unilateral decisions are avoided in the best interests of the child and the family.

Because of the complexity of interaction between these agencies, communication is a crucial element. The following are key components for ensuring clear communication and accountabilities and should provide a structure for those working in the acute setting:

Key components for clear communication and accountabilities

- Take a history from the child where possible, with an interpreter when necessary
- Access previous records and the national child protection register, where available
- Make comprehensive and contemporaneous records of all findings, decisions and communications
- Seek further opinion where needed and allow discharge of the child only by a senior doctor and with a plan for future care
- Have clear lines of responsibility and a single set of hospital records
- Ensure training and updates in child protection for those managing children

---

Doctors may be concerned about sharing information with other professionals because of the ethical consideration of confidentiality. In the UK, the General Medical Council (2012) gives the following advice.

Ask for consent to share information unless there is a compelling reason for not doing so. Information can be shared without consent if it is justified in the public interest or required by law. Do not delay disclosing information to obtain consent if that might put children or young people at risk of significant harm.

Advice on consent will vary from country to country and you should be aware of your own national guidance and advice.

C.6 Medicolegal aspects

Healthcare professionals must be familiar with the medicolegal aspects of their work. These may vary according to the jurisdiction where the clinician practices. They will in most cases cover the following:

- Court orders to enable:
  - Emergency protection
  - Child assessment
  - Residence
  - Police protection
- Consent to examination

In some cases where there is involvement of either a criminal or family court, healthcare professionals may be required to write statements and/or present evidence.

Court reports

When preparing a written report on a child for the court, all healthcare professionals should keep in mind that the written report may be used in subsequent court appearances. Therefore, the report should be confined to the facts. Whenever possible, objective and measurable evidence of the child's health and development should be presented. Where subjective views must be given they should reflect balanced professional judgement. If the report is comprehensive and comprehensible, then the healthcare professional may not be called to give verbal evidence in person. Always keep a copy of your report.

Statements

The purpose of a statement is to provide the court with an informative and relevant account of the medical assessment of the child. The statement will give details of the persons involved, the observations and the findings. Information given by another person should not be included unless this has been requested. In many areas, the prosecutors wish statements to record all information, although hearsay may be excluded before presentation to the court.

A statement is a professional document. It should be well written in clear, readily understandable language. Technical terms should be avoided or, if used, should be followed immediately by appropriate lay terms. Most statements will be for the prosecution and a printed statement form will be provided. The standard sequence of writing a statement is shown in the box below.

Sequence for writing a statement

- Full name with surname in capitals
- Qualifications
- Occupation
- Name of person requesting the assessment
- Date, time and place of the assessment
- Name of person who was examined
- Name of persons present
- Details of the relevant history – if a general history was taken but produced nothing significant then make a general comment including the sight of the detailed notes
- Details of examination – if it was a joint examination then specify who did each part
- Investigations
- Opinion on findings
- The time at which the examination ended

Each page must be signed at the bottom, and the final page must be signed on the line below the final text. Any alterations must be initialled. Always keep a copy of the statement.

Presentation of evidence

Dress in a professional manner. Arrive early in court. Take along all notes relevant to the case. Review these on the day before the court proceedings, as well as your report. With permission from the magistrate or judge, you may refer to contemporaneous notes. However, thorough preparation helps to put the whole picture of the incident into the forefront of your mind so that you can find the appropriate notes more quickly.

When giving evidence stay calm even when challenged. Do not be persuaded to answer questions that are outside your knowledge or experience.

C.7 Summary

- Safeguarding is everyone's responsibility
- If you have concerns that a child is being/has been abused you have an obligation to refer
- Abuse should always be considered as a potential differential diagnosis – it can often be rapidly excluded, but if it is not thought about it will be missed

APPENDIX D
When a child dies

Learning outcomes

After reading this appendix, you will be able to:
- Identify the factors that are important when dealing with the death of a child
- Describe your approach to the death of a child
- Identify your role and that of other agencies

D.1 Introduction

Even with the best preventative measures in place and the use of the most effective resuscitation methods, children will continue to die from serious illness and severe injury. When a death occurs, medical and nursing staff must be able to deal effectively with the child's family and the legal requirements of death as well as cope with their own emotional reactions. Sympathetic and sensitive support of the family at this time can do much to help the grief process and adjustment to the bereavement.

The principles in dealing with a family that has experienced a sudden child death are shown in the box below.

Principles in dealing with a family

- Display caring, kindness and compassion
- Spend as much time as necessary with the family in an unhurried fashion
- Offer information regarding the death as the family requires
- Talk to colleagues later regarding your experience and feelings

Unless a clear care plan indicating 'no resuscitation' has been negotiated in advance with the parents and recorded in the medical records, full resuscitation should be undertaken. Parental presence during resuscitation is increasingly common, and whether this occurs should be a decision made jointly by the child's parents and staff. Although being present at their child's resuscitation is always extremely traumatic for the parents, when it is over they are almost always left with the impression that everything possible was done to save their child. If parents are present during resuscitation, ideally a member of staff will be available exclusively for their support. If the presence of parents is impeding the progress of the resuscitation, they should sensitively be asked to leave.

There may be suspicious circumstances around the death, evidence of abuse or concerns re the family. The response when a child dies unexpectedly should include a multiagency discussion to ensure an appropriate planned response. In some circumstances the police may decide to undertake an immediate criminal investigation. Medical staff will need to cooperate with this investigation.

In all cases, it is important that family are dealt with sensitively and offered appropriate support.

Advanced Paediatric Life Support: A Practical Approach to Emergencies, Sixth Edition. Edited by Martin Samuels and Sue Wieteska.
© 2016 John Wiley & Sons, Ltd. Published 2016 by John Wiley & Sons, Ltd.

D.2 Dealing with the family

Breaking the news

Telling the parents that their child has died is a difficult task and is usually undertaken by a senior and experienced staff member. Before speaking to the parents ensure they are in a private, comfortable environment and that you know the name of the child. Sometimes a bigger family circle may be important and one should invite them, 'Come with the ones you want to be involved'.

A direct and sympathetic approach is best, avoiding euphemisms and clichés. If it is appropriate and you feel comfortable doing it you may show sympathy by holding the parent's hand or putting an arm around them. Usually the parents will turn away towards each other for a while but may wish to ask questions about the cause of death and what they should do now. The parents will often want to know what happened and what treatments were instituted. If you are asked about the cause of death answer as simply and honestly as you can, making it clear that some answers are not yet available.

Caring for the parents

Provide the family with a private room in which they can be alone with their child for as long as they wish. Encourage the family to touch and hold the child. Offer to stay with the family; however, if they wish to be left alone, assure them you will be nearby if they wish to speak with you. In cases where there have been child protection concerns it will be necessary for the parents to be accompanied by a professional when they are with the child.

Accept the family's distress as natural and support them in this by acknowledging their feelings. Be prepared for a variety of responses: there is no 'correct' way to grieve and each person will have a different reaction. Be sensitive to and respectful toward varying cultural norms and rituals surrounding death. Facilitate contact with other family members and friends as required. Even very young children may be included in the grief process right from the start; assist the family in feeling comfortable with this.

Each institution will have its own bereavement support programme: ensure that you are familiar with local resources and that the family is offered ongoing support and medical advice. Remember that if a child dies, most parents/families do not know what will happen or how the procedures work. It is advisable to give them guidance.

D.3 Post-death procedures

Every jurisdiction will have specific legal requirements that need to be adhered to. It is usually necessary for the coroner, the police or another statutory authority to be informed of the death. The requirements for a police or coronial investigation, an autopsy and an inquest will vary from case to case.

A customised checklist is invaluable for ensuring that procedures or information are not forgotten. The box below gives an outline of such a list although local hospital guidelines should be followed even if they are different. In all cases of sudden unexpected death in the UK, there are local procedures for reporting to, and investigation by, a multiagency team led by the Designated Doctor for Unexpected Deaths.

Checklist for post-death procedure

The child

- Full and thorough examination
- Core temperature
- Wrap child in clean warm clothes for parents to see and hold (if consistent with forensic requirements)
- Samples or swabs if agreed as mandatory in local protocol

The parents

- Explain that the child (use name) has died
- Gently get as full a history as possible
- Ask if they would like a priest/religious leader present
- Ask if they want any close relative to be contacted or extended family to be present
- Encourage the parents to see and hold the child

- Let them know if a post-mortem examination needs to be carried out and ensure that they understand all that they wish to know about the procedure and have given their written consent where appropriate. Explain the full process of a post-mortem and what will be done with the dead child. Remember that sometimes a post-mortem might not include the whole body, but may be limited to specific regions, depending on pre-mortem illness, etc.
- Let them know that the police and coroner are always informed of sudden unexpected deaths and will need to ask a few simple questions of the carers
- Ask what address the family will be going to on leaving the hospital
- Arrange transport from the hospital to home and, if alone, make sure they are accompanied on the journey and not left alone at home
- Be gentle, unhurried, calm and careful
- Do not guess at the diagnosis

Details to be obtained

- Child's and parents' names
- Child's date of birth
- Address at which death occurred
- Time of arrival in department
- Time last seen alive
- Usual address if different from above

Inform

- GP – advise of child's death and give the address to which the parents will be going from hospital
- Health visitor
- Social worker
- Any relative as requested by the family
- Coroner – who will need to know the full name and address and date of birth of the child, time of arrival, place of death, brief recent history and any suspicious circumstances

D.4 Take care of the staff

The sudden and unexpected death of a child is extremely distressing for all involved. Some staff members may be profoundly affected. Encourage staff members to talk about the event and their feelings in private soon afterwards with a colleague. Formal staff counselling should be available if needed.

D.5 Summary

When a death occurs, medical and nursing staff must be able to deal effectively with the child's family and the legal requirements of death as well as cope with their own emotional reactions. Sympathetic and sensitive support of the family at this time can do much to help the grief process and adjustment to the bereavement.

You should now be able to:

- Identify the factors that are important when dealing with the death of a child
- Describe your approach to the death of a child
- Identify your role and that of other agencies

APPENDIX E
General approach to poisoning and envenomation

Learning outcomes

After reading this chapter, you will be able to:
- Describe the approach to the management of poisoning in children
- Describe the approach to the management of envenomation in children

E.1 Poisoning: introduction

Deaths from ingested poisons are uncommon (globally in 2012 there were 35 205 – only 4.7% of the number of deaths caused by injury). They are due to therapeutic (especially tricyclic antidepressants) or 'recreational' drugs, household products and, rarely, plants. Infrequently, groups of children may be exposed to inhalational toxins such as chlorine gases in the event of accidents (or occasionally deliberate attempts to cause harm).

In some parts of the world poisoning with agricultural products such as organophosphates and carbamates may also be a significant problem and in others children ingest corrosives from time to time and end up with severe oesophageal burns and complications.

Incidence

There has been a steady decline in the number of childhood deaths from poisonings globally from 52 149 in 2000 to 35 205 in 2012 (WHO data). The selective introduction of child-resistant containers, together with other measures, has reduced the number of poisonings and hospital attendances. It should be remembered, however, that 20% of children under the age of 5 years are capable of opening child-resistant containers!

The decrease in deaths from the inhalation of toxic fumes may be related to the gradual effect of legislation in some countries on the banning of toxic substances in furnishing items. The continued substantial death rate from carbon monoxide poisoning is disappointing but may be related to the fact that although smoke alarms are more readily found in dwellings, they are often non-functional. The decline in mortality from drug poisoning may be due both to more effective treatment and possibly to the more widespread use of less toxic antidepressant drugs.

Accidental poisoning

This is usually a problem of the young child or toddler, with a mean age of presentation of 2.5 years. Accidental poisoning usually occurs when the child is unsupervised, and there is an increased incidence in poisoning following recent disruption in households, such as a new baby, moving house or where there is maternal depression.

Advanced Paediatric Life Support: A Practical Approach to Emergencies, Sixth Edition. Edited by Martin Samuels and Sue Wieteska.
© 2016 John Wiley & Sons, Ltd. Published 2016 by John Wiley & Sons, Ltd.

Intentional overdose

Suicide or parasuicide attempts are usually made by young people in their teens; however, sometimes they may be as young as 8 or 9 years. These children or adolescents should undergo psychiatric and social assessment.

Drug abuse

Alcohol and solvent abuse are among the commonest forms of drug abuse in children.

Iatrogenic drugs

The commonest offender is diphenoxylate with atropine (Lomotil). This combination is toxic to some children at therapeutic doses. The most frequently fatal drug is digoxin.

Deliberate poisoning

Rarely, symptoms are induced in children by adults via the administration of drugs. A history of poisoning will often not be given at presentation.

Most poisoning episodes in childhood and adolescence are of low lethality and little or no treatment is required. This appendix will not address the milder cases but will enable the student to develop an approach to the seriously ill poisoned child, with additional advice on the management of specific poisons.

E.2 Primary assessment and resuscitation in poisoning

- Respiratory rate: the rate may be increased in poisoning from amphetamines, ecstasy, salicylates, ethylene glycol and methanol.
- Acidotic sighing respirations: this may suggest metabolic acidosis from salicylates or ethylene glycol poisoning as a cause for the coma.
- Heart rate: tachycardia is caused by amphetamines, ecstasy, β-agonists, phenothiazines, theophylline and tricyclic antidepressants (TCAs); bradycardia is caused by β-blockers, digoxin and organophosphates.
- Blood pressure: hypotension is commonly seen in serious poisoning; hypertension is caused by ecstasy and monoamine oxidase inhibitors.
- If heart rate is above 200 beats/min in an infant or above 150 beats/min in a child, or if the rhythm is abnormal, perform cardiac monitoring. QRS prolongation and ventricular tachycardia are seen in TCA poisoning.
- Depression of conscious level suggests poisoning with opiates, sedatives (such as benzodiazepines) antihistamines and hypoglycaemic agents.
- Pupillary size and reaction should be noted. Very small pupils suggest opiate or organophosphate poisoning; large pupils amphetamines, atropine and TCAs.
- Note the child's posture. Hypertonia is seen in amphetamine, ecstasy, theophylline and TCA poisoning.
- The presence of convulsive movements should be sought. Convulsions are associated with any drug that causes hypoglycaemia (ethanol) and with TCA poisoning.
- A fever suggests poisoning with ecstasy, cocaine or salicylates.
- Hypothermia suggests poisoning with barbiturates or ethanol.

Airway

- A patent airway is the first requisite. If the airway is not patent it should be opened and maintained with an airway manoeuvre and the child ventilated by bag–valve–mask oxygenation. An airway adjunct can be used. The airway should then be secured by intubation with experienced senior help.
- Management of the airway may be particularly challenging in situations such as: corrosive ingestion; patients with cardiac arrhythmia related to medication such as TCAs; or in patients with profuse respiratory secretions as may occur following organophosphate ingestions.
- If the child has an AVPU score of 'P' or 'U', his or her airway is at risk. It should be maintained by an airway manoeuvre or adjunct and senior help requested to secure it.

Breathing

- All children with respiratory abnormalities, shock or a decreased conscious level should receive high-flow oxygen through a face mask with a reservoir as soon as the airway has been demonstrated to be adequate.
- A number of agents taken in overdose (particularly narcotics) can produce respiratory depression. Oxygen should be given, but it is important to remember that these patients may have an increasing carbon dioxide level despite a normal oxygen saturation whilst breathing oxygen. Inadequate breathing should be supported using a bag–valve–mask device with oxygen or by intermittent positive pressure ventilation in the intubated patient.

Circulation

- A number of poisons can produce shock, by a number of different mechanisms. Hypovolaemia may be caused by gastrointestinal bleeding from iron poisoning or there may be vasodilatation from barbiturates. Shock should be treated with a fluid bolus, as usual. If possible, inotropes should be avoided in poisoning cases as the combination of toxic substance producing shock and an inotrope may be proarrhythmogenic.
- Cardiac dysrhythmias can be expected in TCA, digoxin, quinine and antiarrhythmic drug poisoning. Some antiarrhythmic treatments are contraindicated with certain poisons. See below for advice on TCA poisoning and contact a poisons centre urgently for other advice.
- Gain intravenous or intraosseous access.
- Take blood for a full blood count, urea and electrolytes, toxicology, paracetamol and salicylate levels (in patients who have taken an unknown drug), glucose stick test and laboratory test.
- Give 2 ml/kg of 10% glucose followed by maintenance glucose infusion to any hypoglycaemic patient.
- Give a 20 ml/kg rapid bolus of crystalloid to any patient with signs of shock.
- If a child has a tachyarrhythmia and is shocked, up to three synchronous electrical shocks at 1, 2 and 2 J should be given. If the arrhythmia is broad-complex and the synchronous shocks are not activated by the defibrillator then attempt an asynchronous shock. A conscious child should be anaesthetised first if this can be done in a timely manner. A DC shock may be dangerous in digoxin poisoning. Antiarrhythmics may be used on advice from a poisons centre.

Disability

- Treat convulsions with either diazepam, midazolam or lorazepam.
- Give a trial of naloxone in cases where depressed conscious level and small pupils suggest opiate poisoning.

> In all cases of serious poisoning early consultation with a poisons centre is mandatory. Such centres have a wealth of expertise in the management of poisoning and will advise on the individual patient's needs.

Monitoring

- Electrocardiogram
- Blood pressure (use appropriate size of cuff)
- Pulse oximetry
- Core temperature
- Blood glucose
- Urea and electrolytes
- Blood gases (where indicated)

Lethality assessment

At the end of the primary assessment it is important to assess the potential lethality of the overdose. This requires knowledge of the substance that has been taken, the time it was taken and the dosage. This information may be unattainable in the unwitnessed poisoning episode of a toddler or that of an unconscious or uncooperative adolescent. Some clues about the drug ingested may be available from physical signs noted during the primary assessment (Table E.1).

Some investigation results can add clues to the diagnosis of an unknown poison (Table E.2).

Table E.1 Diagnostic clues from the primary assessment

Signs	Drug
Tachypnoea	Aspirin, theophylline, carbon monoxide, cyanide
Bradypnoea	Ethanol, opiates, barbiturates, sedatives
Metabolic acidosis (sighing respirations)	Ethanol, carbon monoxide, ethylene glycol
Tachycardia	Antidepressants, sympathomimetics, amphetamines, cocaine
Bradycardia	Beta-blockers, digoxin, clonidine
Hypotension	Barbiturates, benzodiazepines, β-blockers, calcium channel blockers, opiates, iron, phenothiazines, phenytoin, tricyclic antidepressants
Hypertension	Amphetamines, cocaine, sympathomimetic agents
Small pupils	Opiates, organophosphate insecticides, phenothiazines
Large pupils	Amphetamines, atropine, cannabis, carbamazepine, cocaine, quinine, tricyclic antidepressants
Convulsions	Carbamazepine, lindane, organophosphate insecticides, phenothiazines, tricyclic antidepressants
Hypothermia	Barbiturates, ethanol, phenothiazines
Hyperthermia	Amphetamines, cocaine, ecstasy, phenothiazines, salicylates

Table E.2 Clues to the diagnosis of an unknown poison

	Metabolic acidosis	An enlarged anion gap $[(Na + K) - (HCO_3 - Cl)]$ of >18	Hypokalaemia	Hyperkalaemia
Beta-agonists			✓	
Carbon monoxide	✓			
Digoxin				✓
Ecstasy	✓			
Ethanol		✓		
Ethylene glycol	✓	✓		
Iron	✓	✓		
Methanol	✓	✓		
Salicylates	✓	✓		
Theophylline			✓	
Tricyclic antidepressants	✓			

The risks of a particular overdose can be assessed once all the information has been gathered. Complex or life-threatening cases should be discussed with a poisons centre. The poisons centre will require the following information:

- Age and weight of the patient
- Time since exposure
- The substance taken
- Amount taken together with any description or labelling
- Patient's condition

If the nature of the overdose is unknown then a high potential lethality should be assumed. Many childhood poisoning incidents have zero lethality and no treatment is required.

E.3 Emergency treatment in poisoning

Drug elimination

Many children have taken a trivial overdose or an overdose of a non-poisonous substance. If the overdose episode is assessed as having a low lethality, then no treatment is required.

If the drug overdose is assessed as having a potentially high lethality or its exact nature is unknown, then measures to minimise blood concentrations of the drug should be undertaken. In general, this means stopping further absorption. Occasionally measures to increase excretion can be employed and in some circumstances specific antidotes may be available. Seek advice from a poisons centre.

There are a number of active elimination techniques such as haemoperfusion and plasmapheresis; their use is infrequent and should be guided by the advice of the poisons centre.

Activated charcoal

Activated charcoal has a surface area of 1000 m^2/g and is capable of binding a number of poisonous substances without being systemically absorbed. It is now widely used in cases of poisoning. However, there are some substances that it will not absorb. These include alcohol and iron. Repeated doses of activated charcoal are useful in some types of poisoning because they promote drug reabsorption from the circulation back into the bowel and interrupt enterohepatic cycling. These types include aspirin, barbiturates and theophylline.

It is often difficult to give charcoal to children as it is unpalatable. Flavouring may be necessary but can diminish the charcoal's activity. The charcoal can be given via a nasogastric or lavage tube after a gastric washout. The dose is at least 10 times the estimated dose of poison ingested. Children should usually be given 25–50 g.

Aspirated charcoal causes severe lung damage, so airway protection is especially important in the child who is not fully conscious or in whom the predicted trajectory of the poisoning is likely to result in an at-risk airway.

Emesis

Emesis caused by ipecacuanha is now rarely used although for many years it was routinely given for the management of poisoning incidents in children. The dose schedule is 15 ml with water (10 ml in children of 6 months to 2 years), repeated once after 20 minutes if necessary. It must not be used in the child with a depressed conscious level. Evidence now suggests that unless emesis occurs within 1 hour of ingestion of the poison, little of the poison will be eliminated. Only about 30% is retrieved even within the hour.

Emesis should only be used for those poisons requiring removal that are not bound by charcoal, or in children who are at risk from developing symptoms from the poison they have taken, who present within 1 hour of ingestion and who will not take the charcoal. It should not be used in patients who may have ingested corrosive substances.

Gastric lavage

Gastric lavage is rarely required as the benefit rarely outweighs the risk. Advice should be sought from the National Poisons Information Service if a significant quantity of iron or lithium has been ingested within the previous hour.

E.4 Emergency treatment of specific poisons

Iron

Depending on the elapsed time since ingestion, the child with iron poisoning may present with shock, which may be due to gut haemorrhage. If over 20 mg/kg of elemental iron has been taken, toxicity is likely. Over 150 mg/kg may be fatal. Intubation, ventilation and circulatory support are necessary in the severely affected child. Initial symptoms of toxicity are vomiting, diarrhoea and abdominal pain. These may lead on to drowsiness, fits and circulatory collapse.

Whole bowel irrigation can be considered once the airway is secured and circulatory access has been gained. Charcoal is not helpful. Desferrioxamine can be administered orally and left in the stomach, or intravenously and infused at a dose of up to 15 mg/kg/h. This treatment should be given immediately to children with serious symptoms such as shock, coma or fits and to all with a serum iron level (4 hours or more after ingestion) of 3 mg/l and gastrointestinal symptoms, leucocytosis or hyperglycaemia. Note that high levels of iron can itself cause haemolysis, so a haemolysed sample should raise alarm bells.

Radiography of the abdomen can help to show how much iron remains within.

Tricyclic antidepressant poisoning

The toxic effects of these agents result from their inhibition of fast sodium channels in the brain and myocardium – this action is known as 'quinidine-like'. With serious intoxication, the cardiac problems are due to intraventricular conduction delay. This results in QRS prolongation (a QRS of more than four little squares on the ECG paper is predictive of serious effects). TCA poisoning causes anticholinergic effects (tachycardia, dilated pupils, convulsions) and cardiac effects (conduction delay, any arrhythmia). Convulsions should be treated as described in Chapter 9.

In addition, alkalinisation up to an arterial pH of at least 7.45, and preferably 7.5, has been shown to reduce the toxic effects on the heart. This can be achieved by hyperventilation (PCO_2 no lower than 3.33 kPa (25 mmHg)) and by infusing sodium bicarbonate (1–2 mmol/kg). Hypotension should be treated with volume expansion, and if an inotrope is necessary, noradrenaline is preferable to dopamine, dobutamine and adrenaline. Glucagon has an inotropic effect and can be used in this circumstance.

The use of antiarrhythmics should be guided by a poisons centre. Lidocaine and phenytoin may be helpful. Quinidine, procainamide and disopyramide are contraindicated.

Opiates (including methadone)

Following stabilisation of airway, breathing and circulation, the specific antidote is naloxone. An initial bolus dose of 10 micrograms/kg should be given. Naloxone has a short half-life, relapse often occurring after 20 minutes. Larger boluses, or an infusion of 5–20 micrograms/kg/h, may be required.

It is important to normalise CO_2 before the naloxone is given because adverse events such as ventricular arrhythmias, acute pulmonary oedema, asystole or seizures may otherwise occur. This is because the opioid system and the adrenergic system are inter-related. Opioid antagonists and hypercapnia stimulate sympathetic nervous system activity. Therefore if ventilation is not provided to normalise CO_2 prior to naloxone administration, the sudden rise in adrenaline concentration can cause arrhythmias.

Paracetamol

Significant paracetamol poisoning in childhood is almost always intentional; the accidental ingestion of paediatric paracetamol elixir preparations by the toddler very rarely achieves toxicity. Doses of less than 150 mg/kg will not cause toxicity except in a child with hepatic or renal disease.

Current treatment of paracetamol poisoning includes oral charcoal if the assessment occurs within 1 hour of ingestion considered to be of high risk and a paracetamol blood level to be taken at 4 hours or later. In liquid ingestions, because of rapid absorption, no oral charcoal should be given. Figure E.1 shows a nomogram indicating the level of blood paracetamol at which acetylcysteine should be given intravenously. A total dose of 300 mg/kg is given over approximately 24 hours. Contact a poisons centre for individual details.

Salicylates

Aspirin slows stomach emptying, so gastric lavage can be undertaken up to 4 hours after ingestion. Repeated charcoal doses should be given for patients who have ingested sustained-release preparations. The salicylate level can be measured initially at 2 hours. However, repeated measurements are necessary and no reliance should be placed on a single salicylate level. The levels will usually rise significantly over the first 6 hours (longer if an enteric-coated preparation is used). Salicylate poisoning causes a respiratory alkalosis and metabolic acidosis. Arterial blood gas estimation is necessary for managing the patient. Alkalinisation of the patient improves the excretion of salicylate: 1 mmol/kg of sodium bicarbonate should be infused over 4 hours. Forced diuresis is no longer used.

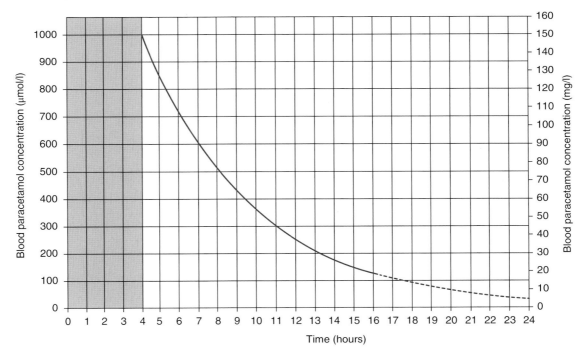

Figure E.1 Nomogram indicating the level of blood paracetamol at which acetylcysteine should be given intravenously. (From Daly *et al.* Guidelines for the management of paracetomol poisoning in Australia and New Zealand: explanation and elaboration. A consensus statement from clinical toxicologists consulting to the Australasian poisons information centres. *Medical Journal of Australia* 2008;188(5):296–301. © 2008 Reproduced with permission from Medical Journal of Australia)

Ethylene glycol

This sweet-tasting substance is available as an antifreeze and de-icer fluid for vehicles. It produces a clinical appearance of inebriation accompanied by metabolic acidosis and causes widespread cellular damage, especially to the kidneys. In unwitnessed ingestions the clue is in metabolic acidosis with an inexplicable anion gap. Activated charcoal is ineffective. Ethanol is a competitive inhibitor of alcohol dehydrogenase and can block metabolism of the ethylene glycol to its poisonous metabolic byproducts. An oral loading dose of 2.5 ml/kg of 40% ethanol (the strength of most spirits) should be started. The aim is to have a blood ethanol concentration of 100 mg/dl. Fomepizole may also be used and haemodialysis may be necessary. Co-factors thiamine and pyridoxine are also recommended.

Cocaine

Cocaine poisoning leads to the local accumulation of the neurotransmitters noradrenaline, dopamine, adrenaline and serotonin. The accumulation of noradrenaline and adrenaline leads to tachycardia, which increases myocardial oxygen demand while reducing the time for diastolic coronary perfusion. Vasoconstriction causing hypertension results from the accumulation of neurotransmitters at the peripheral β-adrenergic receptors, and peripheral hydroxytryptamine (5-HT) receptor stimulation causes coronary artery vasospasm. In addition, cocaine stimulates platelet aggregation. Together, these changes can produce what is effectively a coronary event in a child or an adolescent.

Acute coronary syndrome producing chest pain and varying types of cardiac rhythm disturbances is the most frequent complication of cocaine use, which leads to hospitalisation. Cocaine is also a sodium channel inhibitor, similar to a type I antiarrhythmic agent, and so can prolong the QRS duration and impair myocardial contractility. Through the combination of adrenergic and sodium channel effects, cocaine use may cause various tachyarrhythmias including ventricular tachycardia and ventricular fibrillation. Treatment should be guided by a poisons centre.

Initial treatment of the acute coronary syndrome consists of oxygen administration, continuous ECG monitoring and administration of a benzodiazepine (e.g. diazepam or lorazepam), aspirin and heparin. Hyperthermia should be treated with cooling. Beta-adrenergic blockers are contraindicated in the setting of cocaine intoxication. Ventricular tachycardia should be treated with DC shock as antiarrhythmic drugs may cause further proarrhythmic effects. Since cocaine is a sodium channel blocker, administration of sodium bicarbonate in a dose of 0.5–1 mmol/kg should be considered in the treatment of ventricular arrhythmias.

Ecstasy

Most ecstasy tablets contain 30–150 mg of 3,4-methylenedioxymethamphetamine (MDMA). This drug, which has a half-life of around 8 hours, most probably stimulates both the peripheral and the central α- and β-adrenergic receptors. Early deaths are usually due to cardiac dysrhythmias, while deaths after 24 hours occur from a neuroleptic malignant-like syndrome.

Mild adverse effects occur at low doses and include increased muscle tone, agitation, anxiety and tachycardia. A mild elevation of temperature may also occur. At higher doses, hypertonia with hyperreflexia, tachycardia, tachypnoea and visual disturbance can be seen. In the worst affected children, coma, convulsions and cardiac dysrhythmias can occur. Hyperpyrexia with increased muscle tone can lead to rhabdomyolysis, metabolic acidosis with acute renal failure and disseminated intravascular coagulation.

Activated charcoal should be given to conscious patients. Blood pressure and temperature must be monitored. Diazepam can be used to control anxiety – major tranquillisers should not be used because they exacerbate symptoms. If core temperature exceeds 39°C then active cooling should be commenced and the use of dantrolene sodium (2–3 mg/kg over 10–15 minutes) should be considered. Some children may require ventilation.

Organophosphate poisoning

In organophosphate poisoning you will note the following signs and symptoms:

- B: dyspnoea
- D: pinpoint pupils
- E: rhonorrhoea

The treatment is according to the algorithm in Figure E.2. Very large doses of atropine (up to 250 mg) may be required.

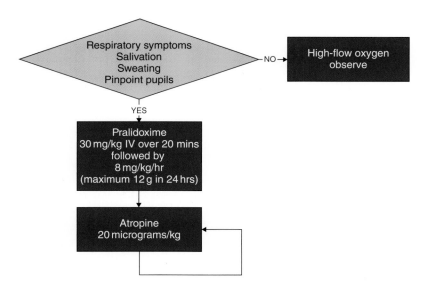

Figure E.2 Algorithm for the management of organophosphate poisoning

E.5   Envenoming (envenomation): introduction

Envenoming may occur as a result of bites or stings from a wide variety of animals, which includes snakes, spiders, insects (e.g. bees, wasps, ants), ticks, jellyfish and fish. The best management of envenoming is prevention, because once major envenoming occurs, reversal through the use of antidotes (antivenoms) may not resolve all medical problems.

Awareness of risk and avoidance of risky behaviour, plus use of even simple clothing such as shoes and pants in potential risk areas, may prevent effective bites/stings or reduce the severity of envenoming. Bites and stings by venomous animals are a risk in both rural and large urban centres.

Symptoms of envenoming may be either the direct result of the venom, or allergic reactions to the venom, or a combination of both. In all cases the principles of management consist of:

- Removal from danger (particularly important for venomous animals)
- Standard resuscitation practice of managing the airway, breathing and circulation
- Limiting the uptake of venom into the circulation where possible
- Administration of antidote (antivenom) where available and appropriate
- Supportive care to the systems affected by the venom
- Management of pain
- Treatment of sites of local injury

Envenoming is not an inevitable consequence of a venomous bite/sting, as the animal can often control how much venom is injected, penetration through clothing may reduce or prevent venom injection into the skin, and the size of the child will affect the concentration of injected venom and so the potential severity of envenoming. The smaller the child, the higher the potential venom concentration after a bite/sting, with consequently greater potential for severe or lethal envenoming. Even for venomous snakebites in small children, a significant number of bites fail to be effective ('dry' bites), and so do not result in envenoming. However, all snakebites should be initially managed as potentially lethal.

The diagnosis of envenoming is crucial and there are three points that are important to consider:

1. Is there a history of exposure to a bite/sting? Even if not, consider envenoming in a child presenting with unexplained paralysis, myotoxicity, coagulopathy, renal failure, collapse or convulsions.
2. Is there an indication of the type of animal involved? Knowing the type of animal can enable prediction of potential risks and targeted therapy. It may help determine if the animal is actually venomous (e.g. in parts of Queensland, python bites are a common, and non-venomous, cause of snakebites).
3. Is there evidence of envenoming or allergic reaction to the bite/sting? This is the key question in determining both emergency and ongoing management.

Determining if envenoming is present may be simple (e.g. the child who screams and then collapses after swimming in areas with box jellyfish, who has numerous adherent jellyfish tentacles – a likely box jellyfish sting with severe envenoming) or complicated (e.g. the child who is bitten by a snake but initially appears well). Considering the setting, history, examination and laboratory findings may all be vital. For snakebites in particular, laboratory testing for coagulopathy (international normalised ratio, activated partial thromboplastin time, D-dimer) and myolysis (creatine kinase) are essential in determining the degree of envenoming, in conjunction with examination looking for paralytic features.

Laboratory tests, conversely, are not important in determining if envenoming is present or the extent of envenoming for spider and tick bites, insect stings (except massive multiple stings) or marine stings.

E.6 Resuscitation and support in envenoming (envenomation)

Danger

A venomous animal can injure multiple humans (although honey bees can sting only once), including first responders (e.g. a box jellyfish in shallow water at a beach, or a cornered snake), so it is important to avoid further bites/stings. In general, attempting to catch or kill the animal entails risks that exceed the benefits, but there are exceptions (e.g. it is important to locate and carefully remove all attached ticks in cases of tick paralysis).

Airway

The airway may be threatened for a number of reasons, including depressed level of consciousness, bulbar palsy, paralysis and swelling of tissues around the airway. The airway must be assessed frequently. Clearance of secretions from the pharynx is the most common problem. Patients who require intubation for reasons other than a depressed level of consciousness require anaesthesia for intubation. It is extremely important to note that a totally paralysed child may be fully conscious.

Breathing

Many venoms cause paralysis, and patients affected by these venoms require ventilatory support. The support must be provided prior to respiratory arrest. As patients may be paralysed but fully awake, anaesthesia for intubation is recommended. Severe muscle spasm or seizures may occur following some types of envenoming, and these patients will require ventilatory support. Also, secretions may contribute to respiratory embarrassment and ventilatory support may prevent the accumulation of secretions.

Circulation

Shock may occur for a variety of reasons including cardiac arrhythmia, bleeding secondary to coagulopathy and massive leakage of fluid into tissues damaged by cytotoxic venoms. Adequate vascular access must be secured with fluid resuscitation appropriate to the clinical situation. Beware fluid overload in children and avoid cannulation/sampling from subclavian, jugular and femoral veins if a coagulopathy is a possibility (snakebites). Some venoms are associated with the development of renal and/or electrolyte problems; fluid and electrolyte therapy must be adapted to the specific venom.

Disability

Assess the child's conscious level, remembering that failure to respond may be a consequence of paralysis and not of the level of consciousness. Look specifically for local neurological problems such as ptosis, ophthalmoplegia and/or bulbar palsy.

Exposure

Full exposure may be required to identify the site of a bite, and in the case of stings it is also important to examine areas of the body covered by hair. The search of cryptic areas such as the scalp and in and behind the ears is particularly important for tick envenoming.

E.7 Specific envenoming issues

Limiting uptake of venom (snakes, funnel web spiders, blue ringed octopus)

Where possible, the rate of uptake of venom into the circulation should be limited. If the bite or sting has affected a limb, it may be possible to slow the rate of absorption of venom from the bite/sting by the application of pressure bandaging and immobilisation (PBI) first aid. PBI is based on limiting lymph transport of the venom, using a broad bandage firmly applied over the bite site, then over the rest of the bitten limb and over the top of clothing, followed by immobilisation of the limb using a splint. To be effective the limb must be immobilised and the patient prevented from moving or walking. The bandage should be as firm as for a sprain, but not so tight as to act as a tourniquet. Crepe bandage has traditionally been recommended, but recent evidence suggests an elasticised bandage is easier to apply effectively and therefore may be preferred. Once applied, PBI should only be discontinued once the child is in a hospital able to treat envenoming with the appropriate antivenom.

> Pressure bandaging and immobilisation is inappropriate for red back spider and tick bites, and stonefish and jellyfish stings.

Inactivating venom locally (jellyfish and fish stings)

Box jellyfish stings are potentially lethal, so inactivating unfired stinging cells on tentacles adherent to the skin is vital. Flooding the tentacles with vinegar is recommended. The application of a cold pack is also recommended by some authorities. For other jellyfish stings and fish/stingray stings, the use of hot water (a shower or immersion at 45°C) is recommended, but ensure the water is not so hot as to cause thermal injury.

Local bite/sting trauma

Stingrays can cause significant local trauma, including the laceration of nerves, tendons and blood vessels, and can penetrate the abdomen or chest wall, including direct injury to the heart. Stingray venom can cause local tissue damage/necrosis. It is therefore important to carefully wash and, where appropriate, debride a stingray wound and control excessive bleeding. For stings penetrating near the heart, incautious removal of the sting may result in lethal injury.

Venom sprayed or spat into the eyes may cause intense pain, temporary blindness and corneal injury, but is not likely to cause envenoming. Urgent irrigation of the eyes is required, then examination of the cornea and appropriate treatment if there is a corneal injury.

All bites/stings have the potential to introduce tetanus or other infections. Tetanus immune status should be ensured, but not until after any acute envenoming coagulopathy (snakebite cases) has fully resolved. Antibiotics should only be used if there is acute infection, not as routine prophylaxis.

Antidotes (antivenom)

Antivenom consists of immunoglobulin G (IgG) antibodies (or fractions thereof) raised in animals against selected venoms. Each antivenom is specific for a particular species or group of animals only. Antivenoms can cause both early (rash, febrile, anaphylactic) and late (serum sickness) adverse reactions. Antivenoms will only bind to their target venoms, not other venoms, and may neutralise venom action but cannot reverse damage caused by venom. It is therefore crucial: (i) that the correct antivenom is used; (ii) that antivenom is only used when clearly indicated; and (iii) that everything is to hand to treat an acute adverse reaction, before antivenom is infused.

Indications for antivenom vary depending on the type of animal/antivenom involved:

- For Australian snakebites antivenom is indicated if there is evidence of significant systemic envenoming, including coagulopathy, myolysis, paralysis, renal damage and collapse/convulsions, but excluding children who have only general symptoms (headache, vomiting, abdominal pain) without evidence of the foregoing problems.
- For funnel web spider bites any evidence of systemic envenoming is an indication to give antivenom.
- For red back spider bites the use of antivenom is more controversial, but most experts would consider it if there is intractable regional envenoming or any degree of systemic envenoming.
- For stonefish stings any significant local pain is an indication to use antivenom.
- For box jellyfish stings the role and indications for antivenom are currently unclear, but it should be used in any patient with life-threatening envenoming.

The choice of antivenom will be determined by the type of venomous animal involved. For snakes there are five different 'specific' antivenoms plus a polyvalent antivenom covering all five types of snake. Currently, the 'specific' antivenoms are polyvalent but the doses are specific for the species indicated. For lower volume 'specific' antivenoms (brown snake and tiger snake in particular), it is preferable to use the correct 'specific' antivenom rather than the 'polyvalent' product, for safety and cost reasons. A snake venom detection test is available to help choose the appropriate 'specific' antivenom, but should be used in conjunction with diagnostic algorithms. Snake venom detection is not a screening test for snakebites and a negative result does not exclude snakebite.

Antivenom should be given as soon as indicated, by the intravenous route. The intramuscular route has traditionally been used for red back spider and stonefish antivenoms, and is anecdotally effective, but the intravenous route is more likely to give a rapid, effective response. For all other antivenoms, the intravenous route is mandatory. The dose is based on quantity of venom injected, not the size of the patient. Therefore, there is no paediatric dosing and children receive the same dose as adults. Intravenous antivenom is usually infused as a dilute solution in 0.9% saline or similar, but the degree of dilution should be carefully adjusted in children to avoid volume overload.

> The use of premedication prior to giving antivenom is no longer accepted practice, but adrenaline must **always** be immediately available before giving antivenom.

Drugs

In addition to antivenom (where available and appropriate), there are a number of problems that may require symptomatic therapy.

Analgesia

Pain may be a major feature of envenoming and adequate analgesia is critical. For painful marine stings, hot water (45°C, but avoid thermal injury) may be effective. Antivenom can be the most effective treatment for pain caused by stonefish stings, red back spider bites and possibly box jellyfish stings. If these treatments are not appropriate or insufficient in cases with severe pain, then consider intravenous opioids titrated to effect or regional nerve block (for marine fish stings).

Sedation

Bites and stings may be associated with extreme anxiety. Reassurance and supportive care is the basis of therapy, but sedation and anxiolysis may be helpful, particularly if patients require transportation. However, be cautious sedating patients with potential for developing neurotoxic paralysis.

Coagulation factor therapy

Antivenom can neutralise venom components attacking the haemostasis system if given early enough, but cannot replace consumed clotting factors. In cases with consumptive coagulopathy (defibrination, venom-induced consumptive coagulopathy) following snakebite, it may take many hours for key clotting factors to return to 'safe' levels. If there is also significant active bleeding, then, once appropriate antivenom has been given, clotting factor replacement therapy (fresh frozen plasma, cryoprecipitate) should be considered.

Monitoring

Many cases of bites/stings by potentially dangerous animals – including snakes, funnel web spiders, box jellyfish and blue ringed octopuses – may result in either no or only minor envenoming, not requiring antivenom. (There is no antivenom available for the blue ringed octopus anyway.) These cases of 'dry' or minor bites/stings require an adequate period of observation, including recurrent examination and blood testing (snakebites only) to ensure late developing envenoming is not missed.

- For snakebites monitoring should be for at least 12 hours if there is no evidence of envenoming or if only minor envenoming is present. In remote areas it might be wise to monitor the patient for longer before sending them home. Blood tests should be performed on presentation, 1 hour after PBI is removed and at 6 and 12 hours post bite.
- For suspected funnel web spider bites (='big black spider' bite) monitor for at least 4 hours post bite; in significant funnel web spider bites envenoming develops within 4 hours.
- For red back spider bites only symptomatic patients require hospital assessment.
- For marine envenoming the requirement for hospital monitoring is determined by the type of bite/sting and symptomatology. Severe or life-threatening envenoming generally occurs very early after exposure, within the first hour or less, and always within the first 4 hours. The exception is stingray wounds to the trunk, which may seem initially alright but should always be fully assessed and observed for a longer period.

Table E.3 contains a summary of the major types of venomous animals, with clinical effects of envenomation, first aid and primary treatments.

Table E.3 Major types of venomous animals injuring humans with a summary of clinical effects, first aid and treatment

Type of animal	Major clinical effects	First aid	Prime treatment
Venomous snakes			
Brown snake	Coagulopathy (defibrination), renal damage, paralysis (rare)	PBI	Brown snake AV, 1–2 vials IV
Tiger snake, rough scaled snake	Coagulopathy (defibrination), paralysis, myolysis, renal damage	PBI	Tiger snake AV, 1–2 vials IV
Copperheads	Paralysis	PBI	Tiger snake AV, 1–2 vials IV
Broad headed, pale headed and Stephen's banded snakes	Coagulopathy (defibrination)	PBI	Tiger snake AV, 1–2 vials IV
Red bellied and blue bellied black snakes	Myolysis, coagulopathy (anticoagulant)	PBI	Tiger snake AV, 1–2 vials IV
Mulga and Collett's snakes	Myolysis, coagulopathy (anticoagulant)	PBI	Black snake or polyvalent AV, 1 vial IV
Taipan	Coagulopathy (defibrination), paralysis, myolysis, renal damage	PBI	Taipan or polyvalent AV, 1 vial IV
Death adder	Paralysis	PBI	Death adder or polyvalent AV, 1 vial IV

Type of animal	Major clinical effects	First aid	Prime treatment
Arthropods			
Funnel web spider	Neuroexcitatory envenoming, catecholamine storm effects, pulmonary oedema	PBI	Funnel web spider AV, 2–4+ vials IV
Red back spider	Neuroexcitatory envenoming, pain, sweating, hypertension, nausea	No first aid is effective	Red back spider AV, 2 vials IV or IM
Paralysis tick	Progressive flaccid paralysis (ascending)	No specific first aid; respiratory support	Respiratory support, remove all ticks
Bee, wasp and ant stings	Anaphylaxis in susceptible individuals	PBI, cardiorespiratory resuscitation, EpiPen®	Adrenaline, cardiorespiratory support
Marine			
Box jellyfish sting	Local pain, skin damage, cardiorespiratory collapse (rare severe cases only)	Flood tentacles with vinegar before removing, cardiorespiratory support (if indicated)	Supportive and symptomatic care, box jellyfish AV IV in selected cases
Irukandji syndrome	Neuroexcitatory envenoming, catecholamine storm effects, intense pain in limbs and back, hypertension, sweating, rash	Flood sting area with vinegar, supportive care	Opioid analgesia, supportive care, consider magnesium sulphate infusion
Other jellyfish stings	Local pain, erythema	Hot water shower or immersion of stung area (45°C, but avoid thermal injury)	Hot water shower or immersion of stung area (45°C, but avoid thermal injury)
Stonefish sting	Local pain	Hot water shower or immersion of stung area (45°C, but avoid thermal injury)	Hot water shower or immersion of stung area (45°C, but avoid thermal injury), stonefish AV IV or IM
Other fish stings	Local pain	Hot water shower or immersion of stung area (45°C, but avoid thermal injury)	Hot water shower or immersion of stung area (45°C, but avoid thermal injury)
Stingray sting	Local pain, local trauma, potential necrosis	Hot water shower or immersion of stung area (45°C, but avoid thermal injury), staunch active bleeding, supportive care	Hot water shower or immersion of stung area (45°C, but avoid thermal injury), supportive care, manage open wound
Blue ringed octopus bite	Rapid flaccid paralysis, collapse	PBI, respiratory support if paralysis develops	Cardiorespiratory support

AV, antivenom; IM, intramuscular; IV, intravenous; PBI, pressure bandaging and immobilisation.

For all cases of envenoming seek **urgent expert advice** from your National Poisons Centre.

E.8 Button battery ingestion

Disk or button batteries are small, coin-shaped batteries used within watches, calculators and many children's toys. The batteries can contain a number of different metals (such as mercury, silver and lithium) along with sodium or potassium hydroxide to facilitate the chemical reaction. Whilst in 2008 24% of ingested batteries were lithium, lithium cells were associated with 92% of fatal ingestions (2000–2009).

Pathophysiology

The harm due to the ingestion of button batteries is as a result of the electric current discharged from the battery, rather than leakage. The current causes liquefaction necrosis of the tissues due to the generation of sodium hydroxide. Severe burns can occur within 2 hours of contact if lodged in areas such as the oesophagus. Damage continues for days to weeks due to residual alkali or weakened tissues. Complications can include perforation, distillation in adjacent structures such as major vessels or the trachea, vocal cord paralysis, and strictures.

Epidemiology and symptoms

Most ingestions occur in children, with the peak incidence in those aged 1 to 3 years; 85% of cases with major problems, and all fatalities between 1985 and 2009, were in children younger than 4 years. More than half of ingestions are unwitnessed, and only 10% of patients will have symptoms. The types of symptoms described include vomiting ± haematemesis, refusal to take anything orally, increased salivation, dysphagia and even airway compromise. If identified and lodged, removal should be considered an emergency. In an older child, self-harm should be considered, with urgent removal plus referral to mental health specialists.

Investigation

Important radiological characteristics suggestive of a button battery include:

- Radiopaque foreign body
- The halo effect/double rim
- Step off on lateral X-ray

X-rays should include the entire oesophagus and abdomen.

Management

- If ingestion of a button battery is suggested and it is within the oesophagus, surgical referral is indicated and the battery should be removed as an emergency.
- If the battery has passed into the stomach and was ingested alone (without a magnet) and there are symptoms, the child should again be referred as an emergency.
- If the battery is >15 mm and has been swallowed by a child <6 years, a repeat X-ray should occur within 4 days. If it remains within the stomach removal is recommended (see http://www.poison.org/battery/guideline).

E.9 Summary

You should now be able to:

- Describe the approach to the management of poisoning in children
- Describe the approach to the management of envenomation in children

APPENDIX F
Resuscitation of the baby at birth

Learning outcomes

After reading this appendix, you will be able to:
- Describe the approach to the resuscitation of the baby at birth and how this differs from the resuscitation of older children

---

F.1 Introduction

The resuscitation of babies at birth is different from the resuscitation of all other age groups as it usually involves a process of assisted transition from intra- to extrauterine life, rather than recovery of a human with serious illness or injury. Knowledge of the physiology of normal transition, and how interruption to transition leading to hypoxia affects this, is essential to understand the process outlined in the algorithm for resuscitating newborn babies (see Figure F.8). The majority of babies will establish normal respiration and circulation without help. A tiny minority will not, and will require intervention.

As some babies may be born unexpectedly out of hospital or in a non-maternity setting within a hospital, or are unwell as a result of peripartum circumstances, it is important that clinicians working in 'receiving' specialties have an understanding of the differences between resuscitating older children and a baby who has just been born. Ideally, someone trained in newborn resuscitation should be present at all deliveries. It is advisable that all those who attend deliveries regularly should have been on courses such as the Newborn Life Support course, organised by the Resuscitation Council (UK), European Resuscitation Council courses, or the Neonatal Resuscitation Program, organised by the American Academy of Pediatrics.

F.2 Normal physiology

Successful transition at birth involves moving from a fetal state, where the lungs are fluid filled and respiratory exchange occurs through the placenta, to that of a newly born baby whose air-filled lungs have successfully taken over that function. Preparation for this in a pregnancy progressing without incident is thought to begin in advance of labour, with detectable cellular changes occurring that may subsequently prime the lung tissues for reabsorption of the intra-alveolar fluid.

After delivery, a healthy full-term baby usually takes his or her first breath within 60–90 seconds. Stimuli for this first breath include exposure to the relative cold of the *ex utero* environment, the physical stimulus of being handled at delivery, and hypoxia resulting from obstruction of the umbilical cord during clamping. In a term baby, approximately 100 ml of fluid is cleared from the airways and alveoli, initially into the interstitial pulmonary tissue, and then later into the lymphatic and

---

Advanced Paediatric Life Support: A Practical Approach to Emergencies, Sixth Edition. Edited by Martin Samuels and Sue Wieteska.
© 2016 John Wiley & Sons, Ltd. Published 2016 by John Wiley & Sons, Ltd.

capillary systems. During vaginal delivery, around 35 ml of fluid from the uppermost airways will be displaced by physical forces experienced by the baby during passage through the birth canal.

The respiratory pattern in newborn mammals has specifically evolved to efficiently replace the fluid in the airways and alveoli with air during the first few breaths. Animal studies show that at initiation of breathing, the inspiratory phase is longer than the expiratory phase (expiratory braking) and, in humans, expiration occurs against a partially closed glottis creating backpressure (producing crying or sometimes a grunting sound). In a healthy baby the first spontaneous breaths may generate a negative inspiratory pressure of between −30 and −90 cmH$_2$O. This pressure is 10–15 times greater than that needed for later breathing but is necessary to overcome the viscosity of the fluid filling the airways, the surface tension of the fluid-filled lungs and the elastic recoil and resistance of the chest wall, lungs and airways. These powerful chest movements also aid displacement of fluid from the airways into the interstitial tissue before subsequent clearance into the lymphatics and ultimately the circulation. The combined effect of these events is to establish the baby's functional residual capacity (FRC).

Neonatal circulatory adaptation commences at the same time as the pulmonary changes. Lung inflation and alveolar distension releases vasomotor compounds that reduce the pulmonary vascular resistance as well as increasing oxygenation. Evidence shows that as pulmonary vascular resistance falls during establishment of the FRC, significant changes in stroke volume can be seen in the heart. Where the umbilical cord has been clamped prior to the first breath, a decrease in heart size is immediately seen, followed by return to its original size. This observation suggests a 'sink' effect, with blood being rapidly drawn into the pulmonary vessels as the lungs inflate with air during the first breaths, without access to placental blood to fill the emptied heart quickly, and hence the observed decrease in size. The increase in size subsequently seen is likely due to the same large volume of blood returning to the left side of the heart from the expanded pulmonary circulation. Bradycardia has been noted in these babies consistent with the observed changes and, importantly, is not seen in babies who take their first breath before cord clamping. Circulatory adaptation proceeds with closure of the interatrial foramen due to pressure changes as the pulmonary venous return to the left atrium increases and finishes with functional, then permanent, closure of the ductus arteriosus over the following days.

F.3 Pathophysiology

The approach to resuscitating newborn humans evolved from observation of the pathophysiology of induced, acute, fetal hypoxia during pioneering mammal-based research in the early 1960s. The results of these experiments, which followed the physiology of newborn animals during acute, total, prolonged asphyxia and subsequent resuscitation, are summarised in Figure F.1.

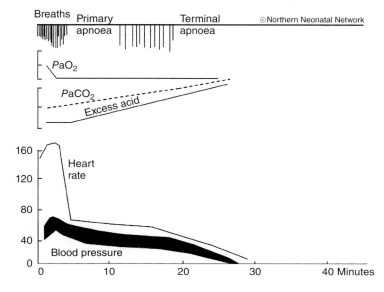

Figure F.1 Response of a mammalian fetus to total, sustained asphyxia starting at time 0. (Reproduced with permission from the Northern Neonatal Network)

When the placental oxygen supply is interrupted or severely reduced, the fetus will initiate respiratory movements (i.e. attempt to breathe) in response to hypoxia. If the interruption of oxygen from the placenta continues and these attempts at breathing fail to provide an alternative oxygen supply – as they will inevitably fail to do so *in utero* surrounded by amniotic fluid – the baby will become unconscious. If hypoxia continues, the higher respiratory centre becomes inactive and unable to continue to drive respiratory movements. The breathing therefore stops, usually within 2–3 minutes. This cessation of breathing is known as **primary apnoea** (Figure F.1).

In the presence of hypoxia, a marked bradycardia will occur quickly. Intense peripheral vasoconstriction helps to maintain blood pressure with diversion of blood away from non-vital organs. The reduced heart rate also allows a longer ventricular filling time, and thus an increased stroke volume, which also helps maintain blood pressure.

As hypoxia continues, primary apnoea is broken: loss of descending neural inhibition by the higher respiratory centre allows primitive spinal centres to initiate forceful, gasping breaths. These deep, irregular gasps are easily distinguishable from normal breaths as they only occur 6–12 times per minute and involve all accessory muscles in a maximal, 'whole body', inspiratory effort. If this fails to draw air into the lungs and hypoxia continues, even this reflexive activity ceases and **terminal apnoea** begins. Without intervention, no further innate respiratory effort will occur. The time taken for such activity to cease is longer in the newly born baby than at any other time in life, taking up to 20 minutes.

The circulation is almost always maintained until **after** all respiratory activity ceases. This resilience is a feature of all newborn mammals at term and is largely due to the reserves of glycogen in the heart permitting prolonged, anaerobic generation of energy in the cardiomyocytes. Resuscitation is therefore relatively uncomplicated if undertaken before all respiratory activity has stopped. Once the lungs are aerated, oxygen will be carried to the heart and then to the brain provided the circulation is still functional (Figure F.2). Recovery will then be rapid. Most babies who have **not** progressed to terminal apnoea will resuscitate themselves if their airway is open. Once gasping ceases, however, the circulation starts to fail and resuscitation becomes more difficult. Support for the circulation is then required in addition to support for the breathing (Figure F.3).

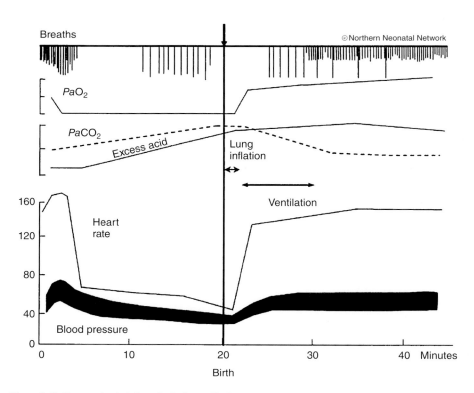

Figure F.2 Effects of lung inflation and a brief period of ventilation on a baby born in early terminal apnoea but before failure of the circulation. (Reproduced with permission from the Northern Neonatal Network)

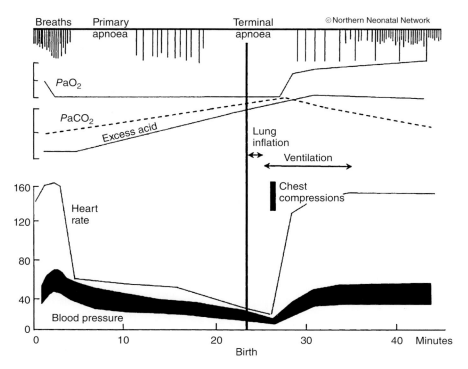

Figure F.3 Response of a baby born in terminal apnoea. In this case lung inflation is not sufficient because the circulation is already failing. However, lung inflation delivers air to the lungs and then a brief period of chest compressions delivers oxygenated blood to the heart, which then responds. (Reproduced with permission from the Northern Neonatal Network)

F.4 Equipment

For many newborn babies, especially those born outside the delivery room, the need for resuscitation cannot be predicted. It is therefore useful to plan for such an eventuality. Equipment that may be required to resuscitate a newborn baby is listed in the box below. As a minimum, most babies can be resuscitated if there is access to: a firm, flat surface; warmth; a way to deliver air or oxygen to the lungs in a controlled fashion to displace the fluid present in the airways at delivery if the baby does not breath itself (ranging from using mouth-to-mouth to equipment-based techniques); and guidance from someone who is familiar with the process of newborn resuscitation (either as part of the resuscitation team or by telephone at the time of need).

- A flat surface
- Radiant heat source and dry towels
- Plastic bag for term and preterm babies
- Suitable hats
- Suction with catheters of at least 12 French gauge
- Face masks
- Bag–valve–mask or T-piece with pressure-limiting device
- Source of air and/or oxygen
- Oropharyngeal (Guedel) airways
- Laryngoscopes with straight blades, 0 and 1
- Nasogastric tubes
- Cord clamp
- Scissors
- Tracheal tubes sizes 2.5 to 4.0 mm
- Umbilical catheterisation equipment
- Adhesive tape
- Disposable gloves
- Saturation monitor/stethoscope

F.5 Strategy for assessing and resuscitating a baby at birth

Resuscitation is likely to be rapidly successful if commenced before the baby has progressed beyond the point at which its circulation has started to fail. Babies in primary apnoea can usually resuscitate themselves if they have a clear airway. Unfortunately it is not possible, during the initial assessment, to reliably distinguish whether an apnoeic, newborn baby is in primary or terminal apnoea. A structured approach that will work in either situation must therefore be applied to **all** apnoeic babies. The structured approach is outlined below. In reality the first four steps (up to and including assessment) are completed simultaneously. After this, appropriate intervention can begin following an ABC approach.

- Call/shout for help
- Start the clock or note the time
- Dry and wrap the baby in warmed dry towels. Maintain the baby's temperature
- Assess the situation
- Airway
- Breathing
- Chest compressions
- (Drugs/vascular access)

Call for help

Ask for help if you expect or encounter any difficulty or if the delivery is outside the labour suite.

Start the clock

Start the clock, if available, or note the time of birth.

At birth

There is no need to rush to clamp the cord at delivery. It can be left unclamped while the following steps are completed. Dry the baby quickly and effectively. Remove the wet towel and wrap the baby in a fresh, dry, warm towel. (For very small or significantly preterm babies it is better to place the wet baby in a food-grade plastic bag – and later under a radiant heater.) Put a hat on **all** babies regardless of gestation. Assess the baby during and after drying: decide whether any intervention is going to be needed. If your assessment suggests that the baby is in need of resuscitation, clamp and cut the cord. If the baby appears well, wait for at least 1 minute from the complete delivery of the baby before clamping the cord.

If the baby is assessed as needing assistance/resuscitation then this becomes the priority. There is not yet sufficient evidence for advocating active resuscitation of the newborn baby while still attached to the placenta by a functioning umbilical cord. Thus, the cord needs to be clamped and cut in order to deliver assistance/resuscitation.

Keep the baby warm

The normal temperature range for a newborn baby is 36.5–37.5°C. For each 1°C decrease in admission temperature below this range in otherwise healthy term newborn babies there is an associated increase in mortality of 28%. In environments likely to receive sick babies or infants the room temperatures should be kept, as a baseline, as close as possible to the recommended minimum for term babies. Where delivery or admission of a newborn baby is imminent **outside** these environments, anticipation and active management of room temperature to achieve this baseline as quickly as possible is required: eliminate any draughts from the room (close window and doors where possible) and heat the room to above 23°C (term babies) or 25°C (preterm babies).

Once delivered, dry the baby immediately and then wrap in a warm, dry towel. In addition to increased mortality risk, a cold baby has an increased rate of oxygen consumption and is more likely to become hypoglycaemic and acidotic. If this is not addressed at the beginning of resuscitation it is often forgotten. Most heat loss at delivery is caused by the baby being wet (evaporation) and in a draught (convection). Babies also have a large surface area to weight ratio, exacerbating heat loss. Ideally an overhead heater or external heat source should be available and switched on, but drying effectively and wrapping the baby in a warm, dry towel with the head covered, ideally by a hat, is the most important factor in avoiding hypothermia. A naked dry baby can still become hypothermic despite a warm room and a radiant heater, especially if there is a draught.

In all babies, the head represents a significant part of the baby's surface area (see Section F.8) so attention to providing a hat is invaluable in maintaining normothermia.

Out of hospital: Babies of all gestations born outside the normal delivery environment may benefit from placement in a food-grade polyethylene bag or wrap after drying and then swaddling. Alternatively, well, newborn babies of more than 30 weeks' gestation who are breathing may be dried and nursed with skin-to-skin contact (or kangaroo mother care) to maintain their temperature whilst they are transferred. Exposed skin should be covered to protect against cooling draughts.

Assessment of the newborn baby

During and immediately after drying and wrapping the baby, make a full assessment as outlined below.

A/B	Breathing	Regular, gasp, none
C	Heart rate	Fast, slow, very slow/absent
C	Tone	Well flexed, reduced tone, floppy

Unlike resuscitation at other ages, **all** three items need to be assessed in parallel to be able to **then** decide on the need for resuscitation and to begin treatment and then assess its effect. This is different to the linear hierarchy of assessment and treatment used at other ages. In the newborn baby, heart rate and breathing provide the most useful information and are the **only** items that need regularly reassessing during resuscitation to assess effectiveness of intervention. At the initial assessment, however, taking note of the baby's tone can also be informative: a baby who is very floppy is likely to be unconscious, suggesting that the baby may have been subject to hypoxia.

Colour, while no longer formally assessed, is still a potentially useful indicator of status. Normal babies are born 'blue' and become 'pink' in the first minutes of life. A baby who is pale and white ('shut down' due to intense peripheral vasoconstriction) is more likely to be acidotic: this sort of appearance suggests significant cardiovascular response to peripartum compromise.

Breathing movements and colour can be determined by observation during drying; tone can be evaluated whilst in the act of drying the baby. Heart rate is determined by auscultation of the heart using a stethoscope which can be done during the drying by a second person or immediately afterwards if the responder is on their own.

Breathing

Most well, term babies will take their first breath 60–90 seconds after delivery and establish spontaneous, regular breathing sufficient to maintain the heart rate ≥100 beats/min within 3 minutes of birth. If there is no breathing (apnoea), gasping or irregular, ineffective breathing that persists after drying, intervention is required.

Heart rate

In the first couple of minutes, auscultating at the cardiac apex is the best method to assess the heart rate. Palpating peripheral pulses is not practical and is not recommended. Palpation of the umbilical pulse can only be relied upon if the palpable rate is ≥100 beats/min. A rate less than this should be checked by auscultation. It may not be possible to feel a cord pulse when there **is** a heart rate that can be detected by auscultation.

In delivery suites, saturation monitors using Masimo (or similar) technology are now widely used by neonatal intensive care unit (NICU) teams when resuscitation is required at term, or when preterm babies have been delivered. However, applying a saturation monitor should not interrupt the process of resuscitation. It is also good practice to correlate the probe reading (heart rate), once good detection signal strength is achieved, with the auscultated heart rate. An ECG, if available, can give a rapid, accurate and continuous heart rate reading during newborn resuscitation. In low-resource or non-specialist settings (especially if the only saturation monitor probe available is designed to fit a larger child or adult), the use of a stethoscope is recommended to allow resuscitation to proceed without delay.

The probe for the saturation monitor must be applied to the **right** (not left) hand or wrist in order to accurately reflect the pre-ductal saturations (which are most likely to reflect the oxygenation of blood returning to the left atrium and which is being distributed to the coronary arteries and cerebral circulation). A correctly applied pulse oximeter can give an accurate reading of heart rate and saturations within 90 seconds of application. Oxygen saturation levels in healthy babies in the first few minutes of life may be considerably lower than at other times (see box). Attempting to judge oxygenation by assessing colour of the skin or mucous membranes is not reliable, but it is still worth noting the baby's colour at birth as well as whether, when and how it changes later in the resuscitation. Very pale babies who remain pale and bradycardic after resuscitation may be hypovolaemic as well as acidotic. Similarly, tone immediately at birth should be assessed, and changes noted as resuscitation progresses.

Time from birth	Acceptable pre-ductal SpO_2 levels
2 min	60%
3 min	70%
4 min	80%
5 min	85%
10 min	90%

An accurate and prompt initial assessment of heart rate is vital because an increase in the heart rate will be the first sign of success during resuscitation.

Outcome of the initial assessment

Initial assessment will categorise the baby into one of the three following groups.

1. Vigorous breathing or crying; good tone; heart rate ≥100 beats/min.
    These are healthy babies. They should be dried and kept warm but there is no need for immediate cord clamping. They can be given to their mothers and nursed skin-to-skin if this is appropriate and the baby can be protected from drafts by covering. The baby will remain warm through skin-to-skin contact under a cover and may also be put to the breast at this stage.

2. Irregular or inadequate breathing or apnoea; normal or reduced tone; heart rate <100 beats/min.
    If gentle stimulation (drying will be an adequate stimulus in this situation) does not induce effective breathing, the cord will need to be clamped and cut to allow resuscitation to commence. After drying and wrapping are completed, the airway should be opened. Most of these babies will improve with inflation of the lungs using a mask and the heart rate should be used to assess the effect of this intervention. Some babies in this group will then require a period of ventilation by mask until they recover respiratory drive and are able to breathe for themselves.

3. Breathing inadequately, gasping or apnoeic; globally floppy; heart rate very slow (<60 beats/min) or absent and colour blue or pale (pale often suggests poor perfusion).

Whether an apnoeic baby is in primary or terminal apnoea (see Figure F.1) the initial management is the same although it will be quickly apparent that in this case delayed cord clamping is not appropriate. Cord milking ('stripping') has sometimes been advocated as an alternative to delayed cord clamping in babies who are in need of immediate assistance. However, the benefits of this have yet to be fully evaluated and thus it cannot be recommended except in the context of a properly conducted prospective study.

Dry and wrap the baby, assessing as you go, and then commence resuscitation. Open the airway and then inflate the lungs. A reassessment of heart rate response then directs further resuscitation. In parallel, continued efficacy of mask ventilation should be monitored by watching for chest movement. After assessment, resuscitation follows the broad categories of the structured approach seen in the algorithm (see Figure F.8):

- Airway
- Breathing
- Circulation
- Use of drugs in a few selected cases

Resuscitation of the newborn baby

Airway

To achieve an open airway, the baby should be positioned with the head in the neutral position (Figure F.4; see also Chapter 19). A newborn baby's head has a large, often moulded, occiput which tends to cause the neck to flex when the baby is supine on a flat surface. A 2 cm folded towel placed under the neck and shoulders may help to maintain the airway in a neutral position and a jaw thrust may be needed to bring the tongue forward and open the airway, especially if the baby is floppy (Figure F.5). However, overextension may also collapse the newborn baby's pharyngeal airway, leading to obstruction. If using a towel under the shoulders, care must be exercised to avoid such overextension of the neck.

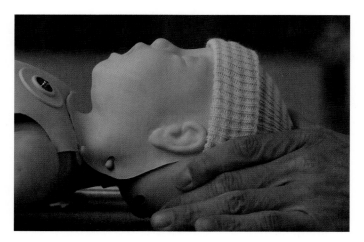

Figure F.4 Neutral position in babies

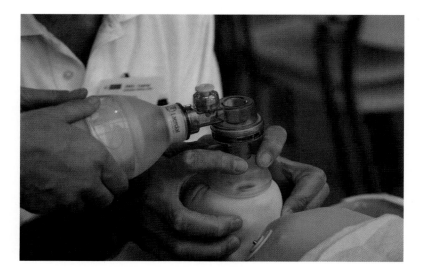

Figure F.5 Jaw thrust

Most secretions found in and around the oropharynx at birth are thin and rarely cause airway obstruction. Priority should be given in **all** babies to the application of a well-fitting mask and inflating the lungs once airway position and control is established. If, during resuscitation, there is concern that there might be an airway obstruction (e.g. if the heart rate is poor and the chest does not move with appropriately applied mask ventilation), the oropharynx can be directly visualised using a laryngoscope. Any obvious material obstructing the airway should be removed by gentle suction with a large-bore suction catheter. Deep pharyngeal suction without direct visualisation should not be performed as it may cause extensive soft tissue injury, vagal nerve-induced bradycardia and laryngospasm. Suction, if it is used, should not exceed −150 mmHg (−20.0 kPa).

Meconium aspiration

Meconium-stained liquor (light green tinge) is relatively common and occurs in up to 10% of births. Meconium aspiration is a **rare** event. Meconium aspiration usually happens *in utero* as the fetus approaches term. It requires fetal compromise severe enough to cause both the reflexive passage of meconium and the onset of gasping respiratory movements.

That meconium has been inhaled before delivery means that the previously widely advocated and used combined obstetric–neonatal strategy of suctioning the airways after delivery has not been shown to be of use. Firstly, one large randomised trial has shown no advantage to suctioning the airway whilst the head is on the perineum. Secondly, another randomised trial has shown that routine intubation and suctioning of the baby's airway offers no advantage. Thirdly, a recent, small, randomised, controlled trial has also demonstrated no difference in incidence of meconium aspiration syndrome in the most obtunded of babies who were subjected to tracheal intubation followed by suction and those who were not intubated. All that these procedures appear to do is delay the application of appropriate resuscitative measures to the baby in need, in a timely fashion. Thus, when faced with a baby who has been born through meconium-stained liquor, and who needs assistance, initiation of resuscitative measures should be the priority **not** clearance of meconium.

From the perspective of effective resuscitation, the only type of meconium that may cause an immediate issue is that which is thick and viscid and which has the potential to block the airway. The presence of thick meconium should prompt consideration of direct visualisation of the oropharynx to remove any obstruction but, again, the emphasis should be on initiating ventilation within the first minute of life in an apnoeic or ineffectively breathing baby. This should not be delayed, and routine tracheal intubation is not recommended.

Breathing (aeration breaths and ventilation)

The first five breaths in term babies should be 'inflation' breaths in order to replace lung fluid in the alveoli with air. These should be 2–3-second sustained breaths ideally delivered using a continuous gas supply, a pressure-limited device (set at a limit of 30 cmH$_2$O) and an appropriately sized mask. Use a transparent, circular, soft mask big enough to cover the nose and mouth of the baby. If no such system is available then a 500 ml self-inflating bag and a blow-off valve set at 30–40 cmH$_2$O can be used (Figure F.6). This is especially useful if compressed air or oxygen is not available. A smaller size of bag (<500 ml) will not have the capacity to sustain the inflation over 2–3 seconds and thus should not be used by choice unless no alternative exists. During these five breaths, it is important to remember that the chest may not be seen to move during the first three breaths as fluid is displaced and replaced by air. After the five breaths, the first reassessment should be done.

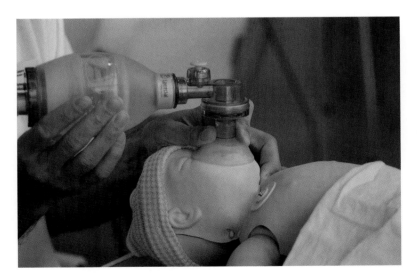

Figure F.6 Bag-and-mask ventilation

Adequate ventilation is usually indicated by either a rapidly increasing heart rate or a heart rate that is maintained at ≥100 beats/min. It is safe to assume the chest has been inflated successfully if the heart rate responds.

Once the chest is inflated and the heart rate has increased **or** the chest has been seen to move, then ventilation should be continued at a rate of 30–40 per minute using shorter breaths (no more than 1-second-long inspiratory time). Continue ventilatory support until regular spontaneous breathing is established.

Where possible, start resuscitation of the newborn baby with air. There is now good evidence for this in term babies and oxygen toxicity causes significant morbidity in premature babies. The use of supplemental oxygen should be guided by pre-ductal pulse oximetry (see above), with reasonable levels listed in the box above on acceptable saturations and on the algorithm (see Figure F.8).

If the heart rate has not responded to the five inflation breaths then check that you have seen chest movement. Auscultation by stethoscope of fluid-filled lungs during the administration of inflation or ventilation breaths may erroneously detect 'breath' sounds even **without** effective lung inflation. Go back and check airway-opening manoeuvres and repeat the inflation breaths.

Circulation

If the heart rate remains very slow (<60 beats/min) or absent, despite adequate lung inflation and subsequent ventilation for 30 seconds (with demonstrable chest movement), then chest compressions should be started.

Chest compressions in the newborn aim to move oxygenated blood from the lungs to the heart and coronary arteries; they are not intended to sustain cerebral circulation as they do in older children or adults. Once oxygenated blood reaches the coronary arteries it will usually result in a change from anaerobic energy generation to aerobic energy generation and, as a result, the heart rate will increase. This will then provide the required cardiac output to perfuse the vital organs. The blood you move using cardiac compressions **can only be oxygenated if the lungs have air in them**. Newborn cardiac compromise is almost always the result of respiratory failure and can only be effectively treated if effective ventilation is occurring.

The most efficient way of delivering chest compressions in the newborn baby is to encircle the chest with both hands, so that the fingers lie behind the baby, supporting the back, and the thumbs are apposed over the lower third of the sternum (Figure F.7). Overlapping the thumb tips is more effective than placing the thumb tips side by side, but is more likely to cause operator fatigue. Compress the chest briskly, **by one-third of the anteroposterior diameter** and ensure that **full recoil of the anterior chest wall is allowed** after each compression, before commencing the next compression. The relaxation phase is when the blood returns to the coronary arteries and therefore is essential to effective technique. Evidence clearly supports a synchronised ratio of three compressions for each ventilation breath (3:1 ratio) as the most effective ratio in the newborn, aiming to achieve 120 events (90 compressions and 30 ventilations) per minute.

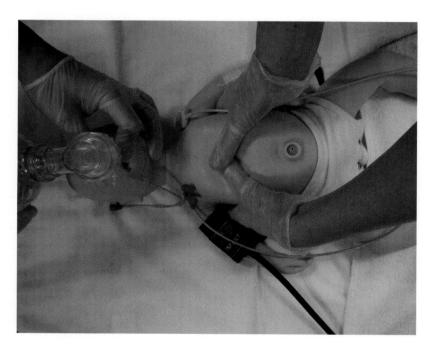

Figure F.7 Hand-encircling technique for chest compressions

The purpose of chest compressions is to move **oxygenated** blood or drugs to the coronary arteries in order to initiate cardiac recovery. Thus there is no point in starting chest compression before effective lung inflation has been established. Similarly, compressions are ineffective unless interposed by ventilation breaths of good quality. Therefore, the emphasis must be upon **good-quality breaths**, followed by effective compressions. Simultaneous delivery of compressions and breaths (otherwise known as chest compression with asynchronous ventilation, and used in older patients with a secure airway) should be avoided even when the baby is intubated, as compressions will reduce the effectiveness of any breath if the two coincide. It is usually only necessary to continue chest compressions for about 20–30 seconds before the heart responds with an increase in heart rate, thus reassessment of the heart rate at regular 30-second intervals is recommended. If chest compressions are required in resuscitation, the inspired concentration of oxygen should be increased if possible.

Once the heart rate is above 60 beats/min and rising, chest compressions may be discontinued. Ventilation breaths will need to be continued, by whichever method has been used effectively thus far, until effective spontaneous breathing commences. In the absence of breathing starting spontaneously, formal mechanical ventilation may need to be instituted. The inspired oxygen concentration should be guided by pulse oximetry.

Drugs

If adequate lung inflation and ventilation with effective cardiac compressions does not lead to the heart rate improving above 60 beats/min, drugs should be considered. The most common reason for failure of the heart rate to respond is failure to achieve or maintain lung inflation, and there is **no point** in giving drugs unless the airway is open and the lungs have been inflated. Airway, breathing (i.e. the observed chest movement) and chest compressions must be reassessed as adequate and effective before proceeding to drug therapy. Drugs are best administered via a centrally placed umbilical venous line or, if this is not possible, an intraosseous needle is an alternative in term babies. The outcome is poor if drugs are required for resuscitation.

Adrenaline   The α-adrenergic effect of adrenaline increases coronary artery perfusion during resuscitation, enhancing oxygen delivery to the heart. In the presence of profound, unresponsive bradycardia or circulatory standstill, 10 micrograms/kg (0.1 ml/kg of 1:10 000) adrenaline may be given intravenously. This **must** be followed by a flush of 0.9% sodium chloride to ensure it reaches the circulation. Further doses of 10–30 micrograms/kg (0.1–0.3 ml of 1:10 000), again with a flush of 0.9% sodium chloride, may be tried if there is no response to the initial bolus. The tracheal route cannot be recommended as there are insufficient data. However, if intratracheal instillation is tried, animal evidence suggests that doses of 50–100 micrograms/kg will be needed. These higher doses must **not** be given intravenously.

Bicarbonate   Any baby in terminal apnoea will have a significant metabolic component to the acidosis present. Acidosis depresses cardiac function. Sodium bicarbonate 1–2 mmol/kg (2–4 ml/kg of 4.2% solution) may be used to raise the pH and enhance the effects of oxygen and adrenaline in prolonged resuscitation, after adequate ventilation and circulation (with chest compressions) has been established. Bicarbonate use remains controversial and it should only be used in the absence of discernible cardiac output despite all resuscitative efforts, or in profound and unresponsive bradycardia. Its use is not recommended during short periods of CPR.

Glucose   Hypoglycaemia is associated with adverse neurological outcomes and worsened cerebral damage in neonatal animal models of asphyxia and resuscitation. Once the neonatal heart has consumed endogenous glycogen supplies, it also requires an exogenous energy source to continue functioning. Therefore, during prolonged resuscitation it is appropriate to consider giving a slow bolus of 2.5 ml/kg of 10% glucose IV. Once a bolus has been given, provision of a secure intravenous glucose infusion at a rate of 100 ml/kg/day of 10% glucose is needed to prevent rebound hypoglycaemia. Clinical evidence from paediatric patients suggests that hyperglycaemia after a hypoxic/ischaemic event is **not** harmful, whereas hypoglycaemia may well be. Many strip glucometers are not reliable in neonates and, wherever possible, should not be used for blood glucose estimation unless using the local laboratory arrangements incurs an excessive delay.

Fluid   Very occasionally hypovolaemia may be present because of known or suspected blood loss (antepartum haemorrhage, placenta/vasa praevia or bleeding from a separated but unclamped umbilical cord). Hypovolaemia secondary to loss of vascular tone following asphyxia is less common. Where a baby remains pale and shocked in appearance, or where there is a persistent bradycardia despite drug administration, intravascular volume expansion may be appropriate. Sodium chloride 0.9% at 10 ml/kg (or other isotonic crystalloid) can be used safely. If blood loss is likely, especially where acute and severe, uncross-matched, cytomegalovirus-negative, O RhD-negative blood should be given in preference. Albumin (and other plasma substitutes) cannot be recommended. However, most newborn or neonatal resuscitations do not require the administration of fluid unless there has been known blood loss or septicaemic shock.

As most newborn babies requiring resuscitation are not hypovolaemic, especially those born preterm, extreme caution should be exercised in order to avoid inappropriately excessive amounts of fluid boluses. Excessive intravascular volume expansion may cause worsened cardiac function in a heart subject to prolonged hypoxia, and is associated with increased rates of (cerebral) intraventricular haemorrhage and pulmonary haemorrhage in preterm babies.

Naloxone **This is not a drug of resuscitation to be given acutely.** Occasionally, a baby who has been effectively resuscitated, is pink, with a heart rate of ≥100 beats/min, may not breathe spontaneously because of the possible effects of maternal opioid medications. If respiratory-depressant effects are suspected the baby should be given naloxone intramuscularly (200 micrograms in a full-term baby). Smaller doses of 10 micrograms/kg will also reverse opioid sedation but the effect will only last a short time (20 minutes compared with a few hours after IM administration). Intravenous naloxone has a half-life shorter than the opiates it is meant to reverse, and there is no evidence to recommend intratracheal administration.

Bicarbonate, glucose, fluid and naloxone should **never** be given intratracheally.

F.6 Response to resuscitation

The first indication of successful progress in resuscitation will be an increase in heart rate. Recovery of respiratory drive may be delayed. Babies in terminal apnoea will tend to gasp first as they recover before starting normal respirations (see Figure F.3). Those who were in primary apnoea are likely to start with normal breaths, which may commence at any stage of resuscitation. Depending on circulatory status, skin colour may recover quickly or slowly, but universally the tone (a proxy for consciousness) of the baby is the last key metric to improve once heart function, circulation and spontaneous, effective breathing are restored.

Discontinuation of resuscitation

The outcome for a baby with no detectable heart rate for more than 10 minutes after birth is likely to be very poor, with death or severe neurodisability the likeliest outcomes. Stopping resuscitation is a decision that should be made by the most senior clinicians present and ideally with input from those experienced in resuscitation of the newborn (which may mean consulting with neonatal teams, in other centres, by telephone or video-conferencing). This decision will depend on a range of variables including parental beliefs and expressed feelings about the potential for significant morbidity, likely aetiology for the presentation, potential reversibility of the cause, and availability of intensive care treatments including therapeutic hypothermia.

Where a heart rate has persisted at less than 60 beats/min without improvement during 10–15 minutes of continuous resuscitation, the decision to stop is much less clear. No evidence is available to recommend a universal approach beyond evaluation of the situation on a case by case basis by the resuscitating team and (ideally) senior clinicians.

A decision to stop resuscitation before 10 minutes, or not starting resuscitation at all, may be appropriate in situations of extreme prematurity (<23 weeks), a birth weight of <400 g or in the presence of lethal abnormalities such as anencephaly or confirmed trisomy 13 or 18. Resuscitation is nearly always indicated in conditions with a high survival rate and acceptable morbidity. Such decisions should be taken by a senior member of the team, ideally a consultant, in consultation with the parents and other team members.

F.7 Tracheal intubation

Most babies can be resuscitated using a mask system. Swedish data suggest that if this is applied effectively, only one in 500 babies actually **need** intubation. Tracheal intubation remains the gold standard in airway management only if the tracheal tube can be correctly placed, without interrupting ongoing ventilation and without causing trauma to the oropharynx and trachea. It is especially useful in prolonged resuscitations, in managing extremely preterm babies and when a tracheal blockage is suspected. It should be considered if mask ventilation has failed, although the most common reason for this is poor positioning of the head with consequent failure to open the airway. It is, however, a common source of task fixation and can result in a significant interruption of resuscitation. It therefore needs experienced operators carefully marshalled to prevent unwarranted delay in moving along the resuscitative algorithm **especially** if mask ventilation is effective prior to the intubation attempt (see Discontinuation of resuscitation above).

The technique of intubation is the same as for older infants and is described in Chapter 21. An appropriately grown, normal, full-term newborn baby usually needs a 3.5 mm (internal diameter) tracheal tube, but 2.5, 3.0 and 4 mm tubes should also be available.

Tracheal tube placement must be assessed visually during intubation and in most cases will be confirmed by a rapid response in heart rate on ventilating via the endotracheal tube. An exhaled CO_2 detection system (either colorimetric or quantitative) is a rapid, and now widely available, adjunct to confirmation of correct tracheal tube placement in the presence of any cardiac output. The detection of exhaled CO_2 should be used to confirm tracheal tube placement but it should not be used in isolation. Listening to air entry in both axillae may help avoid intubation of the right main bronchus, which can give a 'false positive' capnographic test. A number of other false positive reactions can occur with direct contamination of the colorimetric detector by drugs used in the newborn setting.

F.8 Laryngeal mask airway

The laryngeal mask airway (LMA) may be considered as an alternative to a face mask for positive pressure ventilation among newborn babies weighing more than 2000 g or delivered ≥34 weeks' gestation. The LMA should be considered during resuscitation of the newborn baby if face mask ventilation is unsuccessful and tracheal intubation is unsuccessful or not feasible. There is limited evidence evaluating its use for newborn babies weighing <2000 g or delivered <34 weeks' gestation, and none for babies who are receiving compressions.

The insertion of a LMA should be undertaken only by those individuals who have been trained to use it.

F.9 Preterm babies

Unexpected deliveries outside delivery suites are more likely to be preterm. Whilst moderately preterm babies (34–36 weeks' gestation) can be managed in the same way as term babies, many babies born between 31 and 33 weeks' gestation, and **all** babies born before 31 weeks' gestation, need to be carefully supported during their transition to extrauterine life in order to prevent problems, rather than resuscitation, from a hypoxic event.

Premature babies are more likely to get cold (because of a higher surface area to mass ratio), and are more likely to become hypoglycaemic (fewer glycogen stores). There are now several trials that support keeping babies warm through the use of plastic bags placed over babies of <30 weeks' gestation (or <1000 g) without drying the unexposed body parts. Current European guidelines support wrapping the head and body (but not face) of all babies of <32 weeks' gestation in polyethylene wrap or a bag where there is access to a radiant heater. The use of a radiant heater theoretically warms the wet baby through the plastic, trapping a warmed, humidified atmosphere around it to maintain thermal control (box below). In babies of <32 weeks' gestation other interventions may also be needed to maintain temperature such as use of a thermal mattress and warmed humidified respiratory gases when ventilated. After 30 weeks' gestation, an alternative is to dry and wrap the baby in a dry, warm towel in a similar fashion to babies born at term.

Guidelines for the use of plastic bags for preterm babies (<32 weeks' gestation) at birth

- Preterm babies born before 32 completed weeks of gestation may be placed in plastic bags or wrap for temperature stability during resuscitation. They should remain in the bag until they are on the NICU and the humidity within their incubator is at the desired level. It is a way of preventing evaporative heat loss and cannot replace incubators, etc. Neither should it replace all efforts to maintain a high ambient temperature around babies born outside delivery suites
- At birth the baby should not be dried, but should be slipped straight into the prepared plastic bag or wrapping. There is no need to wrap the baby in a towel so long as this is done immediately after birth. This gives immediate humidity. The plastic bag only prevents evaporative heat loss – once in the bag the baby should be placed under a radiant heater
- Suitable plastic bags are food-grade bags designed for microwaving and roasting. They should be large. The bag is prepared with a V cut in the closed end. Purpose-made bags and wraps are also available
- The bag should cover the baby from the shoulders to the feet, with the head protruding through the V cut. This is most easily performed if the hand is placed through the V, the head placed in the hand, and the bag drawn back down over the baby
- The head will stick out of the V cut and should be dried as usual and resuscitation commenced as per standard guidelines. A hat should be placed over the head if practical to further reduce heat loss
- Standard resuscitation can be carried out without any limitations of access, but if the umbilicus is required for any access then a hole can be made above the area and the desired intervention done
- The bag should not be removed unless deemed necessary by the registrar or consultant
- After transfer to a neonatal unit and stabilising ventilation, if required, the baby's temperature should be recorded. The bag is only removed when the incubator humidity is satisfactory, and further care provided as per nursing protocols
- This is a potentially useful technique for keeping larger babies warm when born unexpectedly outside the delivery suite or in the community. However, it should be augmented by also wrapping with warm towels and ensuring a warm environment

The more premature a baby is, the less likely it is to establish adequate spontaneous respirations without assistance. Preterm babies of less than 32 weeks' gestation are likely to be deficient in surfactant especially after unexpected or precipitate delivery. Surfactant, secreted by alveolar type II pneumocytes, reduces alveolar surface tension and prevents alveolar collapse on expiration. Small amounts of surfactant can be demonstrated from about 20 weeks' gestation, but a surge in production only occurs after 30–34 weeks. Surfactant is released at birth due to aeration and distension of the alveoli. Production is reduced by hypothermia (<35°C), hypoxia and acidosis (pH <7.25). Surfactant deficiency can occur at any gestational age but is especially likely in babies born before 30 week's gestation and many units will have a policy to address this issue based on the gestation at birth. Nasal continuous positive airway pressure (CPAP) is now widely used to stabilise preterm babies with respiratory distress and may avoid the need to intubate and ventilate many of these babies. If, however, intubation and ventilation is necessary then exogenous surfactant should be given as soon as possible.

The lungs of preterm babies are more fragile than those of term babies and thus are much more susceptible to damage from overdistension. Therefore, it is appropriate to start with a lower inflation pressure of 20–25 cmH$_2$O (2.0–2.5 kPa), but do not be afraid to increase this to 30 cmH$_2$O (2.9 kPa) if there is no heart rate response. Using a positive end-expiratory pressure (PEEP) helps prevent collapse of the airways during expiration and is normally given using a pressure of 5 cmH$_2$O (~0.5 kPa). In most situations it will not be possible to measure the tidal volume of each breath given and while seeing some chest movement helps confirm aeration of the lungs, very obvious chest wall movement in premature babies of less than 28 weeks' gestation may indicate excessive and potentially damaging tidal volumes. This should be avoided, therefore, especially in the context of a preterm baby who has a heart rate of ≥100 beats/min and in whom there are adequate oxygen saturations.

Premature babies are more susceptible to the toxic effects of hyperoxia. Using a pulse oximeter to monitor both heart rate and oxygen saturation in these babies from birth makes stabilisation much easier. Exposing preterm babies at birth to high concentrations of oxygen can have significant long-term adverse effects. Ranges of pre-ductal oxygen saturation found in the first few minutes of life in well, preterm babies are increasingly being reported; however normal values in well babies born before 32 weeks' gestation are based on small numbers. Trial data have shown clearly that starting resuscitation of the preterm baby in high (>65%) concentration inspired oxygen has no benefit over lower concentrations. The current guidance is that it is acceptable to start resuscitation of a preterm baby at an oxygen concentration between air and 30% as data do not currently exist to refine this range further. Additional oxygen should not be given if the oxygen saturations measured, at the right arm or wrist, are above the values below:

Time from birth	Acceptable (25th centile) pre-ductal saturation above which supplemental oxygen is not needed
2 min	60%
3 min	70%
4 min	80%
5 min	85%
10 min	90%

CPAP via mask versus intubation

As outlined above, tracheal intubation to 'secure' the airway is rarely needed in term babies. In addition, it carries with it the inherent risks of: delaying ongoing resuscitation due to task fixation; causing traumatic injury to oropharyngeal and tracheal tissue; and at worst irreversibly destabilising an otherwise well baby.

In preterm babies there is now good evidence from studies involving nearly 2500 babies under 30 weeks' gestation to suggest that effective initial respiratory support of spontaneously breathing babies with respiratory distress can be given using CPAP. Therefore, CPAP should be considered a first line intervention for ongoing support in this population especially where personnel are not skilled in, or only infrequently practice, tracheal intubation. Where a mask plus T-piece system is being used for initial resuscitation, and a PEEP valve is available on the T-piece, CPAP may be given effectively by mask. Other dedicated CPAP devices utilising small nasal masks or prongs are available and are often found on paediatric high-dependency or level 1 neonatal ('special care') units.

Saturation monitoring

Pulse oximetry gives a quick and relatively accurate display of both heart rate and oxygen saturation that can be easily seen by all involved in the resuscitation. This is particularly useful when stabilising significantly preterm babies or when tempted to give additional oxygen to any baby. Once the oximeter is switched on, a reading can be obtained a few seconds faster if the probe is first attached to the right hand or wrist of the baby and only then connected to the machine. Once the heart rate is displayed with a good trace, it is likely that this will be more accurate than other commonly used methods of assessing heart rate.

Actions in the event of poor initial response to resuscitation

1. Check head position, airway and breathing.
2. Check for a technical fault:
   - Is mask ventilation effective? Is there a significant leak around the mask? Observe chest movement.
   - Is a longer inflation time or higher inflation pressure required?
   - If the baby is intubated:
     - Is the tracheal tube in the trachea? Auscultate both axillae, listen at the mouth for a large leak, and observe movement. Use an exhaled CO_2 detector to ensure tracheal tube position.
     - Is the tracheal tube in the right main bronchus? Auscultate both axillae and observe movement.
     - Is the tracheal tube blocked? Use an exhaled CO_2 detector to confirm tracheal position and patency of the tracheal tube. Remove it and re-try mask support if there is any concern that the tracheal tube is the problem.
   - If starting in air then increase the oxygen concentration. This is least likely to be a cause of poor responsiveness, although if monitoring saturations it could be a cause for a slow increase in observed saturations.
3. Does the baby have a pneumothorax? This occurs spontaneously in up to 1% of newborn babies, but pneumothoraces needing action in the delivery unit are exceptionally rare. Auscultate the chest for asymmetry of breath sounds. A cold light source can be used to transilluminate the chest – the pneumothorax may show as a hyperilluminating area. If a tension pneumothorax is thought to be present clinically, a 21-gauge butterfly needle should be inserted through the second intercostal space in the mid-clavicular line. Alternatively, a 22-gauge cannula connected to a three-way tap may be used. Remember that you may well cause a pneumothorax during this procedure (see Chapter 23).
4. Does the baby remain cyanosed despite a regular breathing pattern, no increased work of breathing and a good heart rate? There may be a congenital heart malformation, which may be duct dependent (see Chapter 6), or a persistent pulmonary hypertension.
5. If, after resuscitation, the baby is pink and has a good heart rate but is not breathing effectively, it may be suffering the effects of maternal opiates. Naloxone 200 micrograms may be given intramuscularly, which should outlast the opiate effect.
6. Is there severe anaemia or hypovolaemia? In cases of large blood loss, 10–20 ml/kg O RhD-negative blood should be given.

Birth outside the delivery room

Whenever a baby is born unexpectedly, the greatest difficulty often lies in keeping him or her warm. Drying and wrapping, turning up the heating and closing windows and doors are all important in maintaining temperature. Special care must be taken to clamp and cut the cord to prevent blood loss.

Hospitals with an emergency medicine department should have guidelines for resuscitation at birth, summoning help and post-resuscitation transfer of babies born in, or admitted to, the department.

Babies born unexpectedly outside hospital are more likely to be preterm and at risk of rapidly becoming hypothermic. However, the principles of resuscitation are identical to the hospital setting. Transport will need to be discussed according to local guidelines.

Communication with the parents

It is important that the team caring for the newborn baby informs the parents of the progress whenever possible. This is likely to be most difficult in unexpected deliveries so prior planning to cover the eventuality may be helpful. Decisions at the end of life must involve the parents whenever possible. All communication should be documented after the event.

F.10 Summary

The approach to newborn resuscitation is summarised in the algorithm in Figure F.8.

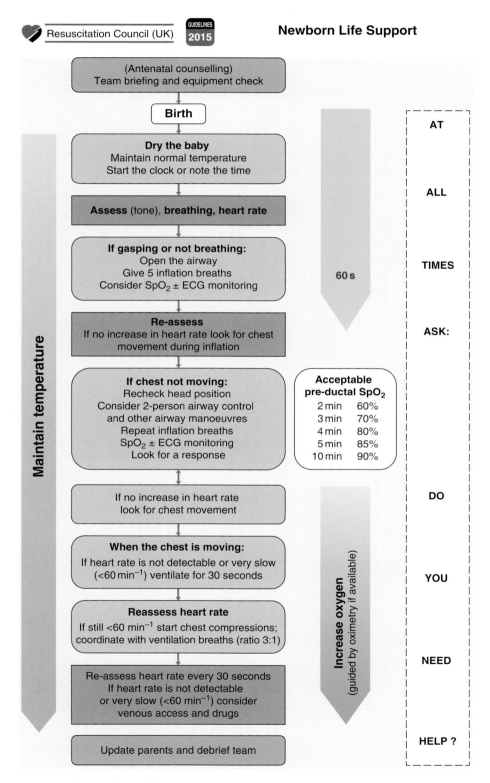

Figure F.8 Newborn resuscitation algorithm. HR, heart rate. (Reproduced with kind permission from the Resuscitation Council (UK))

APPENDIX G
Formulary

This appendix contains drugs mentioned elsewhere in the book, set out alphabetically, along with their routes of administration, dosage and some notes on their use.

G.1 General guidance on the use of the formulary

- When dosage is calculated on a basis of per kilogram and a maximum dose is not stated, then the dose given should not exceed that for a 40 kg child.
- The exact dose calculated on a basis of per kilogram may be difficult to administer because of the make-up of the formulations available. If this is the case the dose may be rounded up or down to a more manageable figure.
- Doses in other formularies are sometimes written as µg or ng. When prescribing such doses these terms should be written in full (micrograms or nanograms, respectively) in order to avoid confusion.
- Although every effort has been made to ensure accuracy, the writers, editors, publishers and printers cannot accept liability for errors or omissions.
- More detailed information about individual drugs is available from the manufacturers, from the British National Formulary for Children, from hospital drug information centres and from the pharmacy departments of children's hospitals.

Abbreviations

The following abbreviations to indicate administration route are used:

ET	endotracheal
IM	intramuscular
IO	intraosseous
IV	intravenous
SC	subcutaneous

The final responsibility for the delivery of the correct dose remains that of the physician prescribing and administering the drug.

Advanced Paediatric Life Support: A Practical Approach to Emergencies, Sixth Edition. Edited by Martin Samuels and Sue Wieteska.
© 2016 John Wiley & Sons, Ltd. Published 2016 by John Wiley & Sons, Ltd.

INDICATION	ROUTE	AGE/WEIGHT				FREQUENCY
			Child 1 month to 18 years			
ACETYLCYSTEINE		**Neonate**	**<20 kg**	**20–40 kg**	**>40 kg (dose as adult)**	
Treatment of paracetamol overdose	First infusion given over 1 hour	150 mg/kg in 3 ml/kg glucose 5%	150 mg/kg in 3 ml/kg glucose 5%	150 mg/kg in 100 ml glucose 5%	150 mg/kg (max. 16.5 g) in 200 ml glucose 5%	Single dose
	Second infusion given over next 4 hours	50 mg/kg in 7 ml/kg glucose 5%	50 mg/kg in 7 ml/kg glucose 5%	50 mg/kg in 25 ml glucose 5%	50 mg/kg (max. 5.5 g) in 500 ml glucose 5%	Single dose
	Third infusion given over next 16 hours	100 mg/kg in 14 ml/kg glucose 5%	100 mg/kg in 14 ml/kg glucose 5%	100 mg/kg in 500 ml glucose 5%	100 mg/kg (max. 11 g) i n 1 litre glucose 5%	Single dose

Notes:
Hypersensitivity reactions managed by reducing or suspending infusion rate until reaction settled.
Rash also managed by giving antihistamine and acute asthma by giving short-acting β2agonist
Sodium chloride 0.9% is an alternative if glucose 5% is unsuitable
May be used up to 24 hours after paracetamol overdose
Caution if patient taking liver enzyme-inducing drugs, e.g. phenytoin
Contraindicated if previous hypersensitivity to any of ingredients
Monitor serum potassium

ACICLOVIR		**Neonate**	**1–3 months**	**3 months to 12 years**	**12–18 years**	
Herpes simplex virus treatment Normal immunity and immuno-compromised	IV infusion	2 mg/kg every 8 hours for 14 days (at least 21 days in CNS involvement)	10 mg/kg every 8 hours for 14 days (at least 21 days in CNS involvement)	250 mg/m^2 every 8 hours for 5 days. Double to 500 mg/m^2 in immunocompromise or in simplex encephalitis (and at least 21 days in CNS involvement)	5 mg/kg every 8 hours usually for 5 days. Double to 10 mg/kg in immuno-compromise or in simplex encephalitis (at least 14 days in encephalitis and at least 21 days in immuno-compromise and encephalitis)	3 times daily

Notes:
In cases of CNS involvement, confirm cerebrospinal fluid is negative for herpes simplex virus before stopping treatment
Reconstitute to 25 mg/ml with water for injections or sodium chloride 0.9% then dilute to a concentration of 5 mg/ml with sodium chloride 0.9% or sodium chloride and glucose and give over 1 hour. Alternatively, may be administered in a concentration of 25 mg/ml using a suitable infusion pump and central venous access and given over 1 hour
To avoid excessive dose in obese patients, parenteral dose should be calculated on the basis of ideal weight for height
Reduce dosage frequency to 12-hourly if estimated glomerular filtration rate is 25–50 ml/min/1.73 m^2 and to once daily if it is 10–25 ml/min/1.73m^2
Maintain adequate hydration

INDICATION	ROUTE	AGE/WEIGHT				FREQUENCY

ACTIVATED CHARCOAL — Neonate | 1 month to 12 years | 12–18 years

		Neonate	1 month to 12 years	12–18 years		
Absorption of poisons	Oral	1 g/kg 1 g/kg every 4 hours	1 g/kg (max. 50 g) 1 g/kg (max. 50 g) every 4 hours	50 g 50 g every 4 hours		Single dose Active elimination technique: repeated doses

Notes:

Do not give to drowsy or comatose child unless airway is safely protected

Not for treating poisoning with petroleum distillates, corrosive substances, alcohols, malathion, cyanide or metal salts including iron and lithium

ADENOSINE — Neonates | 1 month to 1 year | 1–12 years | 12–18 years

		Neonates	1 month to 1 year	1–12 years	12–18 years	
Antiarrhythmic to terminate supraventricular tachycardia and to elucidate mechanism of tachycardia	Rapid IV injection	150 micrograms/kg If necessary repeat every 1–2 minutes increasing the dose by 50–100 micrograms/kg until tachycardia terminated or max. single dose of 300 micrograms/kg given	150 micrograms/kg If necessary repeat every 1–2 minutes increasing the dose by 50–100 micrograms/kg until tachycardia terminated or max. single dose of 500 micrograms/kg given	100 micrograms/kg If necessary repeat every 1–2 minutes increasing the dose by 50–100 micrograms/kg until tachycardia terminated or max. single dose of 500 micrograms/kg given (max. 12 mg)	Initially 3 mg; if necessary followed by 6 mg after 1–2 minutes and then by 12 mg after a further 1–2 minutes In some children over 12 years a 3 mg dose is ineffective, e.g. if small peripheral vein used and higher initial dose may be used	Single dose

Notes:

Drug should be given rapidly over 2 seconds followed by rapid sodium chloride 0.9% flush. A large vein is required

Children who have had a heart transplant are very sensitive to the effects of adenosine

Children receiving dipyridamole should receive a quarter (1/4) of the usual dose of adenosine

ADRENALINE (EPINEPHRINE) — Neonates | <6 years | 6–12 years | 12–18 years

		Neonates	<6 years	6–12 years	12–18 years	
Anaphylaxis treatment by health professionals	Deep IM	150 micrograms	150 micrograms	300 micrograms	500 micrograms	Single dose

Notes:

Repeat the dose at 5–15-minute intervals as clinically needed

Children taking β-blockers may not respond to adrenaline therapy, consider bronchodilator therapy

Children taking non-cardioselective β-blockers may experience severe hypertension and bradycardia with adrenaline

ADRENALINE (EPINEPHRINE) — <6 years | 6–12 years | 12–18 years

		<6 years	6–12 years	12–18 years	
Anaphylaxis treatment by autoinjector	Deep IM	150 micrograms	300 micrograms	500 micrograms	Single dose

Notes:

Repeat the dose at 5–15-minute intervals as clinically needed

Children taking β-blockers may not respond to adrenaline therapy, consider bronchodilator therapy

Children taking non-cardioselective β-blockers may experience severe hypertension and bradycardia with adrenaline

INDICATION	ROUTE	AGE/WEIGHT				FREQUENCY

ADRENALINE (EPINEPHRINE)

INDICATION	ROUTE	Neonates	<6 years	6–12 years	12–18 years	FREQUENCY
Cardiopulmonary resuscitation	ET bolus	30 micrograms/kg	100 micrograms/kg	100 micrograms/kg	100 micrograms/kg	Single dose
		Notes: The use of adrenaline given by ET bolus has not convincingly been shown to be effective. The IV/IO approach is preferred where possible				
	IV/IO	10 micrograms/kg (max. 1 g) repeated every 3–5 minutes if necessary				Single dose
		Notes: In neonates, a higher dose of up to 30 micrograms/kg may be used if the first doses are ineffective Outside the neonatal period, doses over 10 micrograms/kg may be disadvantageous except in the rare circumstances of cardiac arrest following b-blocker overdose				
Prevention of allergic reaction with antivenom in envenomation	Subcutaneous	5–10 micrograms/kg (max. 1 g)				Single dose
Management of croup	Nebuliser	400 micrograms/kg (0.4 ml/kg of 1:1000 adrenaline 1 mg/ml solution) max. 5 mg				Single dose
		Notes: May be repeated after 30 minutes if necessary Effects last for 2–3 hours, monitor carefully				

ALPROSTADIL

INDICATION	ROUTE	Birth to 1 month	FREQUENCY
Duct-dependent congenital heart defects in neonates	IV infusion Then IV infusion	Start at 5 nanograms/kg/min increasing in increments of 5 nanograms/kg/min to 20 nanograms/kg/min Then Decrease to lowest effective dose	Single dose
		Notes: Intensive support required: maximum doses of 100 nanograms/kg/min have been used	

AMINOPHYLLINE

INDICATION	ROUTE	Neonates	1 month to 1 year	1–12 years	12–18 years	FREQUENCY
Severe acute asthma*	IV infusion over 20–30 minutes	N/A		5 mg/kg (max. 500 mg)		Single loading dose over 20–30 minutes
		Notes: Loading dose if no theophylline or aminophylline has been given in the last 24 hours				

AMIODARONE

INDICATION	ROUTE	Neonates	Birth to 18 years	FREQUENCY
Stable supraventricular and ventricular arrhythmias	IV	5 mg/kg over 30 minutes then 5 mg/kg over 30 minutes every 12–24 hours	Initially 5-10 mg/kg over 20 minutes to 2 hours, then by continuous infusion 300 micrograms/kg/h increased according to response to 1.5 mg/kg/h Do not exceed 1.2 g in 24 hours	Single dose
		Notes: Administration by a central line recommended if possible Dilute to a concentration of not less than 600 micrograms/ml with glucose 5% Incompatible with sodium chloride solution		
In CPR: VF and pulseless VT refractory to defibrillation	Rapid IV bolus	N/A	5 mg/kg (max. 300 mg) over 3 minutes	Single dose
		Notes: Should be given over at least 3 minutes Administration by central line recommended if possible		

INDICATION	ROUTE	AGE/WEIGHT			FREQUENCY
ATROPINE SULPHATE		**Neonate**	**1 month to 12 years**	**12–18 years**	
Immediately before induction of anaesthesia	IV injection	10 micrograms/kg	20 micrograms/kg (min. 100 micrograms, max. 600 micrograms)	300–600 micrograms	Single dose
Intraoperative bradycardia	IV injection	10–20 micrograms/kg	10–20 micrograms/kg	300–600 micrograms (larger doses in emergencies)	Single dose

BUDESONIDE		**Neonate**	**1 month to 18 years**	
Croup	Nebuliser suspension	N/A	2 mg	Single dose
		Notes: May be repeated 12-hourly until clinical improvement		

BUPIVACAINE 0.25% (2.5 mg/ml)		**Birth to 12 years**	**12–18 years**	
Long-acting local anaesthetic for nerve blocks	Local infiltration	0.8 ml/kg	0.8 ml/kg up to a max. of 60 ml	Single dose
		Notes: To avoid toxicity in obese patients, use ideal weight Takes 30 minutes for onset Not to be repeated within 8 hours		

CALCIUM GLUCONATE 10%		**Birth to 18 years**	
For acute hypocalcaemia and hyperkalaemia	Slow injection	0.5 ml/kg (max. 20 ml)	Single dose
		Notes: Slow IV injection over 5–10 minutes Ensure there is no extravasation into tissues	

CALCIUM RESONIUM		**Neonate (by rectum)**	**1 month to 18 years (by mouth)**	
Hyperkalaemia associated with anuria or oliguria, or in dialysis patients	See route next to age	0.5–1 g/kg daily (irrigate colon to remove resin after 8–12 hours)	0.5–1 g/kg (max. 60 g) daily in divided doses	Single dose
		Notes: Administer rectally in water or 10% glucose Administer orally in water, not juice/squash which has a high potassium content		

CEFOTAXIME		**Neonate <7 days**	**Neonate 7–21 days**	**Neonate >21 days**	**1 month to 18 years**
Severe infections, including meningitis	IV injection or infusion or IM	50 mg/kg every 12 hours	50 mg/kg every 8 hours	50 mg/kg every 6–8 hours	50 mg/kg every 6 hours (max. 12 g daily) · Single dose

CEFTRIAXONE		**Neonate (IV infusion over 60 minutes)**	**1 month to 12 years (IV infusion)**	**12–18 years (and younger if >50 kg) (IV infusion or IM injection divided between 2–4 sites)**	
Severe infections, including meningitis	See route with age	20–50 mg/kg	80 mg/kg (if <50 kg)	2–4 g daily	Once daily

INDICATION	ROUTE	AGE/WEIGHT				FREQUENCY
CETIRIZINE		**1–2 years**	**2–6 years**	**6–12 years**	**12–18 years**	
Symptomatic relief of allergy	Oral	250 microgram/kg twice daily	2.5 mg twice daily	5 mg twice daily	10 mg once daily	Single dose

INDICATION	ROUTE	AGE/WEIGHT				FREQUENCY
CHLORPHENAMINE (CHLORPHENIRAMINE)		**<6 months**	**6 months to 6 years**	**6–12 years**	**12–18 years**	
Anaphylactic reactions, allergy	IV, IM	250 micrograms/kg (max. 2.5 mg)	2.5 mg	5 mg	10 mg	Single dose
		Notes: May be repeated, if required, up to four times in 24 hours				

INDICATION	ROUTE	AGE/WEIGHT		FREQUENCY
CODEINE PHOSPHATE		**Birth to 12 years**	**12–18 years**	
Moderate pain, short-term use	Oral or IM	Not indicated	30–60 mg every 6 hours where necessary (max. daily dose 240 mg; max. use 3 days)	Single dose
		Notes: Use only if paracetamol or ibuprofen ineffective Significant risk of serious and life-threatening adverse effects in children who undergo tonsillectomy or adenoidectomy for obstructive sleep apnoea Contraindicated in any patient known to be an ultrarapid metaboliser of codeine (CYP2D6 ultrarapid metaboliser) Not recommended in children in whom breathing may be compromised, including those with neuromuscular disorders, severe cardiac or respiratory disorders, respiratory infections, multiple trauma or extensive surgical procedures		

INDICATION	ROUTE	AGE/WEIGHT	FREQUENCY
DANTROLENE		**1 month to 18 years**	
Malignant hyperthermia	IV bolus	2–3 mg/kg initially	Single dose
		Notes: Discontinue trigger agent NB: needs reconstituting from powder, and is slow to dissolve Repeat with 1 mg/kg as required at 5–10-minute intervals to a maximum cumulative dose of 10 mg/kg	

INDICATION	ROUTE	AGE/WEIGHT	FREQUENCY
DESFERRIOXAMINE MESILATE		**1 month to 18 years**	
Acute iron poisoning	IV infusion	Initially up to 15 mg/kg/h Reducing after 4–6 hours as indicated	Continuous
		Notes: If shocked, hypotensive or seriously ill, administer IV Decreased rate of administration after 4–6 hours to ensure that total maximum dose does not exceed 80 mg/kg/day Continue until serum iron is less than total iron-binding capacity Use with caution in patients with renal impairment	

INDICATION	ROUTE	AGE/WEIGHT		FREQUENCY

DEXAMETHASONE

1 month to 2 years

Indication	Route	Dose	Frequency
Croup	Oral	150 micrograms/kg	Twice daily

Notes:
No definitive standard dose has been agreed in the UK
Suggested maximum single dose of 12 mg

Short course to relieve symptoms of brain tumour	IV or oral	500 micrograms/kg	Twice daily

Notes:
Can also be used to reduce oedema around tumours compressing nerves

DIAMORPHINE

		Birth to 1 month	**1 month to 18 years**	
Control of severe pain	Intranasal	Not recommended	0.1 mg/kg	Single dose

Notes:
Dilute with saline to volume of 0.2 ml
Monitor closely for at least 30 minutes and repeat if needed; may repeat 6-hourly
Avoid in acute respiratory depression
Naloxone is an antidote
Use with caution in head injury

DIAZEPAM

Birth to 18 years

Treatment of status epilepticus	Rectal	0.5 mg/kg	Single dose

Notes:
If needed, repeat after 5 minutes
Parenteral and rectal use can depress respiration
Caution with other central nervous system depressants

In place of lorazepam where this is not available	IV or IO	0.25 mg/kg	

DICLOFENAC

		1 month to 2 years	**2–18 years**	
Non-steroidal anti-inflammatory drug (NSAID)	Oral or rectal	<6 months: not recommended >6 months: 300 micrograms to 2 mg/kg	300 micrograms to 2 mg/kg	3 times daily

Notes:
Up to a maximum of 150 mg per day
Caution where there is a history of hypersensitivity and in dehydration (risk of renal failure)

DOBUTAMINE

Birth to 18 years

Provides inotropic support in the treatment of low-output cardiac failure, e.g. in septicaemia	IV infusion	5–20 micrograms/kg/min	Continuous

Notes:
Dose can be increased up to a maximum of 40 micrograms/kg/min in older children, if necessary (20 micrograms/kg/min in newborn infants) but side effects are more likely at this higher dose

INDICATION	ROUTE	AGE/WEIGHT				FREQUENCY

DOPAMINE HYDROCHLORIDE

		Birth to 1 month		1 month to 18 years		
Treatment of low-output cardiac states	IV infusion	Start at 3 micrograms/kg/min, increasing as clinically indicated to a max. of 20 micrograms/kg/min		5–20 micrograms/kg/min		Continuous

Notes:
Direct inotropic effect but vasoconstriction may occur at higher doses

ERYTHROMYCIN

		Neonate	1 month to 2 years	2–12 years	12–18 years	
Upper and lower respiratory tract infections	Oral or IV	10–12.5 mg	12.5 mg/kg (max. 1 g)			4 times daily
	Oral		125 mg	2–8 years: 250 mg 9–12 years: 500 mg	500 mg	4 times daily

Notes: Doses can be doubled in severe infections
Maximum single dose 1 g

FLECAINIDE ACETATE

		Birth to 18 years	
Treatment of resistant re-entry supraventricular tachycardia , ventricular ectopics or ventricular tachycardia	Slow IV bolus	2 mg/kg	Single dose

Notes:
Give over at least 10 minutes with ECG monitoring
Avoid in patients with pre-existing heart block
Maximum dose 150 mg

FLUCLOXACILLIN

		Birth to 1 month	1 month to 2 years	2–12 years	12–18 years	
Treatment of infections due to Gram-positive organisms (anti-staphylococcal)	Oral or IV	<7 days: 25–50 mg/kg	–	–	–	Twice daily
		7–21 days: 25–50 mg/kg	–	–	–	3 times daily
		>21 days: 25–50 mg/kg	–	–	–	4 times daily

Notes:
Dose may be increased to 100 mg/kg per dose IV in severe infection (meningitis, cerebral abscess, staphylococcal osteitis)
Oral route only recommended for minor infection

	IV bolus or IM	–	12.5–25 mg/kg			4 times daily

Notes:
Maximum single dose 1 g
Dose may be doubled in severe infection, maximum single dose 2 g

	Oral	–	<1 year: 62.5 mg >1 year: 125 mg	<5 years: 125 mg >5 years: 250 mg	250 mg	4 times daily

Notes:
Doses may be doubled in severe infection

INDICATION	ROUTE	AGE/WEIGHT				FREQUENCY

FLUMAZENIL

		Birth to 1 month	1 month to 2 years	2–12 years	12–18 years	
Reversal of acute benzodiazepine overdosage	IV bolus over 15 seconds	10 micrograms/kg (max. dose 50 micrograms/kg)	10 micrograms/kg (max. dose 50 micrograms/kg)		200 micrograms (max. dose 1 mg)	Single dose

Notes:
Initial dose as shown
If the desired effect is not achieved, repeat at 1-minute intervals to a max. total dose of 40 micrograms/kg (2 mg maximum dose in 12–18-year-olds)

	IV infusion	2–10 micrograms/kg/h (max. dose 400 micrograms/h)			100–400 micrograms/h	Continuous

Notes:
This should be individually adjusted to achieve the desired level of arousal
There is limited experience of the use of flumazenil in children

FRUSEMIDE (FUROSEMIDE)

		Birth to 12 years	12–18 years	
To induce diuresis in cardiac or renal failure or fluid overload; hypertension	IV bolus	500 micrograms to 1 mg/kg	20–40 mg	Single dose

Notes:
Single doses up to 4 mg/kg have been used. Dose can be repeated every 8 hours

GLUCAGON

		Birth to 1 month	1 month to 2 years	2–18 years	
Severe insulin-induced hypoglycaemia in the treatment of diabetes	IM, SC	Not recommended	500 micrograms	500 micrograms to 1 mg (<25 kg: 500 micrograms >25 kg: 1 mg)	Single dose

Notes:
Should be effective within 10 minutes
Only use when IV glucose is difficult or impossible to administer. If not, give IV glucose 5–10% instead

HYDROCORTISONE

		Birth to 1 month	1 month to 12 years	12–18 years	
Anaphylaxis and emergency treatment of severe acute asthma	IV bolus, IM or IO	2.5 mg/kg Then: 2 mg/kg	4 mg/kg (max. dose 100 mg) Then: 2–4 mg/kg	100–300 mg Then: 100–300 mg	Single dose 4 times daily

Notes:
Maintenance dose may be repeated if necessary every 6 hours
May be given by IO route if IV is not possible

IBUPROFEN

		1 month to 2 years	2–12 years	12–18 years	
Pyrexia, mild to moderate pain	Oral dose by weight	5 mg/kg		–	3–4 times daily
	Oral dose by age	1–2 years: 50 mg	3–7 years: 100 mg 8–12 years: 200 mg	200–600 mg	3–4 times daily

Notes:
Maximum of 20 mg/kg/day up to 2.4 g/day
Avoid where there is a history of hypersensitivity and in dehydration (risk of renal failure)

INDICATION	ROUTE	AGE/WEIGHT				FREQUENCY

INSULIN — **Birth to 18 years**

INDICATION	ROUTE	AGE/WEIGHT	FREQUENCY
Primary treatment for patients with type 1 and 2 diabetes uncontrolled by other means	IV infusion in ketoacidosis	0.05–0.1 units/kg/h Notes: Adjust dose according to blood glucose level	Continuous

IPRATROPIUM

INDICATION	ROUTE	Birth to 1 month	1 month to 2 years	2–12 years	12–18 years	FREQUENCY
Treatment of chronic reversible airways obstruction. May be used with a β_2-agonist in the treatment of severe, acute asthma	Nebulised	25 micrograms/kg	125 micrograms	250 micrograms	500 micrograms	Single dose

Notes:
Can be repeated every 20–30 minutes in the first 2 hours in acute severe asthma
Reduce dose frequency as clinical improvement occurs

LABETALOL

INDICATION	ROUTE	Birth to 1 month	1 month to 12 years	12–18 years	FREQUENCY
Hypertension and hypertensive crises	IV bolus	–	250–500 micrograms/kg	50 mg	Single dose

Notes:
Loading dose

	ROUTE	Birth to 1 month	1 month to 12 years	12–18 years	FREQUENCY
	IV infusion	500 micrograms/kg/h up to a max. of 4 mg/kg/h	1–3 mg/kg/h	120 mg/h	Continuous

Notes:
Start at low dose and titrate according to response, until the blood pressure has been reduced to an acceptable level
Avoid in asthma, heart failure and heart block

LIGNOCAINE (LIDOCAINE)

INDICATION	ROUTE	Birth to 12 years	12–18 years	FREQUENCY
Antiarrhythmic VF or pulseless tachycardia Local anaesthetic	IV/IO	1 mg/kg (max. dose 100 mg)	50–100 mg	Single dose

Notes:
Repeat every 5 minutes if needed to a total maximum of 3 mg/kg
In the 12–18-year age group give 50 mg in lighter patients or those whose circulation is impaired

	ROUTE	Birth to 12 years	12–18 years	FREQUENCY
	IV infusion	Then: 600 micrograms/kg to 3 mg/kg/h	4 mg/min for 30 minutes then 2 mg/min for 2 hours then 1 mg/min	Continuous

Notes:
In the 12–18-year group: reduce concentration further if infusion is continued beyond 24 hours
Maintenance dosing: ECG monitoring with infusion

	ROUTE	Birth to 12 years	12–18 years	FREQUENCY
	Local infiltration	Up to 3 mg/kg	Up to 200 mg	Single dose

Notes:
No more often than every 4 hours
Use fine needles (27–29 gauge)
It is less painful if buffered before use with 8.4% sodium bicarbonate 1 ml to every 10 ml lidocaine 1%

	ROUTE	Birth to 12 years	12–18 years	FREQUENCY
	Intraurethral	3–4 mg/kg	–	Single dose

Notes:
Instillagel (2% gel with chlorhexidine 0.25%) solution
Use prior to urinary catheterisation. Warm the solution to body temperature and inject it very slowly to reduce local stinging

INDICATION	ROUTE	AGE/WEIGHT				FREQUENCY

LORATADINE

| | | Birth to 2 years | 2–12 years | | 12–18 years | |
			Less than 30 kg	Over 30 kg		
Symptoms of allergy in association with anaphylaxis	Oral	–	5 mg	10 mg	10 mg	Once daily

Notes:
Hepatic impairment: reduce dose frequency to alternate days in severe impairment

LORAZEPAM

		Birth to 12 years	12–18 years	
Status epilepticus	IV, rectal or sublingual	100 micrograms/kg (max. dose 4 g)	4 mg	Single dose

Notes:
Generally given as a single dose; may be repeated once if initial dose is ineffective
Limited experience in neonates
May cause apnoea
Flumazenil is an antidote

MAGNESIUM SULPHATE

		Birth to 1 month	1 month to 2 years	2–18 years	
Hypomagnesaemia in septicaemia	IV		0.2 ml/kg 50% mgSO$_4$ over 30 minutes (max. 10 ml)		Single dose

Notes:
Repeat later if serum magnesium remains low

Treatment of asthma	IV	Not recommended	Limited experience	Over 2 years: 40 mg/kg	Single dose over 20 minutes

Notes:
Has been used in infants but experience is limited
Maximum of 2 g

Treatment of torsades de pointes	IV	Not recommended	25–50 mg/kg		Single dose

Notes:
Maximum of 2 g

MANNITOL

		Birth to 18 years	
Treatment of oedematous states, including ascites and treatment of raised intracranial pressure	IV infusion over 30 minutes	250–500 mg/kg (1.25–2.5 ml/kg of 20% solution)	Single dose

Notes:
Cerebral and ocular oedema
May be repeated once or twice after an interval of 4–8 hours if necessary (if serum osmolality <310 mOsm/l)

MIDAZOLAM

		Birth to 1 month	1 month to 2 years	2–12 years	12–18 years	
Status epilepticus	Buccal/ intranasal	–	0.5 mg/kg	0.5 mg/kg	0.5 mg/kg	Single dose
		–	<6 months (dose by weight): 300 micrograms/kg >6 months (dose by age): 2.5 mg	1–4 years: 5 mg 5–9 years: 7.5 mg >10 years: 10 mg	10 mg	Single dose

Notes:
Buccal administration is the preferred route over intranasal administration. The parenteral preparation can be used for this route
The dose by weight for the buccal route is 0.5 mg/kg from 6 months. Maximum dose 10 mg

INDICATION	ROUTE	AGE/WEIGHT				FREQUENCY
MORPHINE		**Birth to 1 month**	**1 month to 2 years**	**2–12 years**	**12–18 years**	
Control of severe pain	IV infusion	Pre-term: 25–50 micrograms/kg	–	–	–	Single dose Loading dose
		Then: 5 micrograms/kg/h	–	–	–	Continuous
		Term: 50 micrograms/kg	–	–	–	Single dose Loading dose
		Then: 10–20 micrograms/kg/h	–	–	–	Continuous
	IV bolus	–	100 micrograms/kg		5 mg every 4 hours adjusted according to response	<6 months: up to 4 times in 24 hours >6 months: up to 6 times in 24 hours

Notes:
Respiratory monitoring is mandatory
Give IV over at least 5–10 minutes
<1 year: use the lower stated dose and consider oxygen saturation monitoring

| | IV infusion | – | 10–30 micrograms/kg/h <6 months: initial rate is 10 micrograms/kg/h >6 months: initial rate is 20 micrograms/kg/h | | | Continuous |

Notes:
Use IV bolus as starting dose first
1 mg/kg body weight in 50 ml saline, infused at 1 ml/h = 20 micrograms/kg/h

| | Oral | – | 1-3 months: 50–100 micrograms/kg every 4 hours adjusted according to response 3–6 months: 100–150 micrograms/kg every 4 hours adjusted according to response 6–12 months: 200 micrograms/kg every 4 hours adjusted according to response 1–2 years: 200–300 micrograms/kg every 4 hours adjusted according to response | 200–500 micrograms/kg (max. 10 mg) | 5-10 mg | Up to 6 times in 24 hours |

Notes:
Starting doses should be reviewed regularly and adjusted according to the patient's response

INDICATION	ROUTE	AGE/WEIGHT				FREQUENCY
NALOXONE		**Birth to 1 month**	**1 month to 2 years**	**2–12 years**	**12–18 years**	
Reversal of opioid-induced central and respiratory depression	IV infusion	10 micrograms/kg Notes: Use 400 micrograms/ml naloxone preparation Gradual onset of action (3–4 minutes) but the effect is prolonged	–	–	–	Continuous
	IV bolus	–	100 micrograms/kg (max. dose 2 mg)		400 micrograms	Single dose
		–	Then, if no response: 100 micrograms/kg at 1-minute intervals to a max. of 2 mg		Then, if no response after 1 minute: 800 micrograms Then, if no response after a further 1 minute: 800 micrograms Then, if no response after a further 1 minute: 2 mg (4 mg may be required in a seriously poisoned child)	Single dose
		Notes: Then review diagnosis; further doses may be required if respiratory function deteriorates Due to short half-life of naloxone, repeat doses as necessary to maintain opioid reversal Observe for recurrence of central nervous system and respiratory depression If IV not possible use IM or SC				
	IV infusion	–	5–20 micrograms/kg/h		Infuse a solution of 4 micrograms/ml at a rate adjusted according to response	Continuous

Notes:

Specifically indicated for the reversal of respiratory depression in a newborn infant whose mother has received narcotics within 4 hours of delivery. It is generally preferred to give an IM injection for a prolonged effect

Do not administer to newborns whose mothers are suspected of narcotic abuse, as a withdrawal syndrome may be precipitated

Always establish and maintain adequate ventilation before administration of naloxone

INDICATION	ROUTE	AGE/WEIGHT				FREQUENCY

NIFEDIPINE

INDICATION	ROUTE	Birth to 1 month	1 month to 18 years	FREQUENCY
Hypertensive crisis	Oral	–	250–500 micrograms/kg	Single dose

Notes:
Administration for rapid effect in hypertensive crisis or acute angina: bite capsules and swallow liquid, or use liquid preparation if 5 or 10 mg dose inappropriate; if liquid form is unavailable, extract contents of capsule via a syringe and use immediately – cover syringe with foil to protect contents from light; capsule contents may be diluted with water if necessary
Modified-release tablets may be crushed although this may alter the release profile; crushed tablets should be administered within 30–60 seconds to avoid significant loss of potency of drug

PARACETAMOL

INDICATION	ROUTE	Birth to 1 month	1 month to 2 years	2–12 years	12–18 years	FREQUENCY
Analgesic/ antipyretic	Oral loading dose	15 mg/kg	15 mg/kg		1 g	Single dose
	Oral maintenance dose	≤32 weeks' gestation: 15 mg/kg	32 weeks' gestation to 12 years: dose by weight, 15 mg/kg	500 mg to max. 1 g	1 g	4–6-hourly, max. 4 doses per day <32 weeks' gestation: 8–12-hourly (max. 60 mg) 32 weeks' gestation to 1 month: 8-hourly (max. 30 mg)

Notes:
Maximum daily dose 60 mg/kg (total 4 g)
Preterm 28–32 weeks: max. daily dose 30 mg/kg

	Rectal loading dose		1–3 months: 30 mg/kg >3 months: 40 mg/kg		1 g	Single dose
	Rectal maintenance dose		15–20 mg/kg; max. 75 mg/kg (or 4 g) per day	500 mg to 1 g	1 g	4–6-hourly <32 weeks' gestation: 12-hourly 32 weeks' gestation to 1 month: 8-hourly

Notes:
Maximum daily dose 60 mg/kg (total 4 g)
Preterm 28–32 weeks: maximum daily dose 30 mg/kg

	IV	7.5 mg/kg 32 weeks' gestation to term: 8-hourly Term infants: 4-6 hourly, give over 15 minutes	10–50 kg: 10 mg/kg >50 kg: 1 g, give over 15 minutes	–		4–6-hourly <32 weeks gestation: 12-hourly 32 weeks' gestation to 1 month: 8-hourly

Notes:
<10 kg: maximum daily dose 30 mg/kg
10–50 kg: maximum daily dose 60 mg/kg
>50 kg: maximum daily dose 4 g

INDICATION	ROUTE	AGE/WEIGHT			FREQUENCY
PARALDEHYDE		**Birth to 18 years**			
Status epilepticus	Rectal	0.8 ml/kg to max. 20 ml			Single dose
		Notes: Doses stated in ml/kg or as ml of paraldehyde Dilute with an equal volume of olive oil before administration, or if using a ready-prepared 'special', remember that it is already diluted and dose accordingly			
PHENOBARBITAL (PHENOBARBITONE)		**Birth to 12 years**	**12–18 years**		
Status epilepticus Respiratory depression especially when used with benzodiazepines	IV slow bolus	20 mg/kg	20 mg/kg		Single
		Notes: Loading dose at 1 mg/kg/min, i.e. over 20 minutes			
		Then: 2.5–5 mg/kg	Then: 300 mg dose		Once to twice daily (once daily in neonatal period)
		Notes: Maintenance at 1 mg/kg/min, i.e. over 20 minutes			
PHENYTOIN		**Birth to 1 month**	**1 month to 12 years**	**12–18 years**	
Antiepileptic	IV	20 mg/kg	20 mg/kg		Single dose
		Notes: Loading dose over 20 minutes Monitor ECG and blood pressure			
	IV	2.5–5 mg/kg		–	Twice daily
		–		100 mg	3–4 times a day
		Notes: Usual maintenance dose over 20 minutes Reduce does in liver disease			
POTASSIUM CHLORIDE		**Birth to 1 month**	**1 month to 18 years**		
Acute hypokalaemia	IV infusion	–	0.1–0.25 mmol/kg/h		Continuous
		Notes: Always check the dose carefully, as an overdose can be rapidly fatal; dilute with at least 50 times its volume and mix well Restrict to critical care areas, store in a locked cupboard and document as for controlled drugs Recheck the potassium level after 3 hours			
PREDNISOLONE		**Birth to 1 month**	**1 month to 12 years**	**12–18 years**	
Acute asthma	Oral	–	1 mg/kg (max. dose 40 mg)	40–50 mg	Once daily
		Notes: Treat for 1–5 days and then stop (no need to taper doses)			
Suppression of inflammatory and allergic disorders	Oral	–	1–2 mg/kg	40–50 mg	Once daily
		Notes: The daily dose can be given in 2–3 divided doses if necessary. Consider alternate-day treatment in long term			
Croup requiring intubation	Oral	–	1 mg/kg	40–50 mg	Twice daily

INDICATION	ROUTE	AGE/WEIGHT			FREQUENCY

PROPRANOLOL		**Birth to 12 years**	**12–18 years**		
Dysrhythmias	IV bolus	25–50 micrograms/kg	1 mg		Single dose
		Notes: Repeat injection as needed up to 4 times daily Give slowly over at least 3–5 minutes; rate of administration should not exceed 1 mg/min			

QUININE		**Birth to 18 years**			
Treatment of *Plasmodium falciparum* malaria	IV infusion over 4 hours at least	20 mg/kg (max. 1.4 g) Notes: For seriously ill patients or those unable to take tablets			Single loading dose
		Then: 10 mg/kg (max. 700 mg) Notes: Maintenance dose can be repeated 3 times daily but change to oral therapy as soon as possible			Then after 8 hours maintenance dose

Notes:
Risk of arrhythmias with amiodarone and flecainide
Side effects are common: tinnitus, headache, visual disturbance and hypoglycaemia
Use glucose 5% to dilute to a concentration of 2 mg/ml (maximum 30 mg/ml in fluid restriction)
Monitor ECG and blood sugar

SALBUTAMOL		**Birth to 1 month**	**1 month to 2 years**	**2–18 years**	
Treatment of asthma	Aerosol inhaler	–	Up to 1 mg		Single dose
		Notes: Asthma reliever given as required; 1–2-hourly initially, then reduce frequency to 4–6-hourly; 1000 micrograms = 10 sprays (each of 100 micrograms)			
	Nebuliser solution	<5 years: 2.5 mg >5 years: 5 mg			Single dose
		Notes: Asthma reliever given as required according to severity and response			
	IV bolus over 5 minutes	5 micrograms/kg		15 micrograms/kg (max. 250 micrograms)	Single dose
		Notes: Status asthmaticus: maximum concentration 50 micrograms in 1 ml			
	IV infusion	1–5 micrograms/kg/min			Continuous
		Notes: Status asthmaticus: doses up to 10 micrograms/kg/min have been used Solution compatible with potassium but not with aminophylline			
Renal hyperkalaemia	IV bolus	4 micrograms/kg			Single dose
		Notes: Repeat if necessary			
	Nebuliser	2.5–5 mg			Single dose
		Notes: Repeat if necessary			

INDICATION	ROUTE	AGE/WEIGHT				FREQUENCY
SODIUM BICARBONATE		**Birth to 18 years**				
Resuscitation	Slow IV	1 ml/kg of 8.4% initially if indicated Followed by 0.5 ml/kg of 8.4% if needed				
Metabolic acidosis	Slow IV	1–2 mmol/kg Notes: Only after attention to ventilation and perfusion Always infuse slowly If acidosis is persistent consider inborn errors or toxins				
Renal hyperkalaemia	Slow IV	1 mmol/kg Notes: Dose adjusted according to plasma bicarbonate level				Single dose

INDICATION	ROUTE	AGE/WEIGHT				FREQUENCY
SODIUM CHLORIDE 3%		**Birth to 18 years**				
Management of raised intracranial pressure	IV	3–5 ml/kg IV over 15 minutes				Single dose

INDICATION	ROUTE	AGE/WEIGHT				FREQUENCY
SODIUM NITROPRUSSIDE		**Birth to 18 years**				
Hypertensive crisis	IV infusion	500 nanograms/kg/min Notes: Initial dose: increase in increments of 200 nanograms/kg/min as necessary to a maximum of 8 micrograms/kg/min Use only with expert advice				Continuous

INDICATION	ROUTE	Birth to 1 month	1 month to 2 years	2–12 years	12–18 years	FREQUENCY
TERBUTALINE						
Relief of bronchospasm in bronchial asthma	Nebulised	–	2.5–5 mg	<5 years: 2.5–5 mg >5 years: 5–10 mg	10 mg	Single dose
		Notes: Reliever doses are repeated as required				

INDICATION	ROUTE	Birth to 1 month	1 month to 2 years	2–12 years	2–18 years	FREQUENCY
VERAPAMIL						
Treatment for supraventricular tachycardia (adenosine first line)	Slow IV bolus	–	<1 year: – >1 year: 100–300 micrograms/kg (max. 5 mg)	100–300 micrograms/kg (max. 5 mg)	5 mg	Single dose over 2–3 minutes
		Notes: ECG and blood pressure monitoring required Dose may be repeated after 30 minutes if necessary. Many cases are controlled by doses at the lower end of the range Caution in liver disease. Do not use with β-blockers Use only with expert advice				

Index

Page numbers in *italics* denote figures, those in **bold** denote tables.

Advanced Paediatric Life Support: A Practical Approach to Emergencies, Sixth Edition. Edited by Martin Samuels and Sue Wieteska.
© 2016 John Wiley & Sons, Ltd. Published 2016 by John Wiley & Sons, Ltd.